AF667267

# The Unstable Elbow

Robert Z. Tashjian
Editor

# The Unstable Elbow

## An Evidence-Based Approach to Evaluation and Management

Springer

*Editor*
Robert Z. Tashjian, MD
Department of Orthopedics
University of Utah School of Medicine
Salt Lake City, UT, USA

Videos can also be accessed at
http://link.springer.com/book/10.1007/978-3-319-46019-2

ISBN 978-3-319-46017-8 ISBN 978-3-319-46019-2 (eBook)
DOI 10.1007/978-3-319-46019-2

Library of Congress Control Number: 2016959757

© Springer International Publishing Switzerland 2017
This work is subject to copyright. All rights are reserved by the Publisher, whether the whole or part of the material is concerned, specifically the rights of translation, reprinting, reuse of illustrations, recitation, broadcasting, reproduction on microfilms or in any other physical way, and transmission or information storage and retrieval, electronic adaptation, computer software, or by similar or dissimilar methodology now known or hereafter developed.
The use of general descriptive names, registered names, trademarks, service marks, etc. in this publication does not imply, even in the absence of a specific statement, that such names are exempt from the relevant protective laws and regulations and therefore free for general use.
The publisher, the authors and the editors are safe to assume that the advice and information in this book are believed to be true and accurate at the date of publication. Neither the publisher nor the authors or the editors give a warranty, express or implied, with respect to the material contained herein or for any errors or omissions that may have been made.

Printed on acid-free paper

This Springer imprint is published by Springer Nature
The registered company is Springer International Publishing AG
The registered company address is: Gewerbestrasse 11, 6330 Cham, Switzerland

# Foreword

The field of elbow surgery has continued to advance tremendously over the last two decades. Instability represents one of the most frequent clinical problems in elbow surgery. Traumatic elbow injuries oftentimes carry an element of instability. Chronic instability can be the result of traumatic injuries, throwing sports, or developmental disorders (coronoid hypoplasia, distal humerus varus malunion). Surgical techniques to reconstruct the various elements involved in elbow stability have improved substantially. However, salvage procedures are still occasionally required when instability surgery goes wrong.

Although isolated pieces of information about various aspects of elbow instability can be gathered from scientific manuscripts, it is difficult to find a single source that provides an updated, comprehensive review of the unstable elbow. Dr. Tashjian has definitely accomplished that task in his book. *The Unstable Elbow* covers the basic science underlying elbow instability, the evaluation and management of both acute and chronic instability, and salvage procedures such as arthroplasty and arthrodesis for persistently unstable elbows.

Dr. Tashjian has become a very active academic shoulder and elbow surgeon. I have had the pleasure of getting to know him personally through interactions in various meetings, and I have read a number of his publications. He has a great writing style and the innate ability to compile and summarize large collections of data into meaningful manuscripts. With a list of peer-reviewed articles close to 100, and experience in various teaching courses, some specifically on elbow instability, Dr. Tashjian has the required perspective on elbow instability to serve as Editor of such a great monograph.

The lead authors for all chapters in this book are true experts in elbow surgery. Dr. Tashjian created a comprehensive table of contents and assigned the various chapters of his book to individuals with sound knowledge, backed up by their own original research. I could not think of a better group of individuals to summarize the state of the art in elbow instability.

In times of quick access to information, mostly through internet-based tools, the foundation provided by a solid book that, when read from beginning to end, will establish an ample frame of reference on a given subject is simply priceless. Hopefully, the content of this book will enable many orthopedic surgeons around the world to help so many patients unfortunate enough to suffer from elbow instability in one form or another.

I feel honored to have been asked to write this Foreword for Dr. Tashjian's book on *The Unstable Elbow*. I am familiar with the extraordinary amount of work and effort required to complete a monograph like this one, and I would like to personally congratulate Dr. Tashjian and his fellow authors in creating a wonderful book.

Rochester, MN, USA

Joaquin Sanchez-Sotelo, MD, PhD
Mayo Clinic and Mayo College of Medicine

# Preface

The understanding of elbow instability has exponentially grown over the past 25–30 years. Very limited knowledge existed prior to that point even with regard to the basic anatomy and mechanics of the various elbow stabilizers. Most injuries were treated conservatively except for highly displaced fractures or grossly unstable joints, and often there was no set algorithm or strategy in treating these injuries leading to unpredictable results. With anatomic and mechanical studies defining the critical stabilizers of the elbow and a more concentrated focus on clinical outcomes and developing protocols for treating certain patterns of elbow instability, the results of nonoperative and operative treatment have improved. Recent refinements of injury and fracture classifications and identification of new injury patterns have increased the percentage of successful results in these often challenging cases. With such a rapid growth in knowledge, it can be extremely challenging for surgeons to have a full understanding of what is the most "up-to-date" treatment for these injuries. Most often this requires searching through the literature and arriving at a conclusion based upon the assimilation of material from several articles. Up until this point, no single resource has distilled this information on the topic of elbow instability in a usable form that can be easily applied to everyday clinical use. This deficiency was the origins of the current textbook.

I am grateful to have recruited a group of experts in the field of elbow surgery to put together a series of manuscripts outlining the current treatment strategies for all aspects of elbow instability. The initial chapters focus on anatomy, biomechanics, and the most currently utilized surgical approaches for the treatment of elbow instability. The following chapters focus on the evaluation and surgical treatments of acute and chronic elbow instabilities. The authors have not only assimilated the data in the literature to make clear recommendations as to the most appropriate treatment for these injuries but also added their own personal "pearls of wisdom" in both their diagnosis and surgical management. I want to individually thank each author for putting the time and effort required to make this project a reality. I hope the readers will find the text a reference that they will return to over and over to help guide them in the management of each of these challenging problems.

Our goal with this text was to put everything regarding elbow instability "under one roof" and thereby making it an almost essential resource for surgeons treating these injuries. I think we have achieved and surpassed these goals beyond my expectations and I hope the readers feel this way as well. Finally, I hope this text is a springboard for further research on the treatment of these injuries. The text allows a "big picture look" at the problem, and this often allows gaps in our knowledge and treatments to be identified. We hope this textbook serves you and your patients well and also provides a platform for identifying areas of treatment that need to be expanded and improved upon in the future.

Salt Lake City, UT, USA Robert Z. Tashjian, MD

# Contents

# Contributors

**Joseph A. Abboud, MD** Department of Orthopedic Surgery, The Rothman Institute, Thomas Jefferson University, Philadelphia, PA, USA

**Alexander W. Aleem, MD** Department of Orthopedic Surgery, The Rothman Institute, Thomas Jefferson University, Philadelphia, PA, USA

**Samuel A. Antuña, MD, PhD, FEBOT** Shoulder and Elbow Unit, Department of Orthopedics, Hospital Universitario La Paz, Madrid, Spain

**April D. Armstrong, BSc(PT), MD, MSC, FRCSC** Penn State Milton S. Hershey Medical Center, Bone and Joint Institute, Hershey, PA, USA

**George S. Athwal, MD, FRCSC** Division of Orthopedic, Department of Surgery, Roth McFarlane Hand & Upper Limb Centre, Western University, London, ON, Canada

**Gregory I. Bain, MBBS, FRACS, PhD** Department of Orthopedic Surgery, Flinders University of South Australia, Adelaide, Australia

**Raul Barco, MD, PhD, FEBOT** Department of Orthopedic Surgery, Hospital Universitario La Paz, Madrid, Spain

**Yehia H. Bedeir, MD, MBBCh, MCh Orth** Department of Orthopedic Surgery, El-Hadara University Hospital, Alexandria, Egypt

Department of Orthopedic Surgery, MedStar Union Memorial Hospital, Baltimore, MD, USA

**John-Erik Bell, MD, MS** Department of Orthopedics, Dartmouth Hitchcock Medical Center, Lebanon, NH, USA

**Theodore A. Blaine, MD, MBA** Department of Orthopedics & Rehabilitation, Yale University School of Medicine, New Haven, CT, USA

**Pieter Caekebeke, MD** Department of Orthopedic, AZ Monica, Deurne, Antwerpen, Belgium

**Ryan P. Calfee, MD, MSc** Department of Orthopedic Surgery, Washington University School of Medicine, St. Louis, MO, USA

**Lawrence Camarda, MD, PhD** Department of Orthopedic Surgery, Università degli Studi di Palermo, Palermo, Italy

**Nicholas M. Capito, MD** Champion Orthopedics, Augusta, GA, USA

**Shannon R. Carpenter, MD** Department of Orthopedic Surgery, MedStar Union Memorial Hospital, Baltimore, MD, USA

**Peter N. Chalmers, MD** Department of Orthopedic Surgery, Washington University in St. Louis, St. Louis, MO, USA

**Aaron M. Chamberlain, MD, MSc** Department of Orthopedic Surgery, Washington University Medical Center, St. Louis, MO, USA

**Kevin Chan, MD, MSc, FRCSC** Division of Orthopedic, Department of Surgery, Roth McFarlane Hand & Upper Limb Centre, Western University, London, ON, Canada

**Emilie V. Cheung, MD** Department of Orthopedic Surgery, Stanford University Hospital and Clinics, Redwood City, CA, USA

Department of Orthopedics, University of Chicago, Chicago, IL, USA

**Megan Anne Conti Mica, MD** Department of Orthopedics, University of Chicago, Chicago, IL, USA

**Kyle R. Duchman, MD** Department of Orthopedics and Rehabilitation, University of Iowa Hospitals and Clinics, Iowa City, IA, USA

**Charles L. Getz, MD** Department of Orthopedic Surgery, The Rothman Institute, Thomas Jefferson University Hospital, Philadelphia, PA, USA

**Andrew Green, MD** Division of Shoulder and Elbow Surgery, Department of Orthopedic Surgery, Warren Alpert Medical School, Brown University, Providence, RI, USA

**Carlos Kalbakdij, MD** Department of Orthopedic Surgery, Hospital Universitario La Paz, Madrid, Spain

**Jay D. Keener, MD** Department of Orthopedic Surgery, Washington University, St. Louis, MO, USA

**David Kovacevic, MD** Department of Orthopedic Surgery, Yale University School of Medicine, New Haven, CT, USA

**Craig J. Macken, BS** ONS Foundation for Clinical Research and Education, Greenwich, CT, USA

**Ana Mata-Fink, MD, MS** Department of Orthopedic Surgery, Yale University School of Medicine, New Haven, CT, USA

**Anand M. Murthi, MD** c/o Lyn Camire, Editor, Department of Orthopedic Surgery, MedStar Union Memorial Hospital, Baltimore, MD, USA

**E. Scott Paxton, MD** Department of Orthopedic Surgery, Warren Alpert Medical School, Brown University, Providence, RI, USA

**Matthew L. Ramsey, MD** Department of Orthopedic Surgery, The Rothman Institute, Thomas Jefferson University, Philadelphia, PA, USA

**Dane H. Salazar, MD** Department of Orthopedic Surgery, Washington University, St. Louis, MO, USA

**Eric J. Sarkissian, MD** Department of Orthopedic Surgery, Stanford University Hospital and Clinics, Stanford, CA, USA

**James M. Saucedo, MD, MBA** Department of Orthopedics, The Hand Center of San Antonio, University of Texas Health Sciences Center of San Antonio, San Antonio, TX, USA

**Paul Sethi, MD** Department of Orthopedic Surgery, ONS Foundation for Clinical Research and Education, Greenwich, CT, USA

**J. Michael Smith, MD** Department of Orthopedics, Dartmouth Hitchcock Medical Center, Lebanon, NH, USA

**Laura E. Stoll, MD** Department of Orthopedic Surgery, Washington University School of Medicine, St. Louis, MO, USA

**Roger van Riet, MD, PhD** Department of Orthopedic Surgery and Traumatology, AZ Monica, Deurne, Antwerpen, Belgium

**Robert W. Westermann, MD** Department of Orthopedics and Rehabilitation, University of Iowa Hospitals and Clinics, Iowa City, IA, USA

**Brian R. Wolf, MD, MS** Department of Orthopedics and Rehabilitation, University of Iowa Hospitals and Clinics, Iowa City, IA, USA

**Justin C. Wong, MD** Department of Orthopedic Surgery, Thomas Jefferson University Hospital, Philadelphia, PA, USA

# Part I

# Anatomy and Biomechanics of the Elbow

# Anatomy of the Elbow

1

J. Michael Smith and John-Erik Bell

## Introduction

The elbow is classified as a trochoginglymoid joint because it has the abilities to both flex and extend as a hinge and to supinate and pronate about an axis. Its motion is coordinated with the shoulder to position the hand in space away from the trunk and therefore is crucial for everything from activities of daily living to professional athletics. The joint itself is composed of a complex balance of bone and soft tissues that contribute to motion and stability. It is one of the most congruous joints of the musculoskeletal system and also one of the most stable based on almost equal contributions from the soft tissue constraints and the articular surfaces [1]. Despite this inherent stability, injuries to the bones or soft tissues of the elbow can ultimately result in an unstable joint prone to subluxation or dislocation.

It has become common practice to categorize key elbow anatomic structures into the broad groups of primary and secondary stabilizers. Figure 1.1 is a classic representation of the interplay of the main anatomic stabilizers. The primary stabilizers of the elbow are the ulnohumeral joint, medial collateral ligament (MCL) complex, and lateral collateral ligament (LCL) complex. These are each functionally static stabilizers with fixed positions relative to one another through the elbow's arc of motion. The secondary stabilizers of the elbow are composed of both static and dynamic structures and include in particular the joint capsule, the radiocapitellar joint, and the surrounding musculature.

J.M. Smith, MD (✉) • J.-E. Bell, MD, MS
Department of Orthopedics, Dartmouth Hitchcock Medical Center, 1 Medical Center Drive, Lebanon, NH 03766, USA
e-mail: judd.m.smith@hitchcock.org; jebell527@yahoo.com; John-Erik.Bell@hitchcock.org

## Primary Stabilizers

### Ulnohumeral Joint

The highly congruent bony architecture of the ulnohumeral joint makes it an inherently stable articulation, particularly at the extremes of flexion and extension. The distal humerus is composed of two columns that flare out from the diaphysis and include the medial and lateral condyles and epicondyles, which serve as important sites of origin for other stabilizing structures of the elbow (See Fig. 1.2). Positioned between the two columns are the hemispherical capitellum on the lateral side and the adjacent trochlea on the medial side, its name derived from a Latin word meaning "pulley." The trochlea is covered by cartilage over an arc of 300–330° and articulates with the semilunar notch of the ulna [1, 2]. The medial contour of the trochlea is more prominent and projects more distally than the lateral portion. The center of rotation of the trochlea lies collinear

© Springer International Publishing Switzerland 2017
R.Z. Tashjian (ed.), *The Unstable Elbow*, DOI 10.1007/978-3-319-46019-2_1

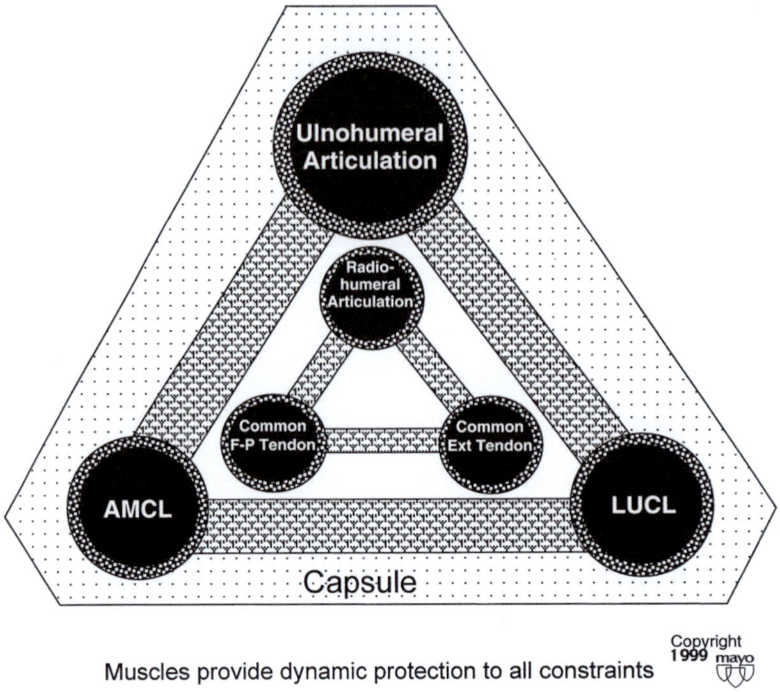


**Fig. 1.1** Illustration showing the static and dynamic constraints to instability. The three primary static constraints to elbow instability are the ulnohumeral articulation, the anterior medial collateral ligament (AMCL), and the lateral collateral ligament, especially the ulnar part of the lateral collateral ligament, which is also referred to as the lateral ulnar collateral ligament (LUCL). The secondary constraints include the radial head, the common flexor and extensor tendon origins, and the capsule. Dynamic stabilizers include the muscles that cross the elbow joint, F-P (flexor-pronator), and produce compressive forces at the articulation. Used with permission of Mayo Foundation for Medical and Educational Research. All rights reserved [47]

**Fig. 1.2** Anatomic features of the distal humerus. This figure republished with permission from The Elbow and Its Disorders, 4th Ed, Morrey BF, 2009, Copyright Elsevier [3]

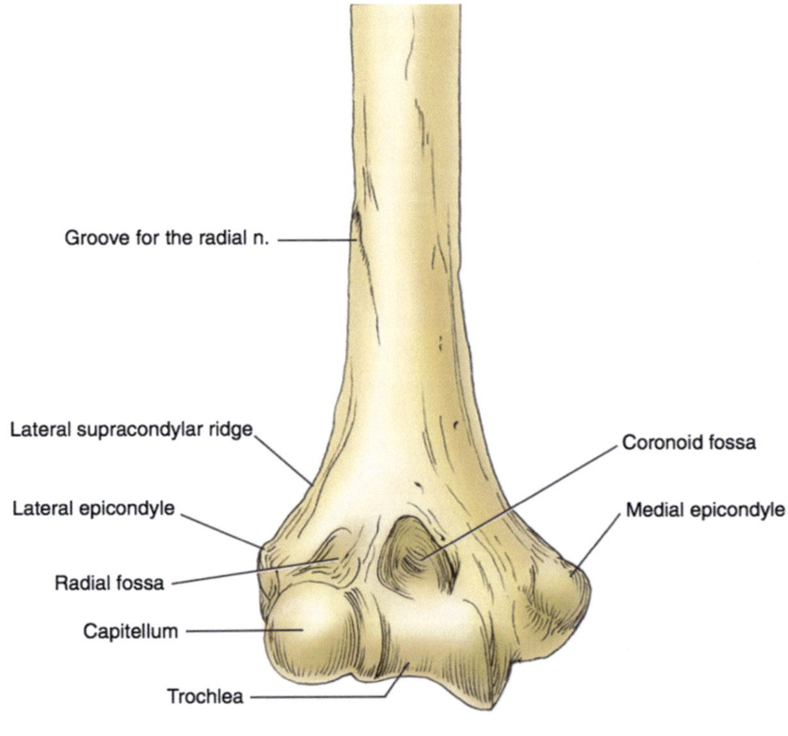

with the anterior cortex of the humerus, rotated about 30° anteriorly with respect to the long axis of the humerus. In the transverse plane, the axis of rotation is rotated internally approximately 5° and in the frontal plane it is in approximately 6° of valgus.

The proximal aspect of the ulna contains the semilunar notch (also known as the greater sigmoid notch or incisura semilunaris), the guiding ridge, and the coronoid process [3]. The trochlear groove on the humerus mates with the guiding ridge of the semilunar notch with a high degree of congruity. To match the anterior position of the trochlea on the humerus, the semilunar notch on the proximal ulna has a posterior inclination of about 30° that promotes bony stability of the elbow in full extension [1]. The ulnohumeral articulation ultimately has its greatest stability at terminal extension and flexion, due to the high degree of conformity between articular surfaces. In extension, the olecranon articulates with the conforming olecranon fossa, while in flexion, the coronoid articulates with the coronoid fossa and the radial head articulates with the radial fossa. In a study designed to remove sequential sections of the ulna while testing the stability of the articulation in extension and at 90° of flexion, it was determined that valgus stress is primarily resisted by the proximal half of the sigmoid notch, whereas varus stress is resisted primarily by the coronoid portion of the articulation [4].

In normal circumstances the range of motion through the ulnohumeral joint is from 0°, or slightly hyperextended, to 150° of flexion [3]. There have been several published analyses of the hinge-like motion of the elbow demonstrating that its rotation occurs through the center of the arcs formed by the trochlear sulcus and capitellum [5, 6]. In several three-dimensional studies of elbow motion, it has been revealed that the elbow has a "helical" type motion with a varying axis of rotation [5, 7]. For practical purposes, the ulnohumeral joint can be assumed to move as a uniaxial articulation.

The coronoid process of the ulna plays a significant role in ulnohumeral stability, and the understanding of its stabilizing role continues to evolve through several recent investigations. Three structures insert on the coronoid: the anterior bundle of the MCL, anterior joint capsule, and the brachialis [8]. The "critical portion" of the coronoid needed for stability has been debated and information on the amount of the coronoid required for stability with or without ligamentous integrity and with and without the radial head is now emerging [9]. As sections of the coronoid are sequentially removed, the elbow becomes progressively unstable. An investigation by Hull et al. has shown that significant varus instability exists after 50 % resection of the coronoid process, particularly in lower flexion angles [10]. Recent attention has been given to the anteromedial facet of the coronoid. O'Driscoll et al. has proposed a new variation to the classic fracture classification of Regan and Morrey attributing more significance to anteromedial facet involvement owing to the facet's significant stabilizing function [11]. Anteromedial facet fractures can involve injury to the anterior bundle of the medial collateral ligament if they involve the sublime tubercle, and are typically associated with disruptions of the lateral ulnar collateral ligament and posterior band of the MCL, leading to varus and posteromedial rotational instability. The importance of the anteromedial facet with regards to varus stability was confirmed in a biomechanical study by Pollock et al. [12].

## Medial Ligaments

The medial collateral ligament (MCL) is a complex of ligamentous structures that together serve as primary stabilizers to valgus and internal rotatory stresses on the joint [13] (See Fig. 1.3). The MCL is composed of three parts: an anterior bundle (anterior oblique), posterior bundle (Bardinet ligament), and a transverse segment (ligament of Cooper) [3, 13–16]. Of these three parts, the anterior bundle is felt to be the component most consistently identified in cadaveric studies while the posterior bundle and transverse bundle are occasionally absent or indistinguishable from the joint capsule [17]. The anterior bundle originates from the anteroinferior medial epicondyle and inserts immediately adjacent to the articular

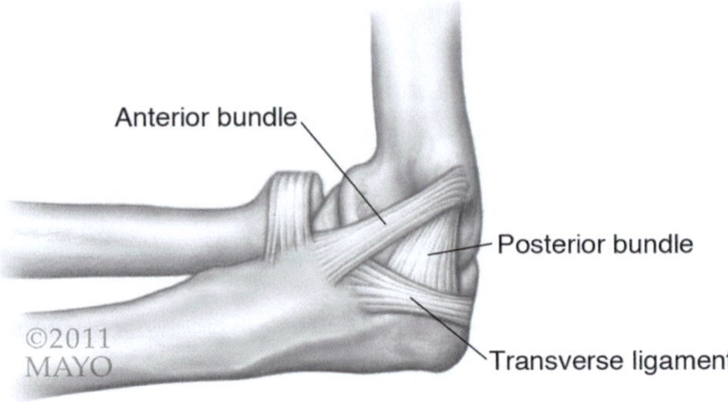


**Fig. 1.3** Medial collateral ligament complex with anterior bundle, posterior bundle, and transverse ligament. Used with permission of Mayo Foundation for Medical and Educational Research. All rights reserved [3]

surface of the ulna at the sublime tubercle [1, 14, 17]. The average area of the origin has been measured as 45.5 $mm^2$, and the average area of the insertion has been measured as 127.8 $mm^2$. The edge of the insertion is separated from the ulna articular margin by an average of 2.8 mm [18]. Biomechanical studies have led to further subdivision of the anterior bundle into an anterior band, a posterior band, and more central isometric "guiding bundle." [19] The posterior bundle is generally described as a fan-shaped thickening of the capsule originating from the inferior medial epicondyle, inserting along the mid-portion of the medial margin of the semilunar notch [3] and forming the floor of the cubital tunnel [14]. The transverse ligament is composed of horizontal fibers from the coronoid to the tip of the olecranon [17]. Of the aforementioned structures, the anterior bundle has been identified as the most important structure for valgus elbow stability with the posterior bundle a distant second. The transverse ligament has no measurable impact on elbow stability [14, 20].

The anterior bundle of the MCL does not originate precisely at the center of rotation of the ulnohumeral joint, thus the tension within the ligament varies from flexion to extension (See Fig. 1.4). Further research into this concept has lead to the description of the separate anterior and posterior bands [21]. The anterior band is under tension in extension while the posterior band is under tension in flexion [14]. The intermediate segment (or guiding bundle) is a small group of fibers that are functionally isometric sitting between anterior and posterior bands [17, 22]. Based on these observations, the anterior and posterior bands appear to have biomechanically different roles.

These three parts of the MCL have been studied in several biomechanical investigations designed to determine their relative contributions to stability. In general, these studies have utilized cadaveric specimens and materials testing instrumentation designed to apply a specific amount of force and then measuring the resultant displacement and angulation. In these models, the ligamentous structures are sequentially cut as force is applied in order to determine relative contributions to valgus stability [13, 14, 23–25]. These investigations agree that the anterior bundle of the MCL is the most important contributor to valgus stability. In an early study by Morrey et al., the MCL was shown to contribute roughly 31 % of total elbow valgus stability in extension and 55 % of the stability in 90° flexion [24]. Follow-up studies by Morrey et al. and Hotchkiss et al. showed that it acts as a primary valgus stabilizer between 20 and 120° of flexion supplying up to 78 % of valgus stability [13, 23]. In similar fashion, Callaway et al. showed that the anterior band of the anterior bundle serves as the primary restraint to valgus rotation at 30, 60, and 90° of flexion while the posterior band is the co-primary restraint at 120° flexion. The posterior bundle is a secondary restraint at 30° only [14]. An intact MCL provides essentially full stability in the absence of the radial head, which becomes significant in surgical decision-making in the setting of isolated comminuted fractures of the radial

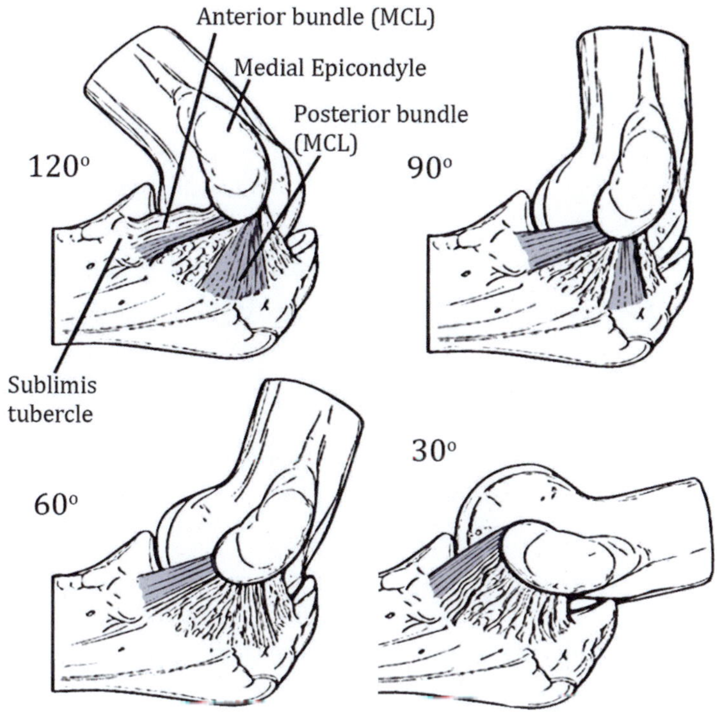


**Fig. 1.4** Dynamic representation of the medical collateral ligament complex at different points of elbow flexion. Areas of tension highlighted by the shaded areas in the figure. Within the anterior bundle, the bands tighten in reciprocal fashion. The anterior band is taught in extension and relaxed in flexion while the posterior band is taught in flexion and relaxed in extension (represented by the *shaded areas*). Tension in the posterior bundle increases with elbow flexion (Modified with permission from Callaway et al. Biomechanical evaluation of the medial collateral ligament of the elbow. J Bone Joint Surg Am. 1997;79:1223–31 [14])

head where excision may be considered an option with intact ligaments [13]. However in the setting of elbow instability and compromised ligaments, radial head excision is not an option and repair or replacement should be performed.

## Lateral Ligaments

The lateral collateral ligament complex (LCL) contributes to varus and posterolateral stability. The LCL consists of 3 main parts that have been shown to contribute in some measure to elbow stability: the lateral ulnar collateral (LUCL), radial collateral (RCL), and annular ligaments (see Fig. 1.5). Also included in the description of the LCL is the accessory LCL, which functions to stabilize the annular ligament during varus stress [3]. These structures have more anatomic variability and are sometimes difficult to distinguish compared to their medial counterparts [17]. The Lateral Ulnar Collateral Ligament (LUCL) serves as the primary restraint to posterolateral rotatory instability (PLRI) and varus forces [26–28]. Overall LCL complex remains taut throughout the range of motion of elbow flexion and extension [1].

The RCL originates from the lateral epicondyle and is a complex of several components that insert on the annular ligament. It is approximately 20 mm long and 8 mm wide. Its superficial surface is the location of the supinator muscle origin [3]. It is nearly isometric throughout elbow flexion and extension with its greatest contribution to stability in extension [29]. Morrey et al. demonstrated that the RCL contributes 14 % of varus stability in extension and 9 % in 90° flexion [24]. More recent anatomical studies have attributed a

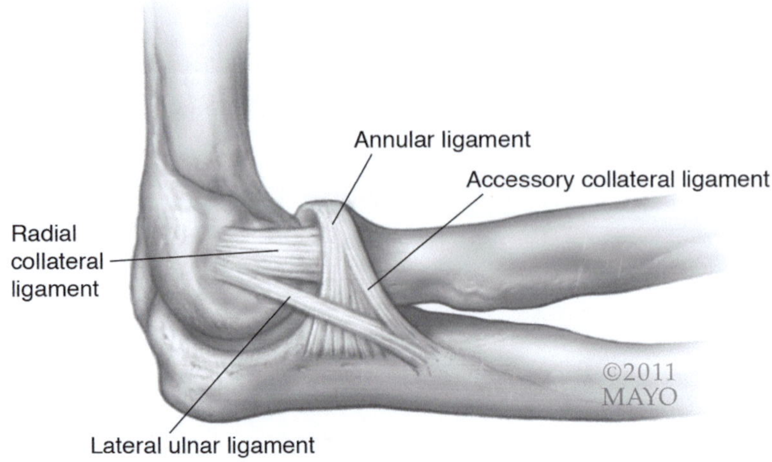


**Fig. 1.5** Lateral collateral ligament complex with lateral ulnar collateral, radial collateral, annular and accessory collateral ligaments. Used with permission of Mayo Foundation for Medical and Educational Research. All rights reserved [3]

more significant role to the RCL in preventing PLRI [30].

The LUCL was originally described by Morrey and An [17]. It is a thickening of the ligamentocapsular complex that originates from the lateral epicondyle, blends into the fibers of the annular ligament and terminates on the supinator crest, deep to the fascia surrounding the extensor carpi ulnaris and supinator muscles [3, 31]. The humeral attachment of the LUCL is a well-defined area on the lateral side of the elbow at the isometric point [32]. Its biomechanical role is to stabilize the elbow during varus stress as well as serving as a posterior buttress to prevent radiocapitellar subluxation [31]. O'Driscoll described the role of the LUCL as preventing ulnohumeral rotation along the long axis of the ulna [28]. Investigations have shown that isolated lateral ulnar collateral or radial collateral ligament injuries do not result in instability but rather, combined injuries are necessary to create functional instability [30, 33].

Lastly, the annular ligament is an important stabilizer of the proximal radioulnar and radiocapitellar joints. It originates and inserts on the anterior and posterior margins of the lesser sigmoid notch, encircling the radius but not attaching to it [3, 31]. The more distal aspect of the ligament has a smaller radius to more tightly contain the radial neck [31]. It serves as the site of origin for the supinator muscle, with deep muscle fibers intimately fused with the ligament [34]. Transection of the annular ligament results in medial-lateral and anterior-posterior translation of the radial head by 44 % and 24 %, respectively [35]. Dunning et al. demonstrated that when the annular ligament is intact, either the RCL or LUCL can be transected without creating significant PLRI, demonstrating the annular ligament's role as a primary static stabilizer [33].

## Secondary Stabilizers

### Radiocapitellar Joint

The radiocapitellar joint is a secondary stabilizer to valgus stress. The lateral column of the distal humerus terminates with the capitellum and articulates with the radial head. The capitellum is hemispherical in shape and covered with hyaline cartilage. It projects anteriorly from the diaphysis by 30° [3]. The corresponding concave radial head has an angular arc of about 40° and a rim of articular cartilage covering 240° to articulate with the lesser sigmoid notch of the proximal ulna [3]. The center of rotation of the radiocapitellar joint moves from anterior on the capitellum in flexion to inferior on the capitellum in full extension. The radial head is directed 15° off the long axis of the radius [3]. There is a combined rotation of approximately 170° through this joint, 90° supination and 80–90°

pronation [1]. With loading of the elbow, it has been demonstrated that 60 % of axial loads are imparted through the radiocapitellar joint and 40 % are through the ulnohumeral joint [36].

Valgus stability comes primarily from the medial collateral ligament, and when the MCL is intact, the radial head does not offer any significant additional valgus constraint. This is of particular importance in the setting of isolated comminuted radial head fractures. The radial head may be resected without altering the stability of the otherwise normal elbow in the setting of these isolates comminuted fractures [37]. With a released or compromised medial collateral ligament, the radial head provides some resistance to valgus stress [1]. Thus, the radial head is important as a secondary valgus stabilizer, contributing an additional 30 % of valgus stability through both flexion and extension and is crucial for stability in the setting of damaged medial ligaments [13, 17].

## Joint Capsule

The joint capsule of the elbow is a thin layer of tissue that surrounds the entire joint and lies in close association with the ligamentous stabilizers. The anterior capsule inserts proximally on the humerus above the coronoid and radial head fossae. Distally, the capsule attaches to the anterior margin of the coronoid medially as well as to the annular ligament laterally. Posteriorly, the capsule attaches above the olecranon fossa, along the supracondylar columns. Distally, the attachment is along the medial and lateral articular margin of the sigmoid notch of the ulna [3]. The capsule is maximally distensible at around 70–80° of flexion with a volume of 25–30 ml [1]. In extension, the anterior capsule contributes about 70 % of the soft tissue restraint to distraction but far less in flexion [24]. The joint capsule has also been shown to be an independent stabilizer of the elbow. In the classic study by Morrey et al., valgus stability is equally divided among the medial collateral ligament, anterior capsule, and bony articulation in full extension [24]. At 90° of flexion, the contribution of the anterior capsule is assumed by the MCL [24]. In the same study, varus stress was noted to be resisted primarily by the anterior capsule (32 %) and the joint articulation (55 %) with the elbow in extension [24]. At 90° of flexion the anterior capsule offers only 13 % of resistance to varus stress [24].

## Musculature

The primary muscles that provide flexion of the elbow include the brachialis, biceps, and brachioradialis. The primary elbow extensor is the triceps. The flexor-pronator group of muscles originates from a common tendon on the medial condyle and includes the flexor carpi radialis (FCR), palmaris longus (PL), pronator teres (PT), flexor digitorum superficialis (FDS), and flexor carpi ulnaris (FCU). The forearm extensors arise from the lateral condyle and include brachioradialis (BR), extensor carpi radialis longus (ECRL), extensor carpi radialis brevis (ECRB), extensor carpi ulnaris (ECU), extensor digiti minimi (EDM), and extensor digitorum comminus (EDC). The anconeus also has its origin at the lateral condyle, and it inserts proximally on the posterior ulna providing a stabilizing role against PLRI. The supinator has a dual origin, with one head from the lateral condyle and another from the proximal ulna.

The elbow flexors assist joint stability primarily by augmenting the ulnohumeral joint. Morrey et al. [13] simulated muscles in a cadaveric model and showed that the biceps, brachialis, and triceps contribute to joint stability through a compression effect on the ulnohumeral joint, augmenting the inherent boney stability of the congruent articulation [13, 38]. The brachialis inserts on the coronoid and acts as a buttress to restrain posterior subluxation [39].

The contributions of elbow musculature to elbow stability have been studied in several models. In cadaveric studies, the ultimate failure of the MCL occurs at an average of 34 Nm of force [40], while professional pitchers can generate up to 120 Nm of valgus torque about the elbow [41]. Many investigators have used this information to generate hypotheses about how the contracted muscles around the elbow must be secondarily supporting the ligaments to prevent injury. Studies have come to different conclusions. One study, using electromyographic evidence showed that the flexor pronator mass did not provide a significant amount of support to the medial side of the elbow [42]. In contrast, An et al. [43] theorized a role for the flexor-pronator mass in dynamic stabilization using a biomechanical model that took into account the moment arm of each muscle and cross sectional area and postulated that the FDS provided the greatest varus moment. Davidson et al. [44] suggested in an anatomic study that the FDS and FCU both contributed to dynamic valgus stability of the elbow, with the FCU hypothesized as having the greatest contribution given its anatomic position in line with the MCL. A model by Park et al. [38] was designed to test elbows in 30 and 90° of flexion with a simulated MCL tear and simulations of flexor-pronator muscle contraction. Their study showed that the flexor-pronator muscles had a measurable independent role on valgus stability with the FCU having the greatest contribution followed by FDS and PT, respectively. This effect was due to direct muscle action with muscle force vectors resisting valgus torque. A study by Udall et al. [45] used a different model with a "stretched MCL" rather than a fully cut ligament and found that the FDS provided the greatest amount of active stabilization from the flexor pronator mass. The authors felt that the stretched ligament model better represented a chronic MCL injury state to better represent the injury commonly sustained by baseball pitchers.

The muscles on the lateral aspect of the forearm play their own role in elbow stability. The principal secondary restraints to varus stress are the extensor muscles with their fascial bands and intermuscular septa [27]. Of all the extensors, the ECU has the best mechanical advantage in resisting rotatory instability because of its course. It originates on the most inferior aspect of the lateral epicondyle and inserts on the ulna approximately 5 cm distal to the center of the radial head [27]. In addition, the anconeus is active in extension and pronation and assists in joint stability, being anatomically oriented to provide restraint to PLRI [46].

## Conclusion

An in-depth understanding of elbow joint anatomy is crucial to diagnosing and treating acute and chronic elbow instability. New discoveries continue to emerge about how key anatomic structures contribute to elbow stability, particularly as experimental models and testing instrumentation become more precise. Future investigations are required to quantify these contributions and determine their overall clinical importance.

## References

1. An K-N, Zobitz ME, Morrey BF. Biomechanics of the elbow. In: Morrey BF, editor. The elbow and its disorders. 4th ed. Amsterdam: Elsevier; 2009. p. 39–63.
2. Guerra JJ, Timmerman LA. Clinical anatomy, histology and pathomechanics of the elbow in sports. Oper Tech Sports Med. 1996;4(2):69–76.
3. Morrey BF. Anatomy of the elbow joint. In: Morrey BF, Sanchez-Sotelo J, editors. The elbow and its disorders. 4th ed. Philadelphia, PA: Saunders; 2009. p. 11–38. The Mayo Clinic Foundation.
4. An K-N, Morrey BF, Chao EY. The effect of partial removal of proximal ulna on elbow constraint. Clin Orthop Relat Res. 1986;209:270–9.
5. Morrey BF, Chao EY. Passive motion of the elbow joint. J Bone Joint Surg Am. 1976;58(4):501–8.
6. London JT. Kinematics of the elbow. J Bone Joint Surg Am. 1981;63(4):529–35.
7. Ishizuki M. Functional anatomy of the elbow joint and three-dimensional quantitative motion analysis of the elbow joint. Nihon Seikeigeka Gakkai Zasshi. 1979;53(8):989–96.
8. Ablove RH, Moy OJ, Howard C, Peimer CA, S'Doia S. Ulnar coronoid process anatomy: possible implications for elbow instability. Clin Orthop Relat Res. 2006;449:259–61.
9. Doornberg JN, Duijn JV, Ring D. Coronoid fracture height in terrible-triad injuries. J Hand Surg Am. 2006;31(5):794–7.
10. Hull JR, Owen JR, Fern SE, Wayne JS, Boardman ND. Role of the coronoid process in varus osteoarticular stability of the elbow. J Shoulder Elbow Surg. 2005; 14(4):441–6.
11. Reichel LM, Milam GS, Hillin CD, Reitman CA. Osteology of the coronoid process with clinical correlation to coronoid fractures in terrible triad injuries. J Shoulder Elbow Surg. 2013;22(3):323–8.
12. Pollock JW. The effect of anteromedial facet fractures of the coronoid and lateral collateral ligament injury on elbow stability and kinematics. J Bone Joint Surg Am. 2009;91(6):1448.

13. Morrey B, Tanaka S, An K-N. Valgus stability of the elbow. Clin Orthop Relat Res. 1991;265:187–95.
14. Callaway GH, Field LD, Deng XH, Torzilli PA, O'Brien SJ, Altchek DW, et al. Biomechanical evaluation of the medial collateral ligament of the elbow. J Bone Joint Surg Am. 1997;79:1223–31.
15. O'Driscoll SW, Jaloszynski R, Morrey BF, An KN. Origin of the medial ulnar collateral ligament. J Hand Surg Am. 1992;17(1):164–8.
16. Brabston EW, Genuario JW, Bell J-E. Anatomy and physical examination of the elbow. Oper Tech Orthop. 2009;19(4):190–8.
17. Morrey BF, An K-N. Functional anatomy of the ligaments of the elbow. Clin Orthop Relat Res. 1985; 201:84–90.
18. Dugas JR, Ostrander RV, Cain EL, Kingsley D, Andrews JR. Anatomy of the anterior bundle of the ulnar collateral ligament. J Shoulder Elbow Surg. 2007;16(5):657–60.
19. Fuss FK. The ulnar collateral ligament of the human elbow joint: anatomy. Function and biomechanics. J Anat. 1991;175:203–12.
20. Eygendaal D, Olsen BS, Jensen SL, Seki A, Sojbjerg JO. Kinematics of partial and total ruptures of the medial collateral ligament of the elbow. J Shoulder Elbow Surg. 1999;8(6):612–6.
21. Schwab GH, Bennett JB, Woods GW, Tullos HS. Biomechanics of Elbow Instability: the role of the medial collateral ligament. Clin Orthop Relat Res. 1980; (146): 42–52.
22. Armstrong A. The medial collateral ligament of the elbow is not isometric: an in vitro biomechanical study. Am J Sports Med. 2004;32:85–90.
23. Hotchkiss RN, Weiland AJ. Valgus stability of the elbow. J Orthop Res. 1987;5(3):372–7.
24. Morrey BF, An K-N. Articular and ligamentous contributions to the stability of the elbow joint. Am J Sports Med. 1983;11(5):315–9.
25. Pribyl CR, Kester MA, Cook SD, Edmunds JO, Brunet ME. The effect of the radial head and prosthetic radial head replacement on resisting valgus stress at the elbow. Orthopedics. 1986;9(5):723–6.
26. McKee MD, Schemitsch EH, Sala MJ, O'Driscoll SW. The pathoanatomy of lateral ligamentous disruption in complex elbow instability. J Shoulder Elbow Surg. 2003;12(4):391–6.
27. Cohen MS, Hastings H. Rotatory instability of the elbow: the anatomy and role of the lateral stabilizers. J Bone Joint Surg Am. 1997;79A(2):225–33.
28. O'Driscoll SW, Bell D, Morrey BF. Posterolateral rotatory instability of the elbow. J Bone Joint Surg Am. 1991;73(3):440–6.
29. Moritomo H, Murase T, Arimitsu S, Oka K, Yoshikawa H, Sugamoto K. The in vivo isometric point of the lateral ligament of the elbow. J Bone Joint Surg Am. 2007;89:2011–7.
30. McAdams TR, Masters GW, Srivastava S. The effect of arthroscopic sectioning of the lateral ligament complex of the elbow on posterolateral rotatory stability. J Shoulder Elbow Surg. 2005;14(3):298–301.
31. Tashjian RZ, Katarincic JA. Complex elbow instability. J Am Acad Orthop Surg. 2006;14:278–86.
32. Driscoll SW, Horii E, Morrey BF, Carmichael SW. Anatomy of the ulnar part of the lateral collateral ligament of the elbow. Clin Anat. 1992;5(4):296–303.
33. Dunning CE, Zarzour ZD, Patterson SD, Johnson JA, King GJ. Ligamentous stabilizers against posterolateral rotatory instability of the elbow. J Bone Joint Surg Am. 2001;83-A(12):1823–8.
34. Bozkurt M, Acar HI, Apaydin N, Leblebicioglu G, Elhan A, Tekdemir I, et al. The annular ligament: an anatomical study. Am J Sports Med. 2005;33(1): 114–8.
35. Galik K, Baratz ME, Butler AL, Dougherty J, Cohen MS, Miller MC. The effect of the annular ligament on kinematics of the radial head. J Hand Surg Am. 2007;32(8):1218–24.
36. Jensen SL, Olsen BS, Seki A, Ole Sojbjerg J, Sneppen O. Radiohumeral stability to forced translation: an experimental analysis of the bony constraint. J Shoulder Elbow Surg. 2002;11(2):158–65.
37. Morrey BF, An K-N. Stability of the elbow: osseous constraints. J Shoulder Elbow Surg. 2005;14(1): S174–8.
38. Park MC, Ahmad CS. Dynamic contributions of the flexor-pronator mass to elbow valgus stability. J Bone Joint Surg Am. 2006;86(10):2268–74.
39. Richards RR, Williams GR, Yamaguchi K, Ramsey ML. Shoulder and elbow arthroplasty. Philadelphia, PA: Lippincott Williams and Wilkins; 2005. p. 279–95.
40. Ahmad CS, Lee TQ, ElAttrache NS. Biomechanical evaluation of a new ulnar collateral ligament reconstruction technique with interference screw fixation. Am J Sports Med. 2003;31(3):332–7.
41. Fleisig GS, Andrews JR, Dillman CJ, Escamilla RF. Kinetics of baseball pitching with implications about injury mechanisms. Am J Sports Med. 1995; 23(2):233–9.
42. Hamilton CD, Glousman RE, Jobe FW, Brault J, Pink M, Perry J. Dynamic stability of the elbow: electromyographic analysis of the flexor pronator group and the extensor group in pitchers with valgus instability. J Shoulder Elbow Surg. 1996;5(5):347–54.
43. An K-N, Hui FC, Morrey BF, Linscheid RL, Chao EY. Muscles across the elbow joint: a biomechanical analysis. J Biomech. 1981;14(10):659–69.
44. Davidson PA, Pink M, Perry J, Jobe FW. Functional anatomy of the flexor pronator muscle group in relation to the medial collateral ligament of the elbow. Am J Sports Med. 1995;23(2):245–50.
45. Udall JH, Fitzpatrick MJ, McGarry MH, Leba TB, Lee TQ. Effects of flexor-pronator muscle loading on valgus stability of the elbow with an intact, stretched, and resected medial ulnar collateral ligament. J Shoulder Elbow Surg. 2009;18(5):773–8.
46. Ring D, Jupiter J. Fracture-dislocation of the elbow. J Bone Joint Surg Am. 1998;80:566–80.
47. O'Driscoll SW, Jupiter JB, King G, Hotchkiss RN, Morrey BF. The unstable elbow. J Bone Joint Surg Am. 2000;82(5):724–38.

# Biomechanics of the Elbow

# 2

Peter N. Chalmers and Aaron M. Chamberlain

## Introduction

The elbow joint is composed of three articulations that share a common joint capsule: the ulnotrochlear joint, the radiocapitellar joint, and the proximal radioulnar joint. Together, these articulations are described as a "trochoginglymoid" joint as they allow two degrees of freedom: elbow flexion and extension and forearm pronation and supination. The elbow thus complements the sphere of motion provided by the shoulder, allowing the hand to be positioned in a wide variety of locations in space. Elbow stiffness and instability can thus lead to substantial functional loss that can threaten a patient's function. The ulnotrochlear joint also provides a fulcrum against which the forearm acts a lever. In this capacity, pressures generated in the elbow can exceed three-times body weight.

The flexion/extension motion of the elbow has been described as a "sloppy hinge" because the axis of rotation moves up to 3–4° and 2.5 mm when ranging from a fully extended to a fully flexed position. This is due to obliquity in the trochlear groove and corresponding sigmoid notch [1]. The flexion-extension axis of the joint does not lie within any cardinal plane of the body as it is 3–8° internally rotated relative to the humeral epicondyles and is in 4–8° of valgus relative to the long axis of the humerus. The valgus obliquity of the flexion-extension axis, combined with obliquity in the humeral and ulnar shafts contributes to the "carrying angle" of the elbow, which is 10–15° in men and 15–20° in women [1, 2]. The combination of internal rotation and valgus in the flexion/extension axis ensures that objects carried in the hand with the elbow extended and the shoulder adducted do not strike the ipsilateral leg and that with flexion the hand naturally comes towards the mouth.

A number of landmarks can be used fluoroscopically to locate the flexion-extension axis of the elbow. On a perfect lateral view of the elbow, this axis should lies at (a) the center of a best-fit circle placed upon the capitellum [1, 3], (b) the center of a best-fit circle placed upon the trochlea [4], and (c) the intersection between the axis of center the radial shaft and the anterior humeral cortical line [5]. The native varus-valgus laxity of the joint has been incorporated into the design of total elbow arthroplasty articulations to create "semi-constrained" implants, which have decreased rates of aseptic loosening [1, 3]. However, apart from the extremes of flexion and extension, the flexion and extension motion of

P.N. Chalmers, MD
Department of Orthopedic Surgery, Washington University in St. Louis, 660 South Euclid Avenue, Campus Box 8233, St. Louis, MO 63110, USA
e-mail: p.n.chalmers@gmail.com

A.M. Chamberlain, MD, MSc (✉)
Department of Orthopedic Surgery, Washington University Medical Center, 660 South Euclid Avenue, Campus Box 8233, St. Louis, MO 63110, USA
e-mail: chamberlaina@wudosis.wustl.edu

© Springer International Publishing Switzerland 2017
R.Z. Tashjian (ed.), *The Unstable Elbow*, DOI 10.1007/978-3-319-46019-2_2

the elbow can basically be considered a simple hinge, allowing the placement of hinged external fixators without significant alteration of joint kinematics [4, 6, 7]. Clinically, accurate location of the axis of rotation is challenging and requires an anatomic reduction and repeated cyclic motion with observation of the articular surfaces for gapping during hinged fixator placement. This must be performed very accurately since malalignments as small as 5° increases energy expenditures for flexion and extension by 3.7-fold [7].

The pronation/supination motion of the elbow takes place through a longitudinal axis that passes through the convexity of the radial head at the proximal radioulnar joint. Although forearm rotation has traditionally been conceptualized as radial rotation around a stable ulna, this axis of rotation is oblique to the axis of the ulna [1, 2]. Thus, some axial ulnar rotation occurs with forearm rotation. In cadaveric studies, up to 6° of ulnar rotation occurs with forearm rotation even with an intact capsule, intact ligaments, and intact articular surfaces [8].

Normal elbow joint range of motion is from 0° of extension to 150° of flexion and from 75° of pronation to 85° of supination. The elbow joint capacity reaches a maximum of 25 mL at 80° [9], which has been suggested as the reason why joint contractures usually center at this position [10]. Classically it has been suggested that only 30° of extension and 130° of flexion are necessary for activities of daily living [11]. Extension loss is often well tolerated because patients can move closer to objects that cannot be reached as a result of an extension loss, while flexion loss is poorly tolerated because it interferes with feeding and head hygiene. Historically, it was suggested that supination loss is more poorly tolerated than pronation loss because pronation loss can be compensated for with shoulder abduction. However, with the advent of keyboards, many patients value pronation over supination as shoulder abduction over an extended period of time rapidly leads to rotator cuff fatigue and pain. A recent study has demonstrated that contemporary tasks such as using a computer mouse or keyboard may require a functional range of motion greater than that reported previously [12].

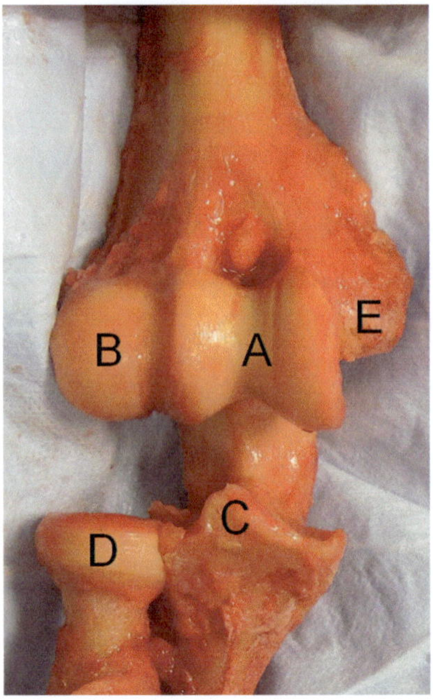


**Fig. 2.1** This clinical photograph with all soft tissues removed from the elbow demonstrates the osseous congruity of the articulation. (*A*) Trochea. (*B*) Capitellum. (*C*) Coronoid. (*D*) Radial head. (*E*) Medial Epicondyle

The articular surfaces of the elbow are among the most highly congruent of any joint within the body and thus significantly contribute to elbow stability. In particular, between the coronoid, sigmoid notch, and olecranon, the proximal ulna provides a 180° arc of articular cartilage that articulates with a 320° of articular cartilage on the trochlea of the distal humerus during flexion and extension motion. The trochlea also has a sulcus that provides a guiding groove for a matching ridge within the sigmoid notch (Fig. 2.1). Numerous cadaveric studies have been conducted to determine the relative contributions of the articular surfaces as compared to the medial and lateral collateral ligaments to elbow stability [5, 13–20]. Regardless of these cadaveric studies, clinically it is known both that (1) in the absence of a periarticular fracture, most elbow dislocations can be treated successfully nonoperatively without recurrence of instability [21, 22] and that (2) in a majority of elbow dislocations both the medial and lateral collateral ligament complexes are completely torn. In many of these cases the entire extensor musculature is avulsed from the humerus as well [23]. Thus, intact articular congruity is sufficient for clinical stability in most cases. These findings are bolstered by a cadaveric study showing that elbow resistance to displacement, torsion, and axial forces in both flexion and extension has an inverse linear relationship to proximal ulnar excision [13].

Muscular forces interact with articular conformity to maintain elbow stability. Coactivation of the agonist–antagonist group (biceps, brachialis, and triceps) acts to center joint forces within the available articular arc of the ulnotrochlear joint [24, 25], while activation of the wrist extensors acts to center the radial head on the capitellum [15, 26]. Both the ulnohumeral and radiocapitellar joints are stabilized via a concavity-compression mechanism. After instability secondary to trauma, elbow rehabilitation regimens have thus focused upon supine active range of motion focusing on coactivation [27]. Electromyographic studies have shown that the anconeus is active during almost all elbow motions, which has led some authors to suggest that this muscle may also serve a role as a dynamic stabilizer [2]. The triceps has more than twice the cross-sectional area of any other muscle crossing the elbow joint and is larger than the biceps and brachialis combined. Of the flexors, the brachioradialis has a larger moment arm than the biceps, which is also larger than the brachialis. Generally, as muscle moment arms increase both muscle force and joint reaction force increase. Thus, those muscles with insertions closest to the articulation have larger moment arms and can produce the largest joint compression forces and thus make the largest dynamic contributions to stability. Moment is affected by joint position. In flexion, the overall potential flexor moment is equal to the potential extensor moment, while in extension the potential extensor moment exceeds the potential flexor moment. This may contribute to a greater propensity for elbow instability in extension as compared to flexion [2]. Muscle moment arms are also affected by humeral length, with potential triceps force production reduced by 20 % with one cm of humeral shortening, 40 % with two cm of humeral shortening, and 60 % with three cm of humeral shortening [28].

Classically, 40 % of axial loads across the elbow are transferred across the ulnohumeral joint and 60 % across the radiohumeral joint. However, load transfer is sensitive to a variety of factors. Changes in varus and valgus positioning of the elbow can lead to large changes in joint loading force. In valgus, 93 % of axial loads are transferred across the radius [29]. In addition, flexion and extension alter loading, with the radiocapitellar joint being more loaded in full extension [30]. This is due to the fact that in this position the muscles passing across the ulnotrochlear joint have the shortest moment arms [24]. The integrity of the interosseous membrane, in particular the central band [31], also alters load transfer, particular with the elbow in varus [29]. Finally, forearm rotational position alters load transfer, with pronation loading the ulnotrochlear joint and supination loading the radiocapitellar joint [29]. Loss of elbow stability can lead to malalignment and overload of one side of the joint, which can lead to accelerated radiocapitellar or ulnotrochlear degenerative changes.

While abundant cadaveric biomechanical studies have been conducted in attempt to understand the contributors to elbow stability [5, 13–20], these experiments are difficult to perform and their findings can be difficult to generalize to biokinematics in the live patient. First, in addition to displacement, instability can occur with rotation in three planes of each of the three bones. Second, cadaveric studies provide incomplete simulation of the contributions from the dynamic stabilizers. Third, while early experiments were performed using mechanical testing equipment, later experiments with electromagnetic tracking equipment have in several cases arrived at very different conclusions [32]. Fourth, forearm rotational position also alters laxity and joint reaction forces, with varus/valgus laxity in general increased in forearm pronation [33, 34], although the medial soft tissues are stressed more in pronation and the lateral soft tissues are stressed more in supination [5, 20, 25, 27, 35]. Finally, the relative contributions of each structure depend upon the deforming force applied, with many early studies applying nonphysiologic forces. As a result, even relatively elementary aspects of elbow biomechanics remain controversial.

## Lateral Elbow Stability

As described by O'Driscoll and colleagues, the most common mechanism for dislocation of the elbow is rotation of the forearm on the humerus into valgus, extension, and external rotation as the forearm supinates off the humerus [36]. As this motion progresses tissue damage progresses from lateral to medial. The lateral collateral ligament complex first tears [37], then the anterior and posterior capsules tear, and finally the ulnar collateral ligament tears [36]. Depending upon the position of the arm and the energy of the trauma during the injury as well as the patient's anatomy, the radial head and coronoid may also be fractured [38–40]. In 66 % of cases there are concomitant tears of the common extensors and in 50 % of cases there are concomitant tears of the anterior band of the ulnar collateral ligament [37]. Dislocation of the elbow without tearing the ulnar collateral ligament is theoretically possible with rotation around an intact ulnar collateral ligament although clinical dislocation without tearing of the ulnar collateral ligament is uncommon [36]. Finally, recent video evidence has suggested valgus may be more common than varus as a mechanism of injury [41].

The articular surfaces provide the majority of the stability to varus stress, supplying 55 % of stability in extension and 75 % in flexion [2]. Among the soft tissues, the lateral collateral ligament complex is the primary stabilizer of the ulnohumeral joint to varus stress [5, 8, 16, 35], with fascial bands within the extensor musculature (in particular the extensor carpi ulnaris, which has the best mechanical advantage) also playing a role resisting varus stress [5]. Clinically, residual lateral instability of the elbow is poorly tolerated because shoulder abduction places a varus stress across the elbow and thus many activities of daily living subject the elbow to varus stress (Fig. 2.2). By the same logic, an external fixation device applied to the lateral elbow for residual instability after instability repair protects the lateral collateral ligament complex by acting as a tension band, while offering relatively less protection to a medial repair or reconstruction [6].

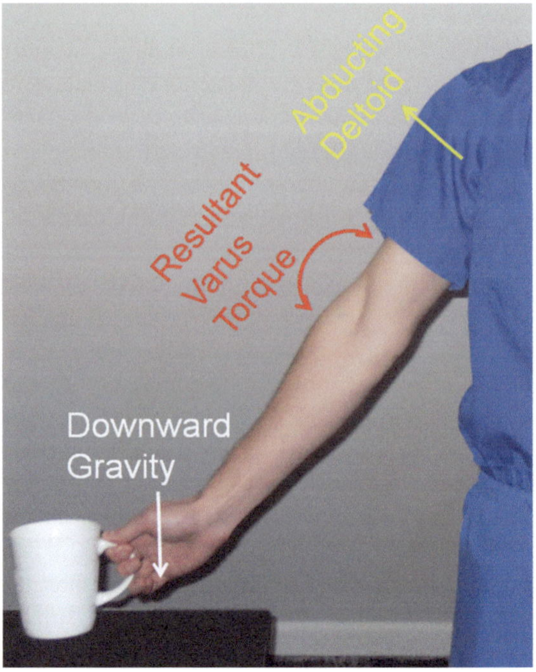


**Fig. 2.2** This clinical photograph demonstrates how activities of daily living subject the elbow to varus stress. In this image, a subject is picking a coffee cup up off of a table. The deltoid (*straight yellow arrow*) pulls through the arm as a lever against gravity on the cup (*straight white arrow*) to create a varus stress across the elbow (*curved red arrow*)

## Lateral Collateral Ligament Complex

The lateral collateral ligament complex is classically thought to be composed of three portions: the lateral ulnar collateral ligament, the radial collateral ligament, and the annular ligament (Fig. 2.3) [5, 16, 42]. These structures are anatomically discrete from one another and from the overlying extensor musculature to a variable degree [5, 43]. Both the lateral ulnar collateral ligament and the radial collateral ligament arise anterior to the lateral epicondyle, with the radial collateral ligament becoming confluent with the fibers of the annular ligament while the lateral ulnar collateral ligament continues to the supinator ridge of the ulna (Fig. 2.4). The lateral collateral ligament complex was classically described to arise from the axis of rotation of the elbow, with the lateral ulnar collateral ligament being

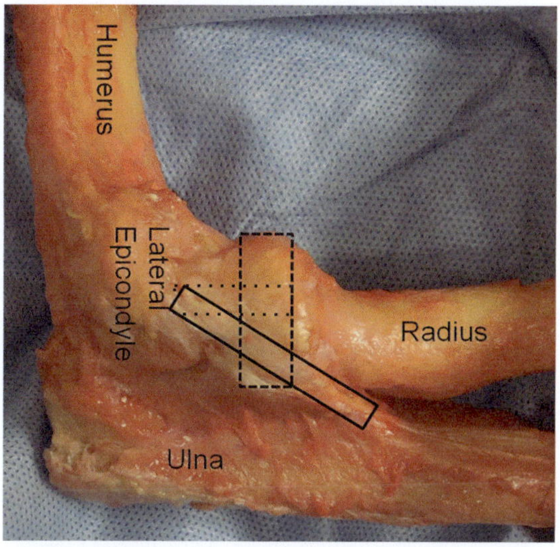


**Fig. 2.3** This clinical photograph of a cadaveric dissection in which all structures aside from the humerus, radius, ulna, joint capsule, and ligaments have been removed demonstrates the lateral collateral ligament complex, including the lateral ulnar collateral ligament (*solid box*), annular ligament (*dashed box*), and radial collateral ligament (*dotted box*)

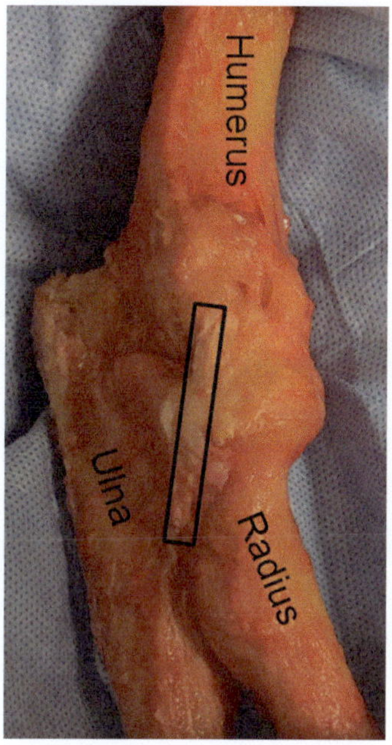


**Fig. 2.5** This clinical photograph demonstrates that, in extension, the lateral ulnar collateral ligament (*solid box*) can be seen to be nearly isometric

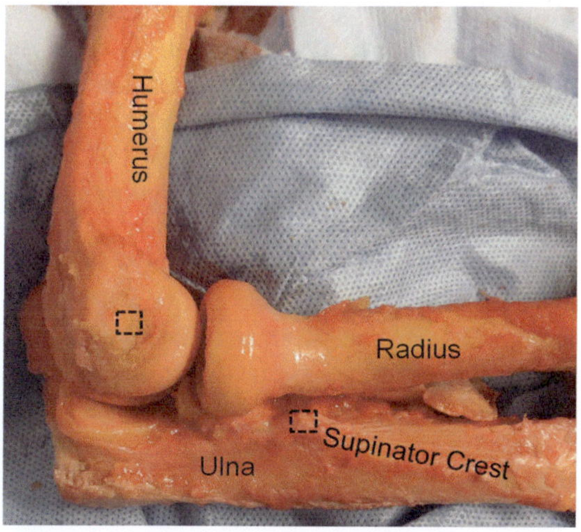


**Fig. 2.4** This clinical photograph with the lateral collateral ligament complex removed demonstrates the attachment sites for the lateral ulnar collateral ligament (*dashed boxes*)

isometric (Fig. 2.5) [2, 42, 44]. However, this remains controversial as both a computer modeling study [45] and a cadaveric study [46] have suggested that the radial collateral ligament is isometric while the lateral ulnar collateral ligament is taut in flexion and loose in extension. The isometric point laterally has been identified 2 mm proximal to the center of the capitellum [45].

Elbow instability is thought to occur in stages such that isolated tears of the lateral collateral ligament complex are possible, leading to a subluxation phenomenon called posterolateral rotatory instability (Fig. 2.6) [47, 48]. Posterolateral rotatory instability is a combination of external rotation/supination of the forearm on the humerus, axial loading, valgus angulation, and posterior displacement of the forearm on the humerus. Clinically, a tear in the lateral ulnar collateral ligament is thought to be the defining pathology to allow this subluxation [44, 48]. However, the Y-shaped configuration of the lateral ulnar collateral ligament and the radial collateral ligament may be structurally self-reinforcing therefore injury of only the lateral ulnar collateral ligament may not lead to gross instability. Cadaver studies have shown that isolated sectioning of either the lateral ulnar collateral ligament or radial collateral ligament is not sufficient to produce posterolateral rotatory instability and requires sectioning of both structures to create instability [18, 49].

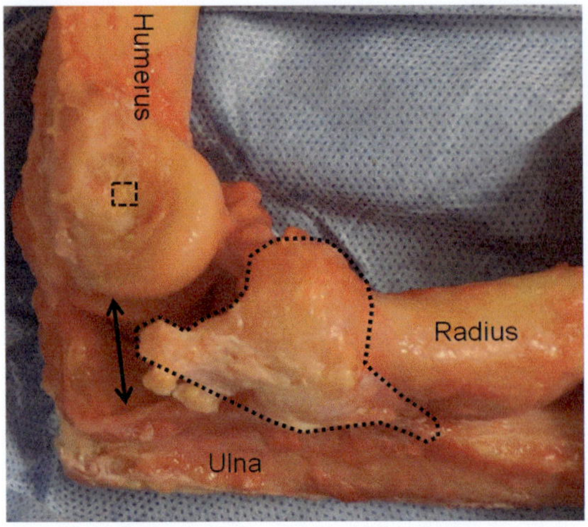


**Fig. 2.6** This clinical photograph demonstrates that after release of the lateral collateral ligament complex (*outlined in dots*) from the humeral attachment (*outlined with a dashed box*) the ulnotrochlear joint gaps (*black double-sided arrow*) with a rotatory stress

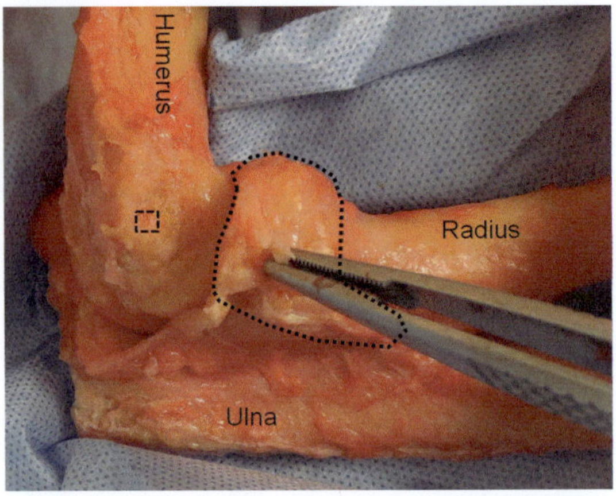


**Fig. 2.7** This clinical photograph demonstrates release of the humeral attachment (*dashed box*) of lateral collateral ligament complex (*outlined in dots* and *gripped by the forceps*), which is the most common anatomic location for ligament tears

Nevertheless, the relative importance of each portion of the lateral collateral ligament complex remains controversial. Olsen and colleagues found that sectioning of the annular ligament while leaving the lateral ulnar collateral ligament intact increased varus opening from 2–3° to 6–11°, suggesting that the lateral ulnar collateral ligament may not be the primary stabilizer and that the annular ligament, which was traditionally thought to be of relatively little importance for stability, may be functionally important [50]. In a sequential sectioning study, Olsen and colleagues found that the radial collateral ligament was the primary stabilizer and that the lateral ulnar collateral ligament was an accessory, while the annular ligament played essentially no role in stabilizing the lateral elbow [8]. Consequently, all components of the lateral complex probably play a role in lateral sided stability and repair of each component will likely maximize stability.

Anatomically, the lateral soft tissues most commonly tear from the humeral origin resulting in tears of both the radial collateral ligament and lateral ulnar collateral ligament. Thus, the preceding debate regarding which portions of the ligament are most important for stability may not be clinically important as both are commonly injured as a unit (Fig. 2.7) [5, 16, 23, 35, 37]. In acute repairs, most surgeons attempt to gather tissue from both from the radial collateral ligament and lateral ulnar collateral ligament [39, 40]. In chronic instability, reconstruction of just the lateral ulnar collateral ligament leads to excellent functional outcomes and reliable restoration of stability [16, 39, 40, 48]. One cadaveric study demonstrated that reconstruction of the lateral ulnar collateral ligament provides equivalent stability to reconstruction of both the lateral ulnar collateral ligament and radial collateral ligament [17]. Thus, regardless of the controversy in cadaveric studies, the lateral ulnar collateral ligament appears to be the most critical part of the lateral collateral ligament complex to reconstruct.

## Coronoid

The coronoid is a critical elbow stabilizer, acting as a buttress against axial loading, rotation, and posterior displacement of the ulna. The coronoid also serves to lengthen the articular surface of the sigmoid notch, improving flexion/extension range of motion. The coronoid is also relatively exposed to shear stress and is thus at risk for fracture. Up to 60 % of the anteromedial facet portion of the coronoid is unsupported by metaphyseal bone placing it at risk for fracture especially during varus posteromedial rotatory dislocations [38]. In one series of operatively treated elbow dislocations, 63 % patients had a coronoid fracture [37].

While all authors agree that the coronoid is an important stabilizer for the elbow, coronoid fracture height varies and the exact height necessitating operative fixation is controversial. One study suggested that loss of as little as 25 % of the coronoid can lead to subluxation of the ulnotrochear joint in midflexion in the absence of the radial head [2]. Another biomechanical study demonstrated that fracture of 40 % of the coronoid increased both varus laxity and internal rotation stress [51]. Still another study found that radial head excision and removal of 30 % of the coronoid could lead to a dislocation even with the medial and lateral ligamentous complexes intact [52]. With an intact radial head, the same study found that 50–70 % coronoid excision was necessary to create a dislocation [52]. Based upon these studies, the threshold that a coronoid surgical repair is indicated remains controversial. The threshold is likely 40–50 % based upon the biomechanical data for fractures in isolation, although it may be as small as 10–15 % depending upon the concomitant injuries and how effectively they can be addressed [38, 52]. As a result, coronoid fracture fixation is a critical portion of the surgical treatment of elbow instability and should be considered as a necessary component of most repairs to maximize stability [38–40]. In cases of instability with coronoid bone loss, several coronoid reconstruction techniques have been described including radial head autograft, olecranon autograft, iliac crest autograft, coronoid allograft, and prosthetic reconstruction emphasizing the importance of restoring the coronoid to achieve stability [51].

## Radial Head and Capitellum

The radial head provides lateral stability through three mechanisms: (1) by acting as a buttress, (2) through the concavity compression mechanism, and (3) by tensioning the lateral ulnar collateral ligament. The radial head is commonly fractured in the setting of elbow instability and in general should be repaired or reconstruction in most cases to maximize stability. Radial head resection increases laxity in multiple directions [52]. In one series of operatively treated elbow dislocations, 58 % of patients had a concomitant radial head fracture [37].

Multiple biomechanical analyses have demonstrated the importance of the radial head in elbow stability. In a cadaveric study, Hotchkiss and colleagues demonstrated that the radial head contributes up to 30 % of stability to valgus torque/displacement in the setting of an intact ulnar collateral ligament [53]. Subsequent cadaveric studies have demonstrated that isolated radial head excision doubles the valgus laxity of the elbow [52] and increases rotatory laxity by up to 145 % [54]. The radial head is particularly important in association with a coronoid fracture—in one cadaveric study when both were absent subluxation occurred even with completely intact ligaments and radial head replacement alone could stabilize the elbow [54]. The mechanism of posterolateral rotatory instability has been suggested to require pathologic external forearm rotation. The radial head serves as a block to excess external rotation, as the anterior radial head must sufficiently externally rotate to clear the distal capitellum to result in posterolateral rotatory instability [55]. Thus even small radial head defects can play an important role in stability if they are inopportunely placed [55]. The capitellum likely plays a similarly important role—in one study after excision of the capitellum -valgus laxity increased 3.1° with active elbow flexion in pronation [56]. Nevertheless, other data supports no change in varus/valgus displacement after capitellar excision in the setting of intact ligaments [57].

In addition to stabilizing the elbow to varus and external rotation, the radial head may also act to tension the lateral collateral ligament complex, as, after excision of the radial head and sectioning of the lateral collateral ligament complex, restoration of both structures is necessary to completely restore elbow laxity [58].

Because the radial head acts as a physical block to dislocation, multiple studies have shown that monoblock radial head replacements provide significantly more stability than bipolar components [15, 59]. In a cadaver study of surgically fixated terrible triad injuries comparing monoblock and bipolar components, 16-fold more force was required to dislocate a monoblock component than a bipolar component [59]. A second, similar study showed that this effect was amplified by the status of the lateral collateral ligament complex and common extensor because the bipolar radial head not only allows posterior translation but it then tilts so that continued force on the radial head now resolves to contain a dislocating shear force vector [60]. Anatomic restoration of radial head height is critical both to restore stability and to avoid altered ulnotrochlear kinematics and accelerated capitellar chondrosis [61]. With excessive radial length the ulna tracks in varus and external rotation, while with inadequate length the ulna tracks in valgus and internal rotation [61]. Even fractures that only involve a portion of the radial head may be plagued by similar issues—in a cadaver study Shukla and colleagues demonstrated that fractures that involved only 30 % of the surface area of the radial head reduced subluxation force by 80 %, even if the fragment was retained but depressed 2 mm or retained but angulated 30°, presumably due to loss of the concavity-compression mechanism [26].

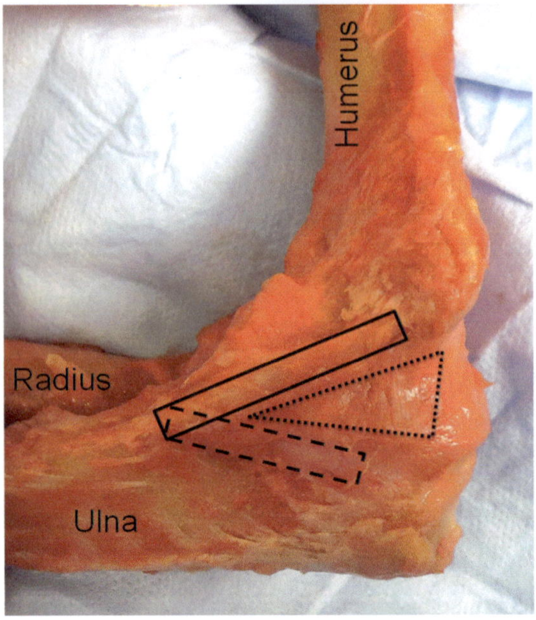


**Fig. 2.8** This clinical photograph of demonstrates the ulnar collateral ligament, including the anterior band (*solid box*), posterior band (*dotted box*), and transverse band (*dashed box*)

## Medial Elbow Stability

The ulnar collateral ligament has three distinct sections: the anterior band, the posterior band, and the transverse band (Fig. 2.8) [19, 42, 62]. The anterior band of the ulnar collateral ligament has been described as isometric in some studies [19, 42, 46] and anisometric in others (Fig. 2.9) [63]. The posterior band is taut from 60 to 120° of flexion and can limit flexion in the stiff elbow and require release [19, 64]. In flexion, the anterior band of the ulnar collateral ligament serves as the primary stabilizer of the elbow to valgus stress (Fig. 2.10) [19, 23, 50, 53, 62, 64], with the radial head serving as a secondary stabilizer [32]. In full extension the anterior capsule and osseous congruity provide valgus stability to the elbow [53],

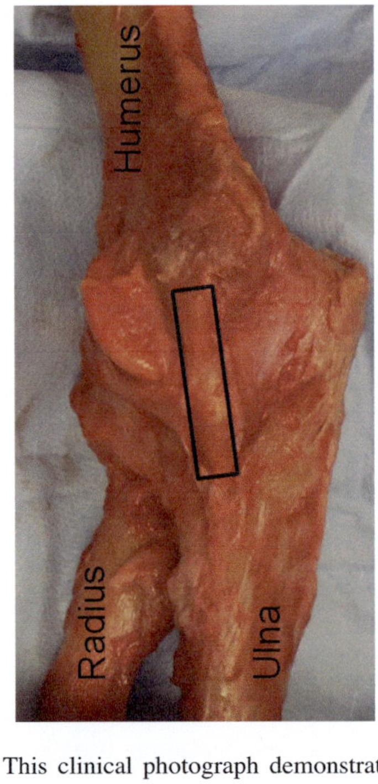


**Fig. 2.9** This clinical photograph demonstrates that, in extension, the anterior band of the ulnar collateral ligament (*solid box*) is nearly isometric

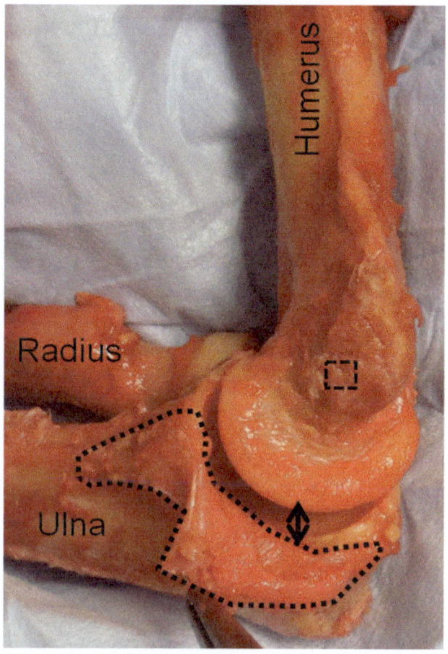


**Fig. 2.10** This clinical photograph demonstrates that, after release of the ulnar collateral ligament (*outlined* in *dots* and *grasped by the forceps*) from the humeral attachment (*dashed box*), the ulnotrochlear joint gaps (*doubled-sided arrow*) to valgus stress

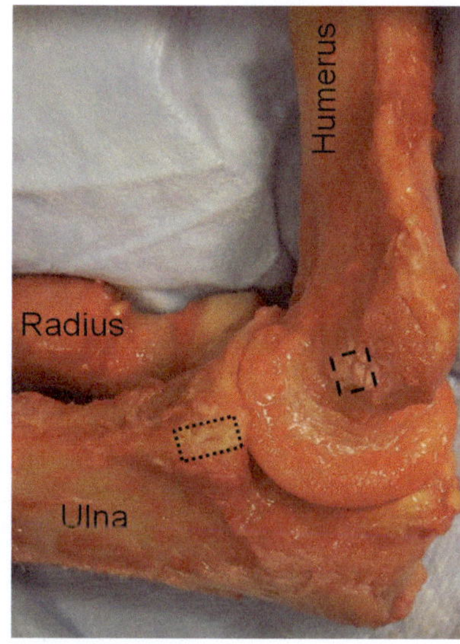


**Fig. 2.11** This clinical photograph with the ulnar collateral ligament removed demonstrates the humeral (*dashed box*) and ulnar (*dotted box*) attachment sites for the ulnar collateral ligament

and thus clinically this ligament must be tested in flexion [20]. The anterior band of the ulnar collateral ligament takes origin from the anterior inferior aspect of the epicondyle proximally and inserts on the sublime tubercle of the ulna distally (Fig. 2.11). The anterior band of the ulnar collateral ligament has a long, thin insertion on the sublime tubercle and the portion immediately adjacent to the articular surface is most critical biomechanically [65].

While the anterior band of the ulnar collateral ligament is the primary valgus stabilizer, the radial head is a secondary valgus stabilizer and can even contribute up to 30 % of the stability with an intact anterior band of the medial collateral ligament [19, 23, 32, 50, 53, 62, 64]. Thus in injuries that affect both structures, the radial head becomes an important stabilizer that must be surgically addressed [32, 61]. If radiocapitellar column length is not restored, the ulnar collateral ligament may not heal at an anatomic length, potentially resulting in chronic valgus instability [32, 61]. However, unlike lateral instability, valgus instability of the elbow can be achieved equally with either monoblock or bipolar radial head arthroplasties [32, 34].

Most symptomatic valgus instability due to an incompetent ulnar collateral ligament is encountered in repetitive trauma in overhead athletes. The overhand pitching motion is one of the fastest human motions, with arm internal rotation velocities exceeding 7000°/s [66–70]. During the late cocking/early acceleration phase, the combination of the internal rotation torque placed on the humerus and the inertia of the forearm, hand, and ball exert a valgus stress on the elbow (Fig. 2.12). This valgus torque exceeds 64–120 Nm [66, 71, 72], which exceeds the 33 Nm capacity of the ulnar collateral ligament [46, 73–76]. As a result, ulnar collateral ligament tears have been frequently described in overhand pitchers, as well as javelin-throwers, quarterbacks, and other overhead athletes [77–82]. While the UCL tear was first documented by Waris in 1946 in javelin throwers [82], an operative reconstruction for this injury was not described until 1986 with Jobe's first cohort of 16 pitchers [79]. Pitchers with complete ulnar collateral ligament tears are frequently (42 %) unable to return to their pre-injury level with nonoperative treatment, but operative reconstruction has return to play rates in excess of 83 % in multiple series [77, 78, 80, 81, 83–87]. Because the valgus torque exerted on the elbow during

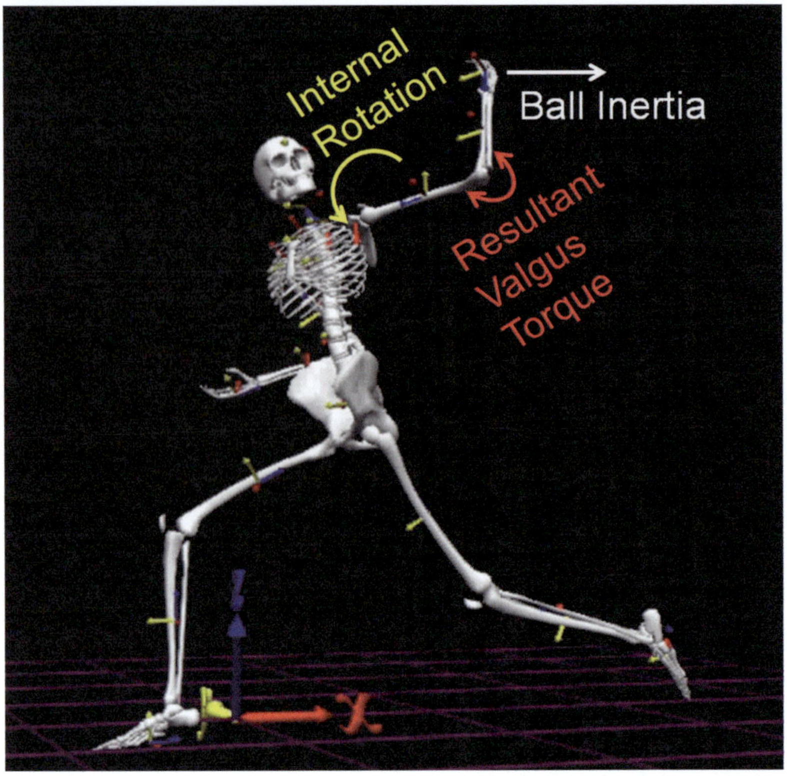


**Fig. 2.12** This schematic of an overhand baseball pitcher demonstrates that during the acceleration phase rapid internal rotation of the humerus (*yellow curved arrow*), works against the inertia of the ball (*white arrow*), to create a valgus torque at the elbow (*red curved arrow*)

high velocity pitches exceeds the load-to-failure of the native ulnar collateral ligament, the flexor-pronator mass is known to act as an important dynamic stabilizer to valgus stress. However, with ulnar collateral ligament injuries, the flexor-pronator mass does not increase activity to compensate and stabilize the elbow, instead flexor-pronator activity is paradoxically decreased [88].

Multiple studies have been conducted comparing varied ulnar collateral ligament reconstruction techniques and this remains an active area of research [63, 65, 89–96]. While these studies have differed in the which reconstruction technique offers to optimal biomechanical characteristics, all studies are in agreement that all current reconstruction techniques for the ulnar collateral ligament are biomechanically inferior the native ligament, which has led to the extended rehabilitation periods necessary after this procedure before overhead throwing can recommence.

## Conclusion

Elbow stability is created by a combination of factors. The osseous congruency of the ulnotrochlear and radiocapitellar joints contributes to overall elbow stability. The dynamic muscular forces provided by the biceps, brachialis, triceps, and wrist extensors interacting to center joint forces within the available articular arc via a concavity-compression mechanism also contribute to stability. The lateral collateral ligament complex is torn with most elbow dislocations and is the primary stabilizer to varus stress. The radial head and coronoid also play a critical role in stability by providing an osseous buttress. The anterior band of the ulnar collateral ligament is the primary stabilizer to valgus stress, with the flexor-pronator mass also playing a valgus stabilizing role. While the ulnar collateral ligament is torn in nearly all elbow dislocations, it infrequently requires surgical treatment. However, the ulnar collateral ligament can be injured in overhead athletes, specifically pitchers, due to chronic valgus stress during the late cocking/early acceleration phase of pitching and often requires surgical treatment in this population for return to pre-injury level of play. Understanding the functional anatomy and biomechanics of elbow instability is critical to successful repair and reconstruction during surgical stabilization of the elbow.

**Acknowledgements** The work for this chapter was performed at Washington University Medical Center in Saint Louis, MO.

## References

1. Morrey BF, Chao EY. Passive motion of the elbow joint. J Bone Joint Surg Am. 1976;58:501–8.
2. An K-N, Zobitz ME, Morrey BF. Biomechanics of the elbow. In: Morrey BF, editor. The elbow and its disorders. 4th ed. Amsterdam: Elsevier; 2009. p. 39–63.
3. Schlein AP. Semiconstrained total elbow arthroplasty. Clin Orthop Relat Res 1976; 222–9.
4. Deland JT, Garg A, Walker PS. Biomechanical basis for elbow hinge-distractor design. Clin Orthop Relat Res. 1987; 303–12.
5. Cohen MS, Hastings H. Rotatory instability of the elbow. The anatomy and role of the lateral stabilizers. J Bone Joint Surg Am. 1997;79:225–33.
6. Sekiya H, Neale PG, O'Driscoll SW, An KN, Morrey BF. An in vitro biomechanical study of a hinged external fixator applied to an unstable elbow. J Shoulder Elbow Surg. 2005;14:429–32.
7. Bigazzi P, Biondi M, Corvi A, Pfanner S, Checcucci G, Ceruso M. A new autocentering hinged external fixator of the elbow: a device that stabilizes the elbow axis without use of the articular pin. J Shoulder Elbow Surg. 2015;24:1197–205.
8. Olsen BS, Søjbjerg JO, Nielsen KK, Vaesel MT, Dalstra M, Sneppen O. Posterolateral elbow joint instability: the basic kinematics. J Shoulder Elbow Surg. 1998;7:19–29.
9. O'Driscoll SW, Morrey BF, An KN. Intraarticular pressure and capacity of the elbow. Arthroscopy. 1990;6:100–3.
10. Morrey BF. Post-traumatic contracture of the elbow. Operative treatment, including distraction arthroplasty. J Bone Joint Surg Am. 1990;72:601–18.
11. Morrey BF, Askew LJ, Chao EY. A biomechanical study of normal functional elbow motion. J Bone Joint Surg Am. 1981;63:872–7.
12. Sardelli M, Tashjian RZ, MacWilliams BA. Functional elbow range of motion for contemporary tasks. J Bone Joint Surg Am. 2011;93:471–7.
13. An KN, Morrey BF, Chao EY. The effect of partial removal of proximal ulna on elbow constraint. Clin Orthop Relat Res. 1986; 270–9.
14. Beuerlein MJ, Reid JT, Schemitsch EH, McKee MD. Effect of distal humeral varus deformity on strain in the lateral ulnar collateral ligament and ulnohumeral joint stability. J Bone Joint Surg Am. 2004;86-A:2235–42.
15. Chanlalit C, Shukla DR, Fitzsimmons JS, Thoreson AR, An K-N, O'Driscoll SW. Radiocapitellar stability: the effect of soft tissue integrity on bipolar versus monopolar radial head prostheses. J Shoulder Elbow Surg. 2011;20:219–25.
16. Cohen MS. Lateral collateral ligament instability of the elbow. Hand Clin. 2008;24:69–77.
17. Dargel J, Boomkamp E, Wegmann K, Eysel P, Müller LP, Hackl M. Reconstruction of the lateral ulnar collateral ligament of the elbow: a comparative biomechanical study. Knee Surg Sports Traumatol Arthrosc. 2015; doi: 10.1007/s00167-015-3627-3.
18. Dunning CE, Zarzour ZD, Patterson SD, Johnson JA, King GJ. Ligamentous stabilizers against posterolateral rotatory instability of the elbow. J Bone Joint Surg Am. 2001;83-A:1823–8.
19. Fuss FK. The ulnar collateral ligament of the human elbow joint. Anatomy, function and biomechanics. J Anat. 1991;175:203–12.
20. de Haan J, Schep NWL, Eygendaal D, Kleinrensink G-J, Tuinebreijer WE, den Hartog D. Stability of the elbow joint: relevant anatomy and clinical implications of in vitro biomechanical studies. Open Orthop J. 2011;5:168–76.
21. Eygendaal D, Verdegaal SH, Obermann WR, van Vugt AB, Pöll RG, Rozing PM. Posterolateral dislocation of the elbow joint. Relationship to medial instability. J Bone Joint Surg Am. 2000;82:555–60.
22. Josefsson PO, Gentz CF, Johnell O, Wendeberg B. Surgical versus non-surgical treatment of ligamentous injuries following dislocation of the elbow joint. A prospective randomized study. J Bone Joint Surg Am. 1987;69:605–8.
23. Josefsson PO, Johnell O, Wendeberg B. Ligamentous injuries in dislocations of the elbow joint. Clin Orthop Relat Res. 1987; 221–5.
24. An KN, Himeno S, Tsumura H, Kawai T, Chao EY. Pressure distribution on articular surfaces: application to joint stability evaluation. J Biomech. 1990;23:1013–20.
25. Seiber K, Gupta R, McGarry MH, Safran MR, Lee TQ. The role of the elbow musculature, forearm rotation, and elbow flexion in elbow stability: an in vitro study. J Shoulder Elbow Surg. 2009;18:260–8.
26. Shukla DR, Fitzsimmons JS, An K-N, O'Driscoll SW. Effect of radial head malunion on radiocapitellar stability. J Shoulder Elbow Surg. 2012;21:789–94.
27. Szekeres M, Chinchalkar SJ, King GJW. Optimizing elbow rehabilitation after instability. Hand Clin. 2008;24:27–38.
28. Hughes RE, Schneeberger AG, An KN, Morrey BF, O'Driscoll SW. Reduction of triceps muscle force

after shortening of the distal humerus: a computational model. J Shoulder Elbow Surg. 1997;6:444–8.
29. Markolf KL, Lamey D, Yang S, Meals R, Hotchkiss R. Radioulnar load-sharing in the forearm. A study in cadavera. J Bone Joint Surg Am. 1998;80:879–88.
30. Morrey BF, An KN, Stormont TJ. Force transmission through the radial head. J Bone Joint Surg Am. 1988;70:250–6.
31. Hotchkiss RN, An KN, Sowa DT, Basta S, Weiland AJ. An anatomic and mechanical study of the interosseous membrane of the forearm: pathomechanics of proximal migration of the radius. J Hand Surg Am. 1989;14:256–61.
32. Morrey BF, Tanaka S, An KN. Valgus stability of the elbow. A definition of primary and secondary constraints. Clin Orthop Relat Res. 1991; 187–95.
33. Pomianowski S, O'Driscoll SW, Neale PG, Park MJ, Morrey BF, An KN. The effect of forearm rotation on laxity and stability of the elbow. Clin Biomech (Bristol, Avon). 2001;16:401–7.
34. Pomianowski S, Morrey BF, Neale PG, Park MJ, O'Driscoll SW, An KN. Contribution of monoblock and bipolar radial head prostheses to valgus stability of the elbow. J Bone Joint Surg Am. 2001; 83-A:1829–34.
35. Safran MR, Baillargeon D. Soft-tissue stabilizers of the elbow. J Shoulder Elbow Surg. 2005;14:179S–85.
36. O'Driscoll SW, Morrey BF, Korinek S, An KN. Elbow subluxation and dislocation. A spectrum of instability. Clin Orthop Relat Res. 1992; 186–97.
37. McKee MD, Schemitsch EH, Sala MJ, O'Driscoll SW. The pathoanatomy of lateral ligamentous disruption in complex elbow instability. J Shoulder Elbow Surg. 2003;12:391–6.
38. Steinmann SP. Coronoid process fracture. J Am Acad Orthop Surg. 2008;16:519–29.
39. Tashjian RZ, Katarincic JA. Complex elbow instability. J Am Acad Orthop Surg. 2006;14:278–86.
40. Wyrick JD, Dailey SK, Gunzenhaeuser JM, Casstevens EC. Management of complex elbow dislocations: a mechanistic approach. J Am Acad Orthop Surg. 2015;23:297–306.
41. Schreiber JJ, Warren RF, Hotchkiss RN, Daluiski A. An online video investigation into the mechanism of elbow dislocation. J Hand Surg Am. 2013;38:488–94.
42. Morrey BF, An KN. Functional anatomy of the ligaments of the elbow. Clin Orthop Relat Res. 1985; 84–90.
43. Murthi AM, Keener JD, Armstrong AD, Getz CL. The recurrent unstable elbow: diagnosis and treatment. Instr Course Lect. 2011;60:215–26.
44. Anakwenze OA, Kancherla VK, Iyengar J, Ahmad CS, Levine WN. Posterolateral rotatory instability of the elbow. Am J Sports Med. 2014;42:485–91.
45. Moritomo H, Murase T, Arimitsu S, Oka K, Yoshikawa H, Sugamoto K. The in vivo isometric point of the lateral ligament of the elbow. J Bone Joint Surg Am. 2007;89:2011–7.
46. Regan WD, Korinek SL, Morrey BF, An KN. Biomechanical study of ligaments around the elbow joint. Clin Orthop Relat Res. 1991; 170–9.
47. O'Driscoll SW, Spinner RJ, McKee MD, et al. Tardy posterolateral rotatory instability of the elbow due to cubitus varus. J Bone Joint Surg Am. 2001; 83-A:1358–69.
48. O'Driscoll SW, Bell DF, Morrey BF. Posterolateral rotatory instability of the elbow. J Bone Joint Surg Am. 1991;73:440–6.
49. McAdams TR, Masters GW, Srivastava S. The effect of arthroscopic sectioning of the lateral ligament complex of the elbow on posterolateral rotatory stability. J Shoulder Elbow Surg. 2005;14:298–301.
50. Olsen BS, Henriksen MG, Sojbjerg JO, Helmig P, Sneppen O. Elbow joint instability: a kinematic model. J Shoulder Elbow Surg. 2009;3:143–50.
51. Gray AB, Alolabi B, Ferreira LM, Athwal GS, King GJW, Johnson JA. The effect of a coronoid prosthesis on restoring stability to the coronoid-deficient elbow: a biomechanical study. J Hand Surg Am. 2013;38:1753–61.
52. Schneeberger AG, Sadowski MM, Jacob HAC. Coronoid process and radial head as posterolateral rotatory stabilizers of the elbow. J Bone Joint Surg Am. 2004;86-A:975–82.
53. Hotchkiss RN, Weiland AJ. Valgus stability of the elbow. J Orthop Res. 1987;5:372–7.
54. Deutch SR, Jensen SL, Tyrdal S, Olsen BS. Elbow joint stability following experimental osteoligamentous injury and reconstruction. Journal of Shoulder and reconstruction. J Shoulder Elbow Surg. 2003;12(5):466–71. doi:10.1016/S1058-2746(03)00062-4.
55. Deutch SR, Jensen SL, Olsen BS. Elbow joint stability in relation to forced external rotation: an experimental study of the osseous constraint. J Shoulder Elbow Surg. 2003;12(3):287–92. doi:10.1016/S1058-2746(02)86814-8.
56. Sabo MT, Shannon HL, Deluce S, Lalone E, Ferreira LM, Johnson JA, King GJW. Capitellar excision and hemiarthroplasty affects elbow kinematics and stability. J Shoulder Elbow Surg. 2012;21:1024–1031.e4.
57. Root CG, Meyers K, Wright T, Hotchkiss R. Capitellum excision: mechanical implications and clinical consequences. J Orthop Res. 2014;32: 346–50.
58. Jensen SL, Olsen BS, Tyrdal S, Søjbjerg JO, Sneppen O. Elbow joint laxity after experimental radial head excision and lateral collateral ligament rupture: efficacy of prosthetic replacement and ligament repair. J Shoulder Elbow Surg. 2005;14:78–84.
59. Chanlalit C, Shukla DR, Fitzsimmons JS, An K-N, O'Driscoll SW. The biomechanical effect of prosthetic design on radiocapitellar stability in a terrible triad model. J Orthop Trauma. 2012;26:539–44.
60. Moon J-G, Berglund LJ, Zachary D, An K-N, O'Driscoll SW. Radiocapitellar joint stability with bipolar versus monopolar radial head prostheses. J Shoulder Elbow Surg. 2009;18:779–84.
61. Van Glabbeek F, Van Riet RP, Baumfeld JA, Neale PG, O'Driscoll SW, Morrey BF, An KN. Detrimental effects of overstuffing or understuffing with a radial head replacement in the medial collateral-ligament

deficient elbow. J Bone Joint Surg Am. 2004;86-A: 2629–35.
62. Schwab GH, Bennett JB, Woods GW, Tullos HS. Biomechanics of elbow instability: the role of the medial collateral ligament. Clin Orthop Relat Res. 1980; 42–52.
63. Armstrong AD, Dunning CE, Ferreira LM, Faber KJ, Johnson JA, King GJW. A biomechanical comparison of four reconstruction techniques for the medial collateral ligament-deficient elbow. J Shoulder Elbow Surg. 2005;14:207–15.
64. Søjbjerg JO, Ovesen J, Nielsen S. Experimental elbow instability after transection of the medial collateral ligament. Clin Orthop Relat Res. 1987; 186–90.
65. Hassan SE, Parks BG, Douoguih WA, Osbahr DC. Effect of distal ulnar collateral ligament tear pattern on contact forces and valgus stability in the posteromedial compartment of the elbow. Am J Sports Med. 2015;43:447. doi:10.1177/0363546514557239.
66. Fleisig GS, Andrews JR, Dillman CJ, Escamilla RF. Kinetics of baseball pitching with implications about injury mechanisms. Am J Sports Med. 1995; 23:233–9.
67. Aguinaldo AL, Chambers H. Correlation of throwing mechanics with elbow valgus load in adult baseball pitchers. Am J Sports Med. 2009;37:2043–8.
68. Anz AW, Bushnell BD, Griffin LP, Noonan TJ, Torry MR, Hawkins RJ. Correlation of torque and elbow injury in professional baseball pitchers. Am J Sports Med. 2010;38:1368–74.
69. Davis JT, Limpisvasti O, Fluhme D, Mohr KJ, Yocum LA, Elattrache NS, Jobe FW. The effect of pitching biomechanics on the upper extremity in youth and adolescent baseball pitchers. Am J Sports Med. 2009;37:1484–91.
70. Dillman CJ, Fleisig GS, Andrews JR. Biomechanics of pitching with emphasis upon shoulder kinematics. J Orthop Sports Phys Ther. 1993;18:402–8.
71. Feltner ME, Dapena J. Three-dimensional interactions in a two-segment kinetic chain. Part 1; General model. Int J Sports Biomech. 1989;5:403–19.
72. Werner SL, Fleisig GS, Dillman CJ, Andrews JR. Biomechanics of the elbow during baseball pitching. J Orthop Sports Phys Ther. 1993;17:274–8.
73. Altchek DW, Hyman J, Williams R, Levinson M, Allen AA, Paletta Jr GA, Dines DM, Botts JD. Management of MCL injuries of the elbow in throwers. Tech Shoulder Elbow Surg. 2000;1:73–81.
74. Dodson CC, Altchek DW. Ulnar collateral ligament reconstruction revisited: the procedure I use and why. Sports Health. 2012;4:433–7.
75. Dodson CC, Thomas A, Dines JS, Nho SJ, Williams RJ, Altchek DW. Medial ulnar collateral ligament reconstruction of the elbow in throwing athletes. Am J Sports Med. 2006;34:1926–32.
76. Morrey BF, An KN. Articular and ligamentous contributions to the stability of the elbow joint. Am J Sports Med. 1983;11:315–9.
77. Bowers AL, Dines JS, Dines DM, Altchek DW. Elbow medial ulnar collateral ligament reconstruction: clinical relevance and the docking technique. J Shoulder Elbow Surg. 2010;19:110–7.
78. Conway JE, Jobe FW, Glousman RE, PINK M. Medial instability of the elbow in throwing athletes. Treatment by repair or reconstruction of the ulnar collateral ligament. J Bone Joint Surg Am. 1992;74:67–83.
79. Jobe FW, Stark H, Lombardo SJ. Reconstruction of the ulnar collateral ligament in athletes. J Bone Joint Surg Am. 1986;68:1158–63.
80. Savoie FH, Morgan C, Yaste J, Hurt J, Field L. Medial ulnar collateral ligament reconstruction using hamstring allograft in overhead throwing athletes. J Bone Joint Surg Am. 2013;95:1062–6.
81. Thompson WH, Jobe FW, Yocum LA, Pink MM. Ulnar collateral ligament reconstruction in athletes: muscle-splitting approach without transposition of the ulnar nerve. J Shoulder Elbow Surg. 2001;10:152–7.
82. Waris W. Elbow injuries of javelin-throwers. Acta Chir Scand. 1946;93:563–75.
83. Dodson CC, Craig EV, Cordasco FA, Dines DM, Dines JS, DiCarlo E, Brause BD, Warren RF. Propionibacterium acnes infection after shoulder arthroplasty: a diagnostic challenge. J Shoulder Elbow Surg. 2010;19:303–7.
84. Petty DH. Ulnar collateral ligament reconstruction in high school baseball players: clinical results and injury risk factors. Am J Sports Med. 2004; 32:1158–64.
85. Podesta L, Crow SA, Volkmer D, Bert T, Yocum LA. Treatment of partial ulnar collateral ligament tears in the elbow with platelet-rich plasma. Am J Sports Med. 2013;41:1689–94.
86. Rohrbough JT, Altchek DW, Hyman J, Williams RJ, Botts JD. Medial collateral ligament reconstruction of the elbow using the docking technique. Am J Sports Med. 2002;30:541–8.
87. Kodde IF, Rahusen FTG, Eygendaal D. Long-term results after ulnar collateral ligament reconstruction of the elbow in European athletes with interference screw technique and triceps fascia autograft. J Shoulder Elbow Surg. 2012;21:1656–63.
88. Glousman RE, Barron J, Jobe FW, Perry J, Pink M. An electromyographic analysis of the elbow in normal and injured pitchers with medial collateral ligament insufficiency. Am J Sports Med. 1992; 20:311–7.
89. Chronister JE, Morris RP, Andersen CR, Buford WL, Bennett JM, Mehlhoff TL. A biomechanical comparison of 2 hybrid techniques for elbow ulnar collateral ligament reconstruction. J Hand Surg. 2014;39:2033–40.
90. Ahmad CS, Lee TQ, ElAttrache NS. Biomechanical evaluation of a new ulnar collateral ligament reconstruction technique with interference screw fixation. Am J Sports Med. 2003;31:332–7.
91. Ciccotti MG, Siegler S, Kuri JA, Thinnes JH, Murphy DJ. Comparison of the biomechanical profile of the intact ulnar collateral ligament with the modified Jobe and the Docking reconstructed elbow: an in vitro study. Am J Sports Med. 2009;37:974–81.

92. Hurbanek JG, Anderson K, Crabtree S, Karnes GJ. Biomechanical comparison of the docking technique with and without humeral bioabsorbable interference screw fixation. Am J Sports Med. 2009;37:526–33.
93. McGraw MA, Kremchek TE, Hooks TR, Papangelou C. Biomechanical evaluation of the docking plus ulnar collateral ligament reconstruction technique compared with the docking technique. Am J Sports Med. 2013;41:313–20.
94. Morgan RJ, Starman JS, Habet NA, Peindl RD, Bankston LS, D'Alessandro DD, Connor PM, Fleischli JE. A biomechanical evaluation of ulnar collateral ligament reconstruction using a novel technique for ulnar-sided fixation. Am J Sports Med. 2010;38:1448–55.
95. Paletta GA, Klepps SJ, Difelice GS, Allen T, Brodt MD, Burns ME, Silva MJ, Wright RW. Biomechanical evaluation of 2 techniques for ulnar collateral ligament reconstruction of the elbow. Am J Sports Med. 2006;34:1599–603.
96. Ruland RT, Hogan CJ, Randall CJ, Richards A, Belkoff SM. Biomechanical comparison of ulnar collateral ligament reconstruction techniques. Am J Sports Med. 2008;36:1565–70.

# Surgical Approaches to the Elbow

# 3

Emilie V. Cheung and Eric J. Sarkissian

## Introduction

Surgical treatment of the unstable elbow requires a thorough understanding of elbow anatomy and the various approaches to the elbow for surgical planning including exposure, repair, and rehabilitation. Often times, multiple superficial or deep approaches are required during the same surgical procedure. Therefore, having knowledge of a variety of approaches will afford the surgeon flexibility during the operation. The close vicinity of neurologic, vascular, and ligamentous structures about the elbow make the various approaches technically challenging. Finally, the surgeon should have a solid understanding of which approaches provide the optimal exposure for each individual pathologic structure in the setting of the unstable elbow to maximize the outcome and minimize surgical morbidity.

Several basic surgical tenets should be followed during any approach to the elbow, but especially in the cases of trauma where the soft-tissue envelope has already been compromised. Full-thickness subcutaneous flaps are preferred to respect skin circulation. Often times minimizing flaps at all may provide the best chance to avoid wound dehiscence or skin edge necrosis especially in patients with poor healing potential. When making multiple incisions, narrow skin bridges should be avoided as well to avoid wound complications. Adhering to internervous anatomic planes will afford improved safety, diminished intraoperative bleeding, and reduced postoperative pain [1]. A sterile tourniquet is routinely recommended and allows ease of removal if more proximal exposure of the humerus becomes necessary. Patient positioning is often dictated by the approach. A posterior or global approach often requires the patient to be lateral, lazy-lateral (bump under ipsilateral shoulder blade with arm across the chest), or prone. Isolated lateral approaches are best treated in the lazy lateral or supine position. Isolated medial approaches are performed in the supine position with abduction and external rotation of the shoulder or prone with abduction and internal rotation of the shoulder.

Approaches to the elbow can be divided into superficial and deep approaches. The three primary superficial approaches in the treatment of elbow instability include posterior, lateral, and medial. Each superficial approach has a variety of deep approaches. The primary deep posterior approaches utilized for elbow instability surgery are the paratricipital approach or triceps reflecting

E.V. Cheung, MD
Department of Orthopedic Surgery, Stanford University Hospital and Clinics, 450 Broadway Street, Pavilion A, Redwood City, CA 94063, USA
e-mail: evcheung@stanford.edu

E.J. Sarkissian, MD (✉)
Department of Orthopedic Surgery, Stanford University Hospital and Clinics, 300 Pasteur Drive, Room R144, Stanford, CA 94305, USA
e-mail: ejsark@stanford.edu

© Springer International Publishing Switzerland 2017

R.Z. Tashjian (ed.), *The Unstable Elbow*, DOI 10.1007/978-3-319-46019-2_3

Bryan-Morrey approach. The lateral deep approaches include Kocher's interval, Kaplan's interval, and the extensor digitorum communis split. The medial deep approaches include flexor carpi ulnaris split, the Hotchkiss over-the-top, the flexor-pronator split, and Taylor-Scham. Posterior pathology primarily addressed through the paratricipital, triceps splitting, or triceps reflecting approach are olecranon fractures associated with fracture-dislocations, total elbow arthroplasty, or global instability patterns requiring medial and lateral access. Pathologies addressed through deep lateral approaches include radial head fractures, capitellar fractures, and coronoid fractures in the absence of radial head and lateral collateral ligament injury. Medial pathologies addressed through the deep medial approaches include the ulnar nerve, coronoid fractures, and ulnar collateral ligament pathology. The lateral and medial deep approaches can be accessed through either lateral or medial superficial approaches respectively or simultaneously through the superficial posterior approach. Each chapter in this textbook outlining the treatment of various injuries associated with the unstable elbow will describe each author's surgical approach.

## Posterior Approaches

Indications for superficial posterior approaches to the elbow include total elbow arthroplasty, open reduction olecranon fracture-dislocations, and global instability requiring medial and lateral simultaneous exposure. The specific deep posterior approaches balance the degree of triceps tendon detachment and the amount of exposure achieved. The three major deep posterior approaches used during the surgical treatment of the unstable elbow are the triceps reflecting, the triceps splitting, and the paratricipital approach. Several other posterior approaches have been described including an olecranon osteotomy or triceps tongue approach but due to the limited use of these approaches during instability surgery, they will not be described in detail.

The standard superficial posterior approach begins with demarcation of the bony landmarks of the elbow including the olecranon and the subcutaneous border of the ulna. Then, a universal posterior skin incision with full-thickness flaps is made. Appropriate management of the ulnar nerve must be considered. The nerve is most easily identified proximally between the medial intermuscular septum and the medial head of the triceps muscle [2]. Iatrogenic nerve injury is not uncommon and may potentially be reduced by leaving the nerve in place therefore limiting the dissection and devascularization of the nerve [3]. Ulnar nerve protection is critical during surgical repair and if ulnar nerve mobilization is deemed necessary for safety, then it should be transposed despite increased dissection in order to prevent injury.

In the triceps-reflecting, or Bryan-Morrey, approach [4] the triceps tendon is sharply detached as a single flap from medial to lateral off the tip of the olecranon (Fig. 3.1). Proximally, the entire extensor mechanism and posterior capsule are reflected as one unit from the distal humerus. As the extensor mechanism is retracted laterally, the elbow is flexed to expose the joint. The ulnar nerve must be monitored closely throughout the procedure to avoid traction injury. Repair of the extensor mechanism to the olecranon at the completion of the procedure is executed with two oblique and one transverse transosseous drill holes. Postoperatively, avoiding active elbow extension against resistance for approximately 6 weeks protects the triceps repair.

For the triceps-splitting approach, a longitudinal incision is made from the proximal triceps muscle to the distal triceps tendon across its insertion on the proximal olecranon [5]. As with the triceps-reflecting approach, ulnar nerve identification and protection is advised prior to the approach. The elbow joint is exposed as the anconeus is reflected subperiostally and laterally, and as the flexor carpi ulnaris (FCU) is reflected medially (Fig. 3.2). The approach may be limited proximally by the location of the radial nerve at the posterior one third of the humeral shaft. The triceps tendon is repaired with nonabsorbable sutures.

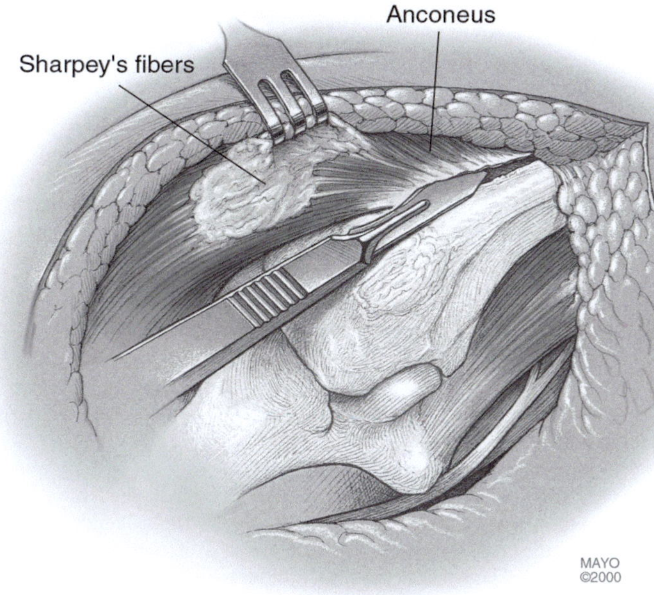


Fig. 3.1 Triceps-reflecting approach. The schematic demonstrates exposure of the distal humerus via subperiosteal reflection of the distal triceps insertion from medial to lateral while maintaining continuity with the forearm fascia and anconeus. Reproduced with permission from © Mayo Foundation for Medical Education and Research. All rights reserved

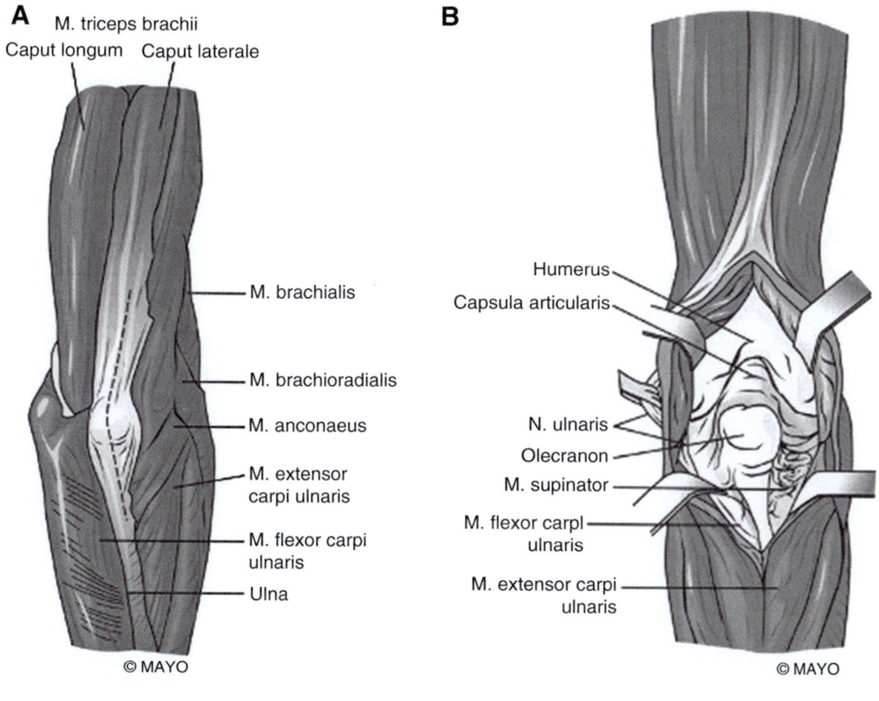


Fig 3.2 Triceps-splitting approach. (**a**, **b**) The illustration depicts exposure of the elbow with distal extension of the incision and retraction of the flexor carpi ulnaris medially and the anconeus laterally (Reproduced with permission from © Mayo Foundation for Medical Education and Research. All rights reserved)

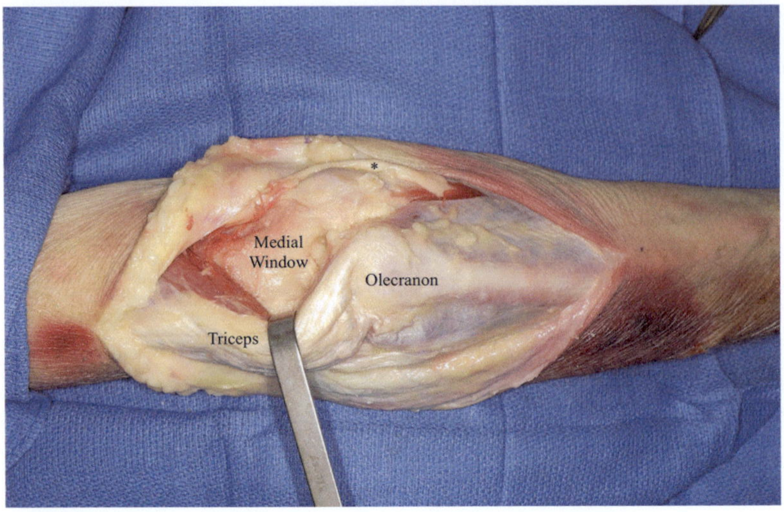


**Fig 3.3** Paratricipital approach. Dissecting free the medial and lateral borders of the triceps from the posterior part of the humerus creates medial and lateral windows to visualize the extra-articular distal humerus while preserving the triceps tendon insertion (* = ulnar nerve; lateral window not seen) (Reprinted with permission from Cheung E, Steinmann S. Surgical Approaches to the Elbow. J Am Acad Orthop Surg. 2009; 17(5): 325–33)

Postoperative protection of active extension against resistance and passive stretching in positions of terminal flexion is instituted.

The paratricipital, or Alsonso-Llames, approach [6] maintains the triceps insertions at the olecranon and eliminates risk of postoperative triceps insufficiency while allowing visualization of the extra-articular distal humerus. The tissue plane between the medial intermuscular septum and the medial side of the olecranon and triceps tendon is developed. Ulnar nerve dissection and protection are recommended to avoid traction injuries. On the lateral side, the plane between the lateral intermuscular septum and the anconeus is developed. Joining the medial and lateral tissue planes to release the triceps from the posterior humeral cortex completes the dissection. Medial and lateral windows are created by retracting the triceps tendon laterally and medially respectively (Fig. 3.3). Distal visualization may be compromised with an intact triceps unit; therefore, the approach is typically utilized for elbow arthroplasty after release of the collateral ligaments or during olecranon fracture dislocations where the distal extent of the approach around the proximal olecranon is utilized. Visualization may be improved by placing the elbow into an extended position to relax the triceps unit.

## Lateral Approaches

Lateral exposures allow access to the lateral column of the distal humerus, radial head, capitellum, and lateral collateral ligament complex. The coronoid process can also be accessed through a lateral approach if the radial head has been fractured or resected. Access to the lateral aspect of the elbow can be achieved through a direct lateral superficial approach or with a posterior superficial approach and elevation of a thick flap until the lateral epicondyle is reached. The presence of associated injuries guides the approach. If medial sided structures (coronoid process, ulnar collateral ligament complex) are likely to require exposure, then a posterior superficial approach is used. If this is unlikely, then a lateral superficial approach can be used. The three primary deep lateral approaches include the Kaplan approach, the Kocher approach, and the extensor digitorum communis split approach.

The Kaplan approach allows for excellent exposure of the radial head without interruption of the lateral ulnar collateral ligament (LUCL) [7] (Fig. 3.4). A skin incision is made with the elbow flexed at 90° from the tip of the lateral epicondyle and extended distally approximately 3–4 cm towards Lister's tubercle of the distal radius. The superficial interval lies between the extensor digitorum communis (EDC) and extensor carpi radialis brevis (ECRB). Special care must be taken to avoid injuring the lateral antebrachial cutaneous nerve, which travels within the adipose tissue at the distal aspect of the incision. The nerve pierces the brachial fascia approximately 3 cm proximal to the lateral epicondyle, and then passes 4.5 cm medial to the lateral epicondyle [8]. Deeper, the approach divides the annular ligament complex but remains anterior to the LUCL along the axis of the radiocapitellar joint.

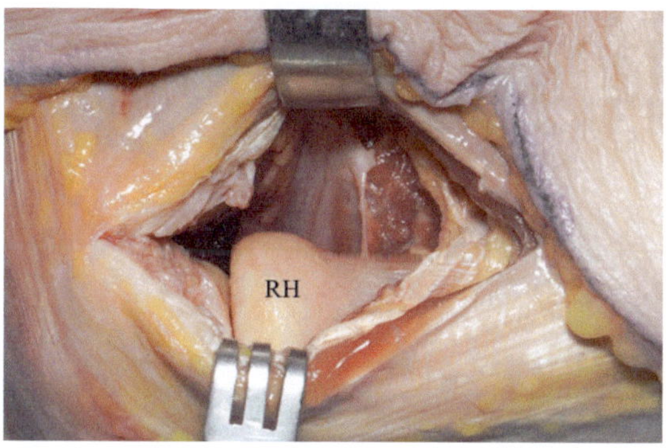


**Fig 3.4** Kaplan approach. The interval between the extensor digitorum communis and extensor carpi radialis brevis provides access to the radial head (RH). Forearm pronation during the approach protects the posterior interosseous nerve (Reprinted with permission from Cheung E, Steinmann S. Surgical Approaches to the Elbow. J Am Acad Orthop Surg. 2009; 17(5): 325–33)

The interval for the Kocher approach is between the anconeus and the extensor carpi ulnaris (ECU) [9]. A fat stripe, often seen, defines the interval. The ECU is retracted anteriorly and the anconeus is retracted posteriorly to allow access to the lateral capsule and ligaments (Fig. 3.5). The capsule is incised along the anterior border of the LUCL. The fibers of the LUCL, if intact, must be recognized and protected to avoid destabilizing the elbow [2]. The Kocher approach may be extended both proximally and distally for LUCL reconstruction and complex radial head fractures, or to the coronoid process in terrible triad injuries primarily if the radial head fragments are removed. Caution must be exercised to avoid injury to the radial nerve. The radial nerve crosses the lateral intermuscular septum from the spiral groove 8–10 cm proximal to the lateral epicondyle [8].

The EDC splitting approach is a direct lateral and alternative safe approach that can provide excellent visualization of the proximal radius (Fig. 3.6). The approach offers more reliable exposure of the anterior half of the radial head while minimizing soft-tissue destruction and reducing the risk of iatrogenic injury to the LUCL compared to the Kocher approach [10]. The EDC splitting approach also reduces risk of iatrogenic injury to the deep branch of the radial nerve. In a cadaveric study, the distance of the deep branch of the radial nerve to the radial head was 20 mm

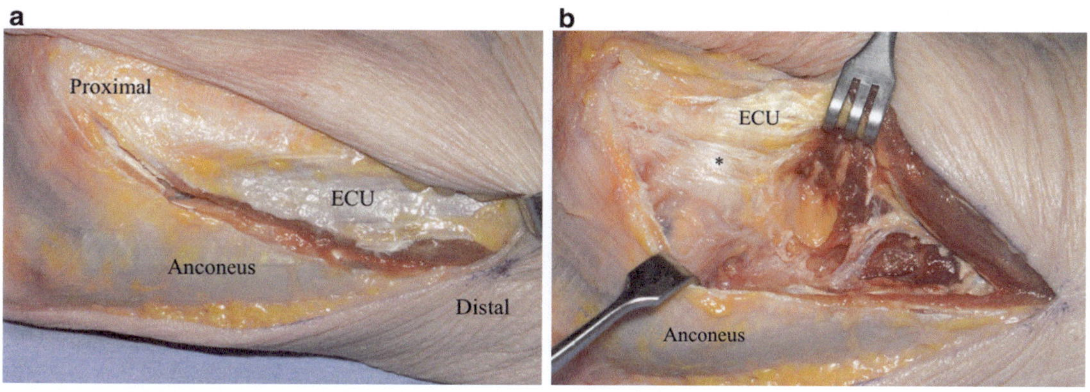


**Fig 3.5** Kocher approach. (**a**) The plane between the anconeus and the extensor carpi ulnaris (ECU) is developed. (**b**) Anterior retraction of the ECU and posterior retraction of the anconeus provides visualization of the lateral capsule (*) and ligaments. The capsule is incised anterior to the equator of the radial head to avoid iatrogenic injury to the lateral ulnar collateral ligament complex (Reprinted with permission from Cheung E, Steinmann S. Surgical Approaches to the Elbow. J Am Acad Orthop Surg. 2009; 17(5): 325–33)

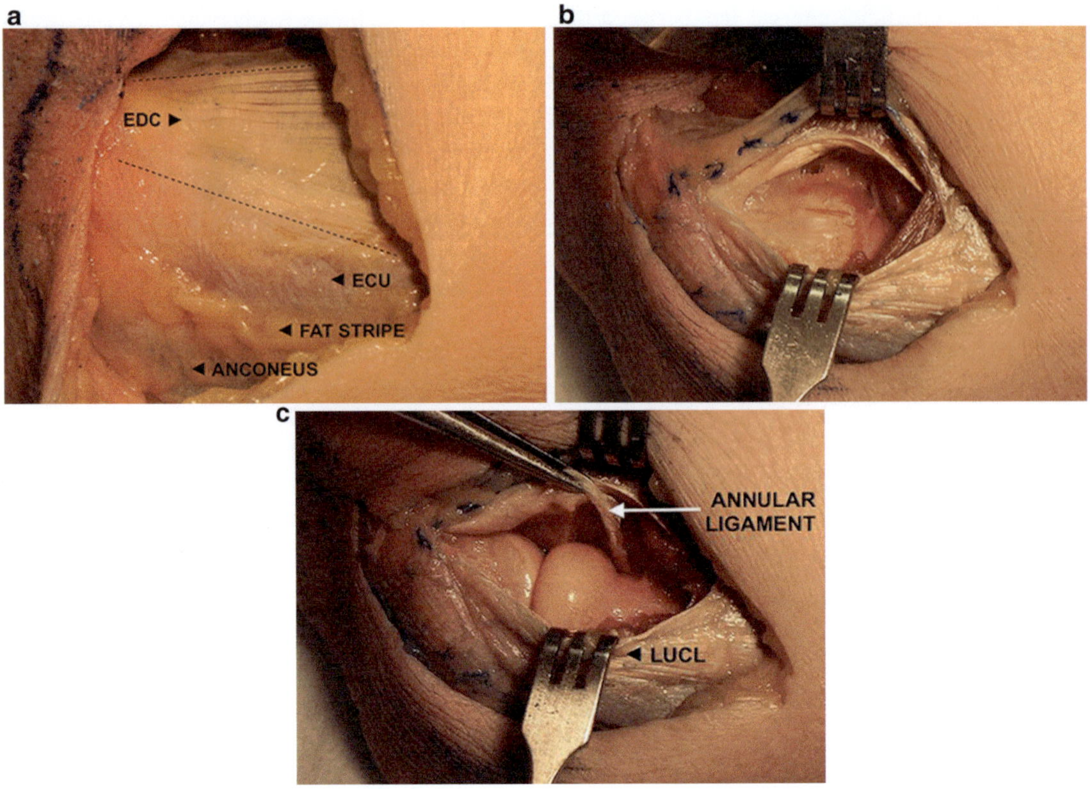


**Fig 3.6** Extensor digitorum communis (EDC) split approach. (**a**) The EDC tendon is identified by its characteristic white tendinous appearance. The borders of the tendon are represented by the dotted lines. (**b**) A longitudinal split of the EDC tendon exposes the lateral radiocapitellar joint capsule. (**c**) The lateral elbow capsulotomy performed anterior to the equator of the capitellum and in line with the EDC split exposes the radiocapitellar joint (ECU = extensor carpi ulnaris, LUCL = lateral ulnar collateral ligament) (Reprinted with permission from Berdusco et al. Lateral elbow exposures: The extensor digitorum communis split compared with the kocher approach. JBJS Essential Surgical Techniques 2015:5(4):e30)

in the EDC splitting approach compared to 7 mm in the Kaplan approach [11]. Once the EDC tendon is identified, the tendon is bisected longitudinally, starting proximally at the lateral epicondylar ridge and extending 25 mm distally from the radiocapitellar joint [10]. After muscle splitting, the capsule and annular ligament are incised anterior to the equator of the capitellum to avoid injury to the LUCL posteriorly and resultant posterolateral rotatory instability. If greater exposure is needed, the anterior half of the EDC and ECRB tendons are detached proximally from the lateral epicondyle. Subsequently, the extensor carpi radialis longus and brachioradialis origins from the supracondylar ridge are detached. The extensile approach allows sufficient access to the ulnar coronoid process, which can be used to treat terrible triad injuries [12].

One of the major pitfalls of the deep lateral approaches is iatrogenic injury to the posterior interosseous nerve (PIN). The distance where the PIN crosses the radius distal to the radiocapitellar joint varies with forearm rotation and alters the surgical safe zone [13–15]. In a cadaveric study utilizing the Kaplan approach, the PIN crossed the radius 4.2 cm distal to the radiocapitellar joint with the forearm in neutral rotation [13]. Supination decreased the distance to 3.2 cm whereas pronation increased the distance to 5.6 cm. Another study utilizing the Kocher approach found pronation of the forearm to safely expose at least 38 mm of the lateral aspect of the radius; supination dwindled the proximal safe zone to as little as 22 mm [14]. In contrast, another study found limited PIN distal translation with pronation and recommended limiting dissection to 4.0 cm from the radiocapitellar joint regardless of forearm rotation during a lateral approach [16]. During the EDC splitting approach, the PIN is generally safe when dissecting up to 29 mm from the radiocapitellar joint and up to 42 mm from the lateral epicondyle with the forearm in pronation [15]. A useful landmark for intraoperative orientation may be the radial tuberosity during a lateral Kocher approach. One study showed the PIN is located a minimum of 2.1 cm distal to the radial tuberosity in pronation at the lateral aspect of the radius and as closed as 7 mm distal to the tuberosity in supination [17]. In general for most lateral approaches if the forearm is kept in pronation, a proximal safe zone of about 4 cm is present from the articular surface of the radial head distally before the PIN is at significant risk for injury.

## Medial Approaches

For the unstable elbow, medial approaches are useful for reconstruction of the ulnar collateral ligament (UCL) complex or coronoid fracture fixation. They may be performed by either a long posterior elbow skin incision, elevating a medial flap, or by a medial incision halfway between the medial epicondyle and the olecranon. The ulnar nerve must be identified and generously mobilized both proximally and distally for protection. A posterior midline skin incision may be preferred to reduce the risk of injury to the medial antebrachial cutaneous nerve [1]. The nerve commonly lies on the fascia anterior to the medial intermuscular septum. Identification of the nerve and protection may prevent formation of a postoperative neuroma. At an average of 14.5 cm proximal to the medial epicondyle, the medial antebrachial cutaneous nerve divides into anterior and posterior branches [8]. The anterior branch crosses the elbow between the medial epicondyle and the biceps tendon. The posterior branch has two or three additional divisions, which typically cross the elbow proximal to the medial epicondyle.

In the FCU split approach, the humeral and ulnar heads of the FCU are divided to expose the coronoid process for visualization of coronoid tip or anteromedial coronoid facet fractures (Fig. 3.7). The exposure is kept anterior to the sublime tubercle and, thus, the UCL so as not to detach the ligament and potentially destabilize the elbow. The capsule is incised parallel and anterior to the UCL, exposing the ulnohumeral joint. Proximal extension is achieved by elevating

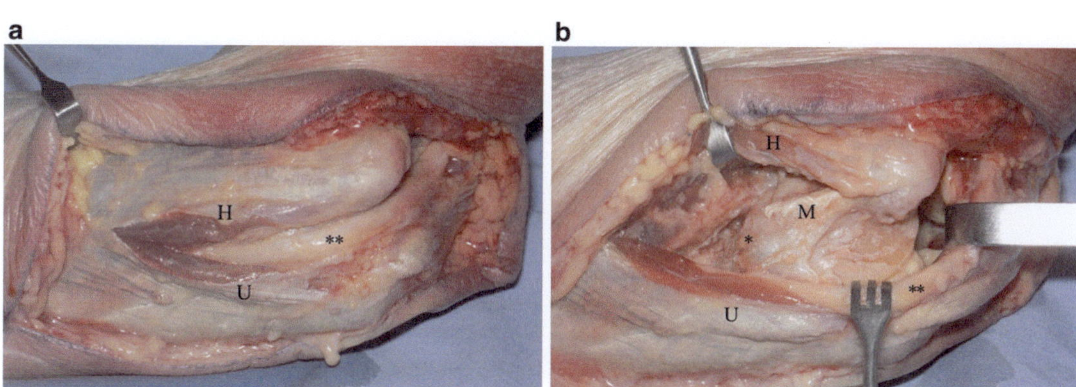


**Fig 3.7** Flexor carpi ulnaris (FCU) split approach. (**a**) The humeral (H) and ulnar (U) heads are divided to enable in situ release of the ulnar nerve (**). (**b**) As the humeral head of the FCU is reflected superolaterally and the ulnar nerve is gently retracted posteriorly, the anterior band of the medial collateral ligament (M) and the coronoid process (*) are exposed (Reprinted with permission from Cheung E, Steinmann S. Surgical Approaches to the Elbow. J Am Acad Orthop Surg. 2009; 17(5): 325–33)

the capsule up to the medial epicondyle. Additional exposure distally is achieved by dissecting the brachialis and the FCU from the ulna, while protecting the ulnar nerve. Transposition of the ulnar nerve may minimize postoperative or posttraumatic ulnar neuritis.

The extended medial, or Hotchkiss, approach [18] provides excellent exposure of the anterior capsule and coronoid process through an approach over the top of the humeral origin portion of the common flexor pronator muscle mass with safe distal extension to the medial ulna. Once the medial intermuscular septum is identified along with the medial supracondylar ridge, the brachial fascia is then incised along the anterior aspect of the septum, and the flexor-pronator group is released from the supracondylar ridge [2]. The flexor group is split longitudinally at the distal aspect. The posterior aspect of the FCU origin is left intact on the medial aspect of the distal humerus to facilitate repair at the end of the procedure. Elevation of the brachialis, flexor carpi radialis, and pronator teres muscles off the anterior capsule allows visualization to the lateral aspect of the anterior elbow joint (Fig. 3.8). The brachialis is released in continuity with the flexor-pronator mass along the medial supracondylar ridge to protect the median nerve, brachial artery, and brachial vein, which lie superficial to the brachialis. The anterior band of the ulnar collateral ligament is preserved beneath the FCU.

The FCU split and the Hotchkiss over-the-top approaches are the two most commonly used surgical techniques to expose medial elbow structures. In one cadaveric study, both were found to provide a comparable area of greater than 800 mm$^2$ of proximal ulna exposure [19]. However, another study using calibrated digital images showed that the FCU split approach may provide enhanced exposure of the osseous and ligamentous structures of the medial elbow [20]. The FCU split approach exposed 13.3 cm$^2$ of average surface area. During the Hotchkiss over-the-top approach, the average surface are exposed was three times less (4.4 cm$^2$) and visualization of the sublime tubercle as well as the anterior and posterior bundles of the UCL was not consistently obtainable [20].

In the throwing athlete, the flexor pronator split approach allows UCL reconstruction with decreased soft tissue trauma in a safe and simple manner. The site of the muscle-split is through the posterior one-third of the common flexor bundle, within the most anterior fibers of the FCU [21, 22]. The anterior bundle of the UCL lies directly deep to this region of the common flexor mass. Additionally, the muscle-split utilizes an internervous plane, as the anterior portion of the

a b

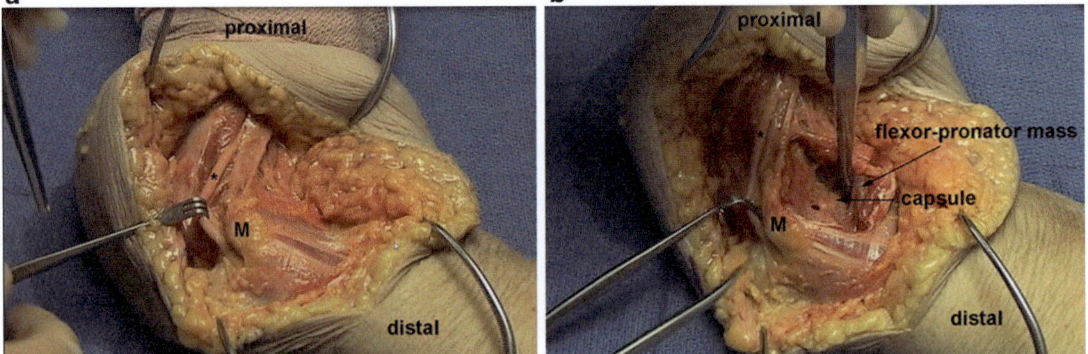


**Fig 3.8** Hotchkiss over-the-top approach. (**a**) The medial intermuscular septum, medial supracondylar ridge of the humerus, and the origin of the flexor-pronator mass are identified while mobilizing and protecting the ulnar nerve. (**b**) Release of the flexor-pronator mass and brachialis from the medial supracondylar ridge allows exposure of the joint (M = medial epicondyle, * = ulnar nerve) (Reprinted with permission from Olson et al. Surgical Approaches to the Elbow. Orthopedic Knowledge Online Journal 2013;11(7))

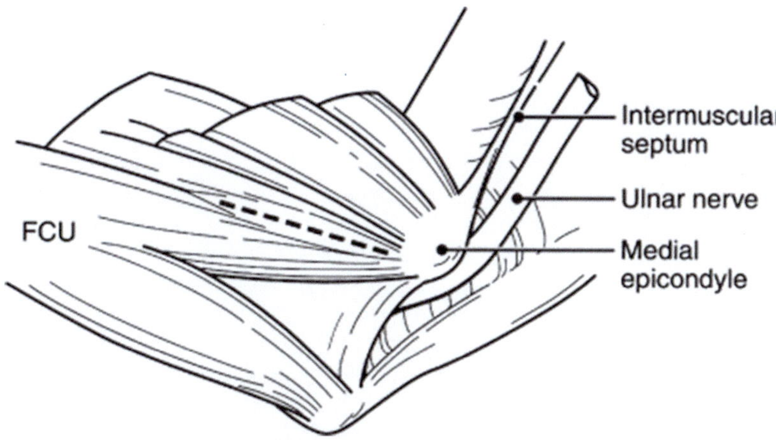


**Fig 3.9** Flexor-pronator split approach. The flexor-pronator mass is split by incising the raphe from the medial epicondyle to the sublime tubercle to expose the ulnar collateral ligament (Reprinted with permission from Conway JE. The DANE TJ procedure for elbow medial ulnar collateral ligament insufficiency. Techniques in Shoulder and Elbow Surgery 2006;7(1):36–43)

flexor bundle is innervated by the median nerve and the posterior portion is innervated by the ulnar nerve (Fig. 3.9). Following the fascial incision from the medial humeral epicondyle to the sublime tubercle approximately 3–4 cm distally, the muscle is bluntly split to the level of the UCL [21]. Safe extension may be performed 1 cm distal to the UCL's insertion on the sublime tubercle. Subperiosteal dissection allows complete exposure of the proximal ulna for placement of bone tunnels, while retractors protect the underlying ulnar nerve [21, 22]. In athletes with medial elbow instability, the muscle-splitting approach without transposition of the ulnar nerve allows excellent results with return to sport and reduced postoperative neurologic complications compared with similar procedures [23].

Fractures of the anteromedial coronoid facet resulting from a varus posteromedial rotational injury force may be repaired via a Taylor-Scham approach. An incision along the subcutaneous border of the ulna is made followed by subperiosteal dissection medially and elevation of the ulnar and deep heads of the flexor digitorum superficialis and pronator teres, respectively (Fig. 3.10). The muscular origin of the flexor digitorum profundus is subsequently elevated, with dissection carried anteriorly until the margin of the coronoid and sublime tubercle are delineated [24, 25]. A variation of this approach has been described using a limited skin incision and elevation of enough of the flexor-pronator mass such that adequate visualization of the anteromedial coronoid facet is achieved [26]. The approach can be extended proximally by transposing the ulnar nerve and then detaching the FCU and part of the flexor-pronator mass as needed creating an L-shaped exposure between the ulnar head of the FCU and the ulna and then proximally up the humeral shaft. A stump of FCU and flexor mass should be left on the humerus for repair at the end of the procedure.

## Preferred Approaches

To expose the different compartments of the elbow, we prefer to utilize separate skin incisions, rather than one large incision. This minimizes the chance of developing a subcutaneous hematoma collection or seroma formation. Traction injuries to the skin are also minimized, which may compromise healthy primary wound healing. For complex elbow fractures and total elbow arthroplasty, we regularly transpose the ulnar nerve anteriorly into a subcutaneous pocket. In contrast, the nerve is preferentially left in situ after decompressing the cubital tunnel retinaculum in the

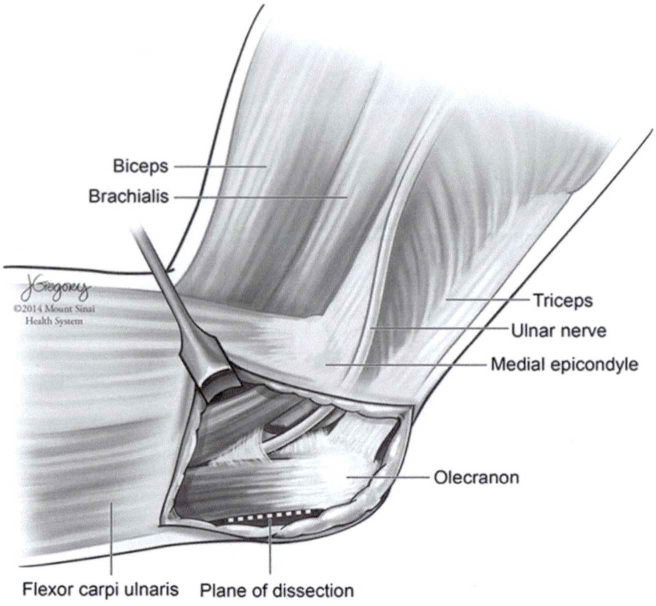


**Fig 3.10** Taylor-Scham approach. Following an incision along the subcutaneous border of the ulna, subperiosteal dissection medially and elevation of the flexor-pronator mass allows access to the anteromedial coronoid facet and sublime tubercle (Reprinted with permission from Shukla et al. A novel approach for coronoid fractures. Techniques in Hand & Upper Extremity Surgery. 2014;18(4):189–193)

setting of posttraumatic contracture release or in some cases of UCL repair or reconstruction.

For terrible triad injuries, we prefer an extended EDC split approach. This provides adequate visualization of the radial head and neck. Often times, the LUCL avulsion is apparent upon entry of the fascia, and the LUCL can be fixed primarily to a suture anchor placed at the isometric point near the lateral epicondyle. Care should be taken to not extend past the radial neck due to the location of the PIN. Proximally, the common extensor group, ECRB and ECRL may also be released along the lateral column such that one may visualize the tip of the coronoid. If the coronoid fracture is small, then suture fixation may be performed through the lateral incision, and transosseous drill holes can be made to secure the suture fixation through the base of the fracture. If, however, the coronoid fracture is large, then an additional medial incision may be made to perform the coronoid fixation through a flexor pronator split approach, making care to avoid injury to the ulnar nerve.

We prefer a flexor pronator split approach for UCL reconstruction. Either retraction of the ulnar nerve posteriorly or anterior transposition minimizes the risk of iatrogenic injury, since the ulnar nerve lies in very close proximity during the approach. Due to the need to place drill holes along the sublime tubercle as well as at the inferior aspect of the medial epicondyle, one must ensure that there is adequate visualization of anchorage of the graft while avoiding injury to the ulnar nerve.

In cases of chronic lateral instability of the elbow requiring LUCL reconstruction, we prefer a Kocher approach, which extends parallel to the course of the LUCL. The approach affords clear visualization of the supinator crest for drilling and fixation of the distal aspect of the graft. The entirety of the lateral epicondyle is also easily visualized through this approach such that the ligament graft may be secured to the most isometric point determined intraoperatively.

## Conclusion

Several surgical approaches exist for addressing elbow instability. The three primary superficial approaches in the treatment of elbow instability include posterior, lateral, and medial. Each superficial approach has a variety of deep approaches. Deep posterior approaches utilized for elbow instability are the triceps reflecting, paratricipital, or triceps splitting. These approaches allow for simultaneous medial and lateral exposure in the setting of global instability. Additionally, the deep posterior approaches are indicated for total elbow arthroplasty and olecranon fracture associated with dislocation. The deep lateral approaches are the Kocher, Kaplan, and the EDC split. Pathology addressed through these approaches include radial head fractures, capitellar fractures, and coronoid fractures in the absence of radial head and LUCL trauma. Deep medial approaches include the FCU-split, the Hotchkiss over-the-top, the flexor-pronator split, and Taylor-Scham. Coronoid fractures and UCL injuries may be addressed through deep medial approaches. Access to deep lateral and medial approaches may be achieved via either lateral or medial superficial approaches respectively, or simultaneously through the superficial posterior approach. Regardless of the approach, a thorough understanding of the anatomy is necessary to determine compromised osseous and ligamentous structures in the unstable elbow for preoperative planning and safe execution of the particular surgical technique.

## References


1. Barco R, Antuña S. Management of elbow trauma: anatomy and exposures. Hand Clin. 2015;31(4):l 509–19.
2. Cheung EV, Steinmann SP. Surgical approaches to the elbow. J Am Acad Orthop Surg. 2009;17(5):325–33.
3. Vazquez O, Rutgers M, Ring DC, Walsh M, Egol KA. Fate of the ulnar nerve after operative fixation of distal humerus fractures. J Orthop Trauma. 2010;24(7):395–9.
4. Bryan RS, Morrey BF. Extensive posterior exposure of the elbow. A triceps-sparing approach. Clin Orthop Relat Res. 1982;166:188–92.
5. Morrey BF, Sanchez-Sotelo J. Approaches for elbow arthroplasty: how to handle the triceps. J Shoulder Elbow Surg. 2011;20(2 Suppl):S90–6.
6. Alonso-Llames M. Bilaterotricipital approach to the elbow. Its application in the osteosynthesis of supracondylar fractures of the humerus in children. Acta Orthop Scand. 1972;43(6):479–90.
7. Kaplan E. Surgical approaches to the proximal end of the radius and its use in fractures of the head and neck of the radius. J Bone Joint Surg. 1941;23(1):86.
8. Adams JE, Steinmann SP. Nerve injuries about the elbow. J Hand Surg Am. 2006;31(2):303–13.
9. Kocher T. Textbook of operative surgery. 3rd ed. London: Adam and Charles Black; 1911.
10. Desloges W, Louati H, Papp SR, Pollock JW. Objective analysis of lateral elbow exposure with the extensor digitorum communis split compared with the Kocher interval. J Bone Joint Surg Am. 2014;96(5):387–93.
11. Han F, Lim CT, Lim JC, Tan BH, Shen L, Kumar VP. Deep branch of the radial nerve in lateral surgical approaches to the radial head - a cadaveric study. Orthop Traumatol Surg Res. 2016;102(4):453–8.
12. Sukegawa K, Suzuki T, Ogawa Y, Ueno K, Kiuchi H, Kanazuka A, et al. Anatomic cadaveric study of the extensile extensor digitorum communis splitting approach for exposing the ulnar coronoid process. J Shoulder Elbow Surg. 2016;25:1268.
13. Calfee RP, Wilson JM, Wong AH. Variations in the anatomic relations of the posterior interosseous nerve associated with proximal forearm trauma. J Bone Joint Surg Am. 2011;93(1):81–90.
14. Diliberti T, Botte MJ, Abrams RA. Anatomical considerations regarding the posterior interosseous nerve during posterolateral approaches to the proximal part of the radius. J Bone Joint Surg Am. 2000;82(6): 809–13.
15. Schimizzi A, MacLennan A, Meier KM, Chia B, Catalano 3rd LW, Glickel SZ. Defining a safe zone of dissection during the extensor digitorum communis splitting approach to the proximal radius and forearm: an anatomic study. J Hand Surg Am. 2009;34(7): 1252–5.
16. Lawton JN, Cameron-Donaldson M, Blazar PE, Moore JR. Anatomic considerations regarding the posterior interosseous nerve at the elbow. J Shoulder Elbow Surg. 2007;16(4):502–7.
17. Hackl M, Wegmann K, Lappen S, Helf C, Burkhart KJ, Muller LP. The course of the posterior interosseous nerve in relation to the proximal radius: is there a reliable landmark? Injury. 2015;46(4):687–92.
18. Kasparyan NG, Hotchkiss RN. Dynamic skeletal fixation in the upper extremity. Hand Clin. 1997;13(4): 643–63.
19. Jost B, Benninger E, Erhardt JB, Kulling FA, Zdravkovic V, Spross C. The extended medial elbow approach-a cadaveric study. J Shoulder Elbow Surg. 2015;24(7):1074–80.
20. Huh J, Krueger CA, Medvecky MJ, Hsu JR. Medial elbow exposure for coronoid fractures: FCU-split versus over-the-top. J Orthop Trauma. 2013;27(12): 730–4.
21. Smith GR, Altchek DW, Pagnani MJ, Keeley JR. A muscle-splitting approach to the ulnar collateral ligament of the elbow. Neuroanatomy and operative technique. Am J Sports Med. 1996;24(5):575–80.
22. Rohrbough JT, Altchek DW, Hyman J, Williams 3rd RJ, Botts JD. Medial collateral ligament reconstruction of the elbow using the docking technique. Am J Sports Med. 2002;30(4):541–8.

23. Thompson WH, Jobe FW, Yocum LA, Pink MM. Ulnar collateral ligament reconstruction in athletes: muscle-splitting approach without transposition of the ulnar nerve. J Shoulder Elbow Surg. 2001;10(2):152–7.
24. Taylor TK, Scham SM. A posteromedial approach to the proximal end of the ulna for the internal fixation of olecranon fractures. J Trauma. 1969;9(7):594–602.
25. Doornberg JN, Ring DC. Fracture of the anteromedial facet of the coronoid process. J Bone Joint Surg Am. 2006;88(10):2216–24.
26. Shukla DR, Koehler SM, Guerra SM, Hausman MR. A novel approach for coronoid fractures. Tech Hand Up Extrem Surg. 2014;18(4):189–93.

# Part II

# Acute Instabilities of the Elbow

# 4 Treatment of Simple Elbow Dislocations

Yehia H. Bedeir, Shannon R. Carpenter, and Anand M. Murthi

## Background

The elbow is the second most commonly dislocated joint [1, 2] representing 11–28 % of total elbow injuries [3, 4], with an annual incidence of 5.21 per 100,000 [5]. Elbow dislocations can be classified based upon the presence or absence of bony injury. Simple elbow dislocations are soft tissue injuries without an associated fracture, whereas complex dislocations have an accompanying fracture. Simple dislocations are much more common, representing approximately 74 % of all elbow dislocations [6].

Elbow stability is maintained by bony, capsuloligamentous, and musculotendinous components. The primary stabilizers of the elbow are the ulnohumeral articulation, the anterior band of the medial collateral ligament (aMCL), and the lateral ulnar collateral ligament (LUCL) complex [7, 8]. The highly congruent anatomy of the distal humerus and the proximal ulna provide inherent stability to the joint. The radial head, along with the MCL complex, contributes to the valgus stability of the elbow. Muscles that cross the elbow are considered dynamic stabilizers that produce joint compressive forces.

Most elbow dislocations occur in the posterior or posterolateral direction. Anterior dislocations are far less common, and divergent dislocations are very rare [9]. Simple elbow dislocations are often caused by falling onto an outstretched hand resulting in a valgus, supinatory, and axially directed load to the elbow [9–11]. Motor vehicle accidents and sports-related injuries are less common causes [11]. The typical injury pattern involves a sequential disruption of anatomic structures from lateral to medial. First, the lateral collateral ligament complex usually avulses off of its origin on the lateral epicondyle of the humerus, resulting in posterolateral instability of the elbow, which may spontaneously reduce. Next, when the anterior and posterior aspects of the capsule are disrupted, the coronoid becomes perched under the trochlea. The anterior bundle of the medial collateral ligament is usually the next to be injured followed occasionally by the entire medial collateral ligament complex and possibly the common flexor origin.

Y.H. Bedeir, MD, MBBCh, MCh Orth
Department of Orthopedic Surgery, El-Hadara University Hospital, El-Mostashfa El-Italy Street El-Hadara, Alexandria 21599, Egypt

Department of Orthopedic Surgery, MedStar Union Memorial Hospital, Baltimore, MD, USA

S.R. Carpenter, MD
Department of Orthopedic Surgery, MedStar Union Memorial Hospital, Baltimore, MD, USA

A.M. Murthi, MD (✉)
c/o Lyn Camire, Editor, Department of Orthopedic Surgery, MedStar Union Memorial Hospital, 3333 North Calvert Street, Suite 400, Baltimore, MD 21218, USA
e-mail: amurthi@hotmail.com; Lyn.Camire@Medstar.net

© Springer International Publishing Switzerland 2017
R.Z. Tashjian (ed.), *The Unstable Elbow*, DOI 10.1007/978-3-319-46019-2_4

Sometimes, the medial collateral ligament complex remains intact, acting as a pivot for a posterolateral dislocation of the elbow [7].

## Evaluation

### History and Physical Examination

The patient usually presents complaining of severe elbow pain after a trauma such as a fall onto an outstretched hand. A general physical examination should always be performed to assess other significant concomitant injuries. Local examination is usually significant for edema and obvious deformity when compared to the contralateral side. The patients' neurovascular status should be assessed carefully before any attempt at a closed reduction is performed. If a compartment syndrome is suspected, emergent fasciotomies of the forearm and hand should not be delayed.

### Diagnostic Imaging

The most valuable investigations performed are plain anteroposterior and lateral radiographs of the elbow [9]. Oblique views can help detect intra-articular fractures [12]. Computed tomography (CT) can be useful in acute simple dislocations if there is any concern for an occult fracture that may be missed on plain radiographs (such as an undisplaced fracture of the coronoid) and to identify intra-articular fracture fragments if there are mechanical symptoms after reduction [13]. Magnetic resonance imaging (MRI) is rarely indicated in an acute simple elbow dislocation. It is more useful in chronic elbow instability to evaluate the integrity of the ligaments [14]. MRI can be helpful in some acute dislocations that early surgical repair is being considered due to persistent instability to evaluate the status of the ligaments as well as any possible interposed tissue (annular ligament) potentially leading to the instability [15]. Diagnostic elbow arthroscopy can be used to detect a radial head subluxation [16], articular damage, or ligamentous disruption [17]. However, the risks and costs of arthroscopy outweigh the benefits in an acute simple elbow dislocation and we do not routinely recommend its use.

## Treatment Algorithm

Once the patient is evaluated clinically and radiographically and emergent situations, such as vascular injury and compartment syndrome, are ruled out or addressed, reduction of the joint should be performed next. Adequate muscle relaxation is required during a reduction attempt. If reduction is difficult or cannot be achieved with analgesics or conscious sedation only, then it can be performed in the operating room with general or regional anesthesia [9]. An intra-articular lidocaine injection may be used to assist in reduction and may reduce the need for sedation or general anesthesia [17]. An image intensifier, if available, can be used to guide the reduction and to assess stability after the reduction [9].

Three different techniques have been described for reducing a posteriorly dislocated elbow. In the first technique, the patient lies supine with the elbow flexed 30° and the forearm supinated. Traction is then applied to the forearm while counter-traction is applied to the arm (Fig. 4.1).

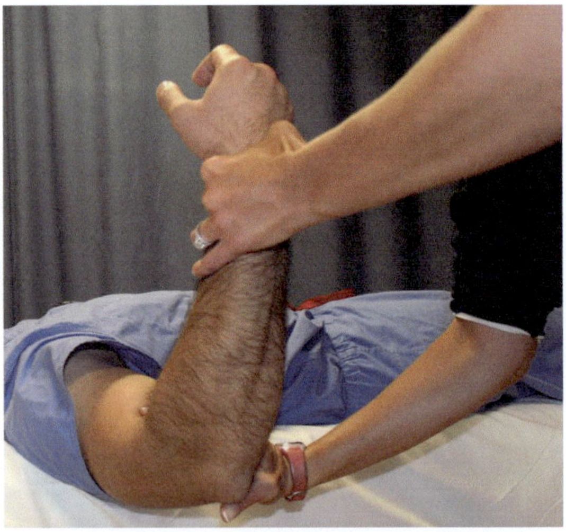

**Fig. 4.1** Supine technique for reducing a posteriorly dislocated elbow

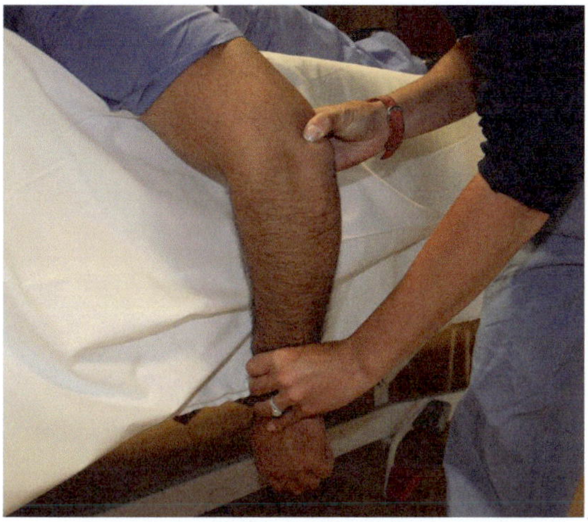

**Fig. 4.2** Prone technique for reducing a posteriorly dislocated elbow

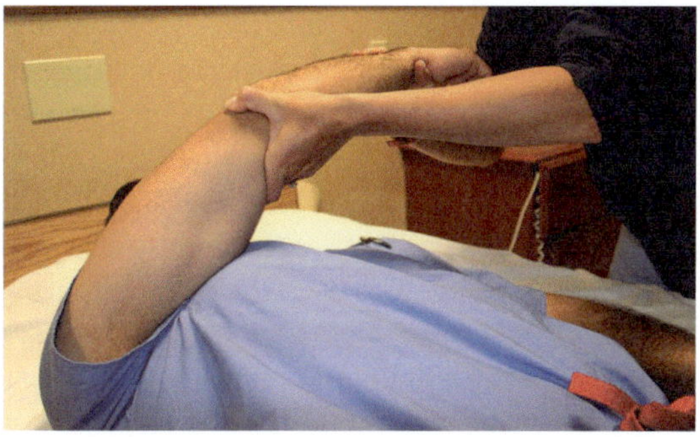

**Fig. 4.3** Alternative supine technique for reducing a posteriorly dislocated elbow

Next, the medial or lateral displacement of the olecranon is corrected. Finally, the olecranon is pushed distally to engage the olecranon fossa of the humerus [7, 9, 18, 19]. An alternative method can be performed with the patient lying prone with the arm and forearm hanging freely over the side of the table. The surgeon applies downward traction to the forearm with one hand, while the other hand pulls the humerus upward and laterally. The thumb of the hand encompassing the arm is used to push the olecranon distally into the olecranon fossa (Fig. 4.2) [20]. A third technique places the patient supine with the arm across the chest, the elbow flexed to 90°, and the forearm fully supinated. The physician applies traction to the forearm with one hand, while the other pulls the arm in the opposite direction. The elbow is gently flexed and the thumb manipulates the olecranon into position (Fig. 4.3) [21].

In all reduction techniques, firm, continuous traction should be applied to overcome the muscle spasms around the elbow that occur after injury. Once these muscles fatigue, the elbow may be more easily reduced. Some surgeons prefer to recreate the deformity by applying a supination, extension, and valgus force with axial traction [22]. This allows the coronoid to clear the distal humerus, and then the olecranon can be manipulated distally. Forearm supination during reduction is important to clear the coronoid under the trochlea, minimizing additional trauma to the intact medial structures [19]. A perched dislocation is reduced by gentle axial distraction and direct pressure over the olecranon while the elbow is slightly extended [23]. A thorough neurovascular examination should always be performed after a reduction attempt.

It is necessary to assess joint stability after reduction. This is performed by moving the elbow through a full range of motion in flexion and extension in neutral rotation. The examiner should note the position where any recurrent subluxation or dislocation occurs. Stability can be confirmed using fluoroscopy during flexion and extension. Valgus stress should be tested with the forearm fully pronated because otherwise posterolateral instability may be mistaken for valgus instability [7]. Full pronation enables the intact medial structures to prevent posterolateral rotatory instability (PLRI). If valgus stability is demonstrated in pronation, the aMCL can be assumed to be intact [19].

Full pronation renders the elbow more stable in an isolated LCL injury by tensioning any intact medial ligaments or any intact lateral musculotendinous (common extensor) origins [19, 24]. On the other hand, in isolated MCL damage, the elbow is usually more stable in supination in which any intact lateral ligaments or medial musculotendinous (flexor-pronator) origins are tightened. Elbow stability is not affected by forearm rotation if both the LCL and the MCL are disrupted [9].

If the elbow is stable throughout an entire arc of motion, a splint is applied in 90° of elbow flexion with whatever forearm rotation achieves the greatest stability [9]. Anteroposterior and lateral radiographs are performed after reduction and splinting. The patient should be seen in the clinic within 7 days to obtain follow-up radiographs. The literature shows a range of recommendations for immobilization. The duration of immobilization in a resting splint should not exceed 2 weeks. It has been shown that immobilization in a splint for 2 weeks enhances comfort and does not have a significantly adverse effect on the final functional outcome [25], whereas longer periods of immobilization can increase elbow stiffness [1]. Because the risk of posttraumatic stiffness after an elbow dislocation is much higher than that of instability in simple elbow dislocations, some surgeons apply a splint for only 1 week [9, 12, 23]. Others just apply a sling for comfort to allow for early active range of motion as soon as pain allows [11]. The argument supporting this protocol is that better final functional outcomes may be seen with the application of a sling and early active mobilization. Maripuri et al. compared the results of a 2-week immobilization followed by physiotherapy versus the application of a sling followed by early active mobilization [26]. They found that early active mobilization provided better functional outcomes, required a shorter duration of physiotherapy, and allowed an earlier return to work. The sling and early active mobilization protocol did not result in any late elbow instability or early recurrent dislocations. Finally, an alternative to the sling is a hinged brace allowing range of motion for therapy while providing varus/valgus stability [17]. Also, a hinged brace is useful when a particular forearm rotation is required to maintain a stable arc of motion or when an extension block is needed to maintain stability [9, 17].

The patient should be seen in clinic within 7 days after injury to recheck a concentric reduction on radiographs and to initiate active range of motion. Follow-up visits are every 5–7 days for a total of 3 weeks after injury [7]. It is important to check for a drop sign on follow-up radiographs. The drop sign is an objective, static, radiographically measurable increase in the ulnohumeral distance noted on the lateral elbow radiograph (Fig. 4.4). A persistent drop sign on both the immediate post-reduction radiographs and subsequent follow-up radiographs should not be overlooked because it may denote the presence of rotational instability. If left untreated, rotational instability may lead to chronic pain with heavy work and sports activities [27]. If the drop sign is persistent, then stress testing should be performed. If stress testing reveals persistent instability, further protection by a hinged brace or repair should be considered [2] (Fig. 4.5). MRI is indicated in the rare cases of an unexplained non-concentric reduction. MRI may reveal incarcerated cartilage fragments or soft tissue [10].

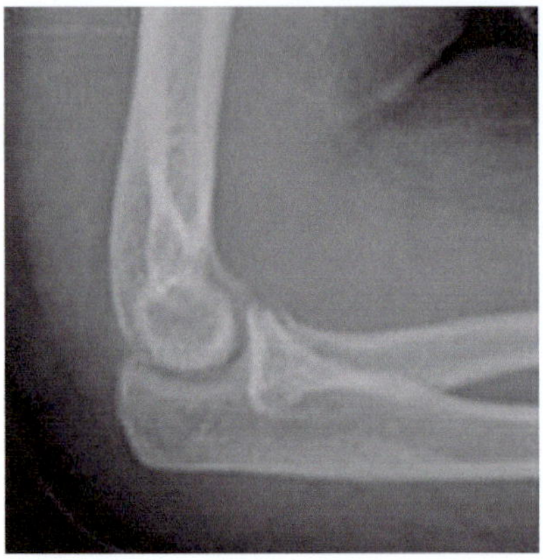

**Fig. 4.4** Lateral X-ray with drop sign

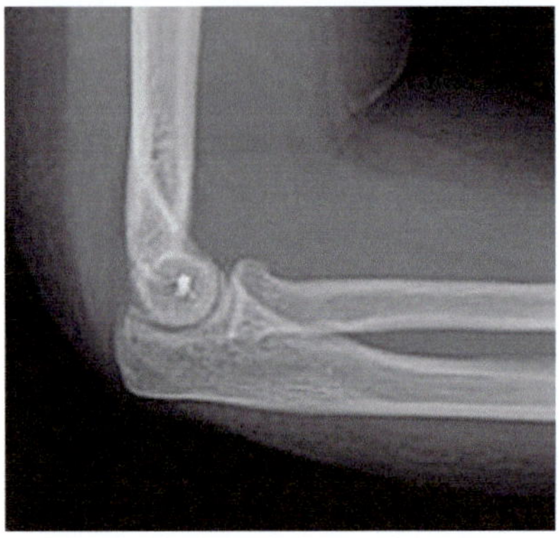

**Fig. 4.5** Lateral X-ray with resolved drop sign

Range of motion is initiated as soon as possible and is preferably active and not passive. Active muscle contraction acts as a stabilizing compressive force across the joint, whereas passive motion may cause distraction and subluxation [17]. Early active mobilization increases the final range of motion, decreases contractures, and improves patient satisfaction and functional outcomes [18].

If subluxation or dislocation in extension is present after reduction, or if subluxation is seen on post-reduction radiographs, then joint stability must be reassessed in full pronation. If forearm pronation eliminates the instability in extension, a hinged brace is applied that allows unlimited flexion and extension while holding the forearm in full pronation. If there is residual instability in full extension or near full extension, an extension block is added [7]. The extension block is adjusted such that it progressively allows more extension. It should be completely removed before 6 weeks after injury and should allow for full range of motion before removal [9]. The elbow should be reassessed similarly in each follow-up visit.

Indications for surgical treatment include residual instability in more than 45° of flexion, joint incongruence on post-reduction radiographs, and/or an open dislocation [17]. Two surgical approaches have been described to address elbow dislocation: the posterior midline incision and the dual-incision approach. A posterior midline skin incision, with full-thickness lateral and medial fasciocutaneous flaps, allows access to both sides of the elbow using a single incision with minimal disruption of local cutaneous nerves [28]. It also avoids different skin incisions in case other elbow procedures are performed later. A dual-incision approach involves a lateral skin incision to address the lateral collateral ligament disruption, with or without a medial incision to address the medial collateral ligament. It provides excellent visualization and avoids the complications of large soft tissue flaps [17] such as hematoma and skin necrosis. The lateral collateral ligament is addressed before operating on the medial side, and stability is reassessed. The medial collateral ligament should be repaired only if there is gross instability after lateral collateral ligament repair [3, 17, 23].

In order to repair the lateral collateral ligament complex, the interval between the extensor carpi ulnaris and anconeus can be utilized. The common extensor origin and lateral capsuloligamentous structures are usually already avulsed from their attachments on the humerus [17, 29, 30], leaving the lateral epicondyle exposed. The LCL, along with the capsule and common extensors, are reattached to the lateral epicondyle using bone tunnels or suture anchors with the elbow in 30° of flexion [17]. Overtensioning of these structures should be avoided [31]. The lateral collateral ligament should be attached to the lateral epicondyle at a point that renders the ligament isometric. The radial collateral ligament is essentially isometric. The lateral ulnar collateral ligament is loose in extension and tightens with elbow flexion. A point 2 mm proximal to the center of the capitellum has been calculated to be the most isometric point of the lateral ulnar collateral ligament and should be the location of the repair [32]. If the lateral collateral ligament tear is intra-substance, it is repaired directly with high-strength, nonabsorbable sutures [4]. The radiocapitellar and ulnohumeral joints should be inspected for soft tissue (annular ligament or capsule) or bony/cartilaginous fragment interposition that may have prevented a complete reduction resulting in persistent instability. More commonly, a persistently unstable simple dislocation is a result of a complete lateral collateral ligament complex avulsion with the extensor tendons and an avulsion of the entire medial collateral ligament complex with the flexor-pronator mass. Isolated lateral collateral ligament and extensor tendon repair is typically enough to restore stability in these severe injuries and medial repair is not typically required.

If instability persists after the lateral repair, the medial collateral ligament and flexor pronator can be repaired. During the approach to the medial collateral ligament, the ulnar nerve must be identified and protected. Transposition of the ulnar nerve is controversial and is not routinely performed by the senior author. The flexor/pronator muscle mass is usually injured in cases where the medial side needs a repair. The medial collateral ligament and flexor/pronator mass are repaired to the medial epicondyle in a similar manner to the lateral structures, with the elbow in 30° of flexion by placing two suture anchors, one anterior and one posterior, to the isometric point to repair the medial collateral ligament and the flexor/pronator mass to the medial epicondyle. Alternatively, the medial collateral ligament can be repaired with a heavy nonabsorbable high-strength suture in a running locked Krackow fashion through a bone tunnel in the medial epicondyle at the isometric point similar to a docking technique. The flexor/pronator mass would still be repaired with anchors as previously described.

If instability persists after medial and lateral collateral ligament repairs, a static or dynamic external fixator should be placed to restore stability. The requirement for an external fixator in cases of persistent elbow instability in cases without fracture is exceptionally rare. Consequently, surgeons should be alerted to potential missed osseous or cartilaginous injuries in cases where medial and lateral collateral ligament repairs are insufficient to restore stability. Rare cases requiring a fixator may be in cases of delayed reductions where the ligaments are compromised and an adequate repair cannot be performed. In these cases, reconstruction should be considered an alternative to external fixation as reconstruction would restore tissue and potentially prevent late instability after the fixator has been removed.

Postoperatively, after a reduction and collateral ligament repair, the elbow is kept in a resting posterior splint in 30° of flexion for 7–10 days [17, 33]. Active assisted range of motion could start at this time. A hinged brace with an extension block (approximately 30°) is used for 6 weeks postoperatively. The extension block is gradually decreased until full extension is allowed by 3 weeks postoperatively. The brace is removed and daily activities are allowed without it at 6 weeks postoperatively. Strengthening is usually initiated 10–12 weeks postoperatively. The patient may participate in sports while in the brace at this time and will continue brace wear with sports activities for a total of 3–6 months postoperatively (Fig. 4.6) [3, 17].

## Published Outcomes and Complications

The prognosis of a simple elbow dislocation is generally good [25]. Simple elbow dislocations that are stable after initial reduction are usually managed with nonoperative treatment and early active mobilization. This provides a high level of patient satisfaction and good functional outcomes [34]. Nonoperative treatment, however, does not lack minor drawbacks. Most patients treated nonoperatively have minor complaints and do not consider themselves fully recovered [11, 27]. More than half of the patients treated nonoperatively complain of residual stiffness and pain in long-term follow-up, especially during heavy work and sports participation [27, 34]. The decrease in the mean flexion arc in the dislocated elbow ranged from 5° to 11° compared to the normal elbow [27, 34, 35]. Josefsson et al. [30], however, showed that surgical management of these elbows is not superior to nonoperative treatment. Although they found that both collateral ligaments were torn in all the studied patients, they still did not recommend early surgical treatment of simple elbow dislocations that can be reduced by closed methods. For a grossly unstable or irreducible elbow dislocation, surgery is the treatment method of choice. Surgical repair of the lateral and/or medial soft tissue stabilizers provides satisfactory outcomes [36]. Primary ligament repair for unstable elbows is superior to nonoperative treatment because it allows early motion, achieves joint stability, and avoids a complicated later ligament reconstruction [33].

Joint contracture is the most common complication of elbow dislocation [17]. Longer periods of immobilization increase the risk and magnitude of a flexion contracture [9, 11, 37, 38]. However, a contracture may be prevented with early active mobilization [11, 37, 38]. Progressive static splinting is started 4–8 weeks after injury if contracture occurs and the range of active motion is less than 30–130° [39]. If no remarkable improvement is achieved (there is less than 10° change over 3 months), then a turnbuckle orthosis can be used [38, 40]. Surgery is indicated

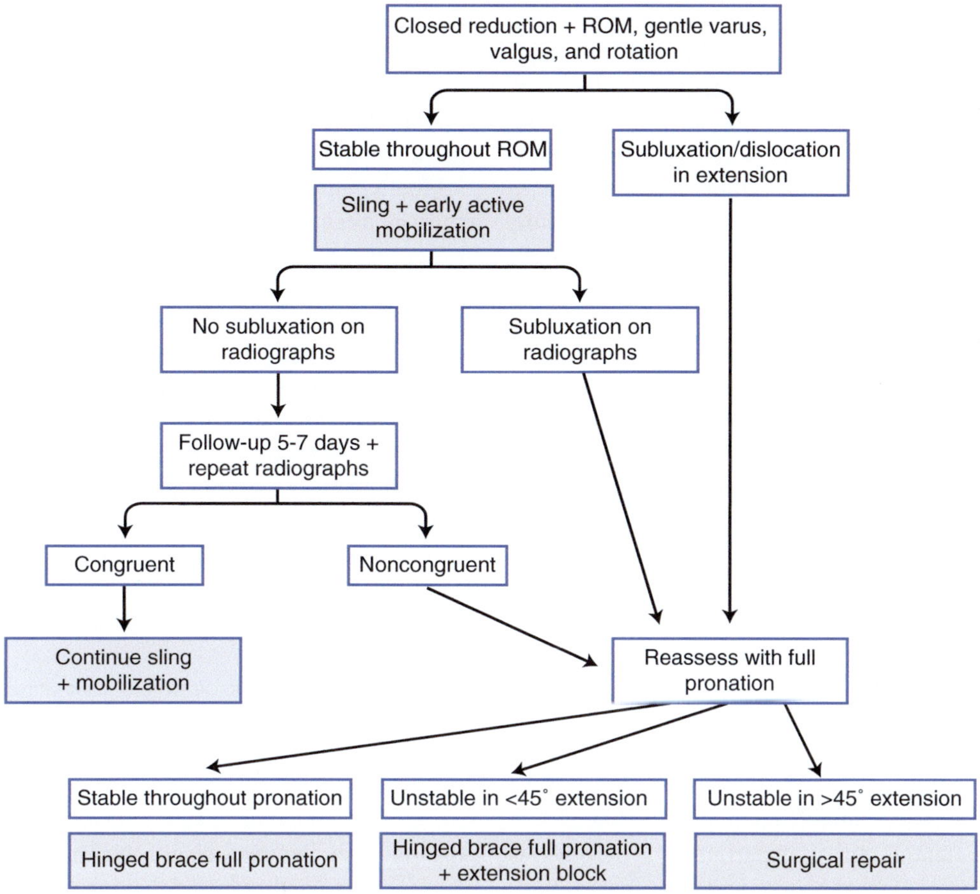


**Fig. 4.6** Treatment algorithm for simple dislocations

if no remarkable improvement occurs despite using a turnbuckle orthosis for 3 months. The choice of surgical procedure depends on the main cause of the decreased range of motion. Many surgical procedures have been described including anterior and posterior capsulectomies, excision of heterotopic ossification, removal of osteophytes, and interpositional or total elbow arthroplasties [41, 42]. The most commonly performed procedure in the case of a stiff elbow after a simple dislocation is a release, either open or arthroscopic, with a capsulotomy or capsulectomy of the both the anterior and posterior compartments. Limitation of rotation is uncommon in these injuries; consequently, only the anterior and posterior capsule typically needs to be addressed. If heterotopic ossification is involved, then removal is required as well typically in an open fashion.

Heterotopic ossification is periarticular calcification that occurs most frequently in the collateral ligaments and is often of limited significance [11, 35]. Significant heterotopic ossification in the ligaments resulting in bridging bone or in cases of significant anterior or posterior heterotopic ossification can dramatically reduce range of motion in flexion and extension and rotation. Heterotopic ossification should be suspected if the patient has remarkable pain and begins to lose range of motion 3–4 weeks after injury [43]. Aggressive stretching increases the risk [9], whereas nonsteroidal anti-inflammatory drugs and external radiation decrease the risk of heterotopic ossification [43]. Significant limitations of range of motion (less than 30–130° of elbow flexion and extension or less than 50° of pronation and/or supination) and neurovascular compression are indications for surgical excision. Excision should be done after maturation, traditionally 12–18 months after injury although excision can be performed as early as 4 months post-injury [44]. Heterotopic ossification is considered mature when bony lesions become stable on sequential plain radiographs.

Neurovascular injury can occur as a result of an elbow dislocation [28]. The ulnar nerve is the most commonly injured nerve, most often due to a valgus stretch [39]. Median nerve injury can occur due to stretch or secondary compression from swelling [28]. Intra-articular nerve entrapment has been reported and can be identified on MRI [45]. Most neurologic injuries are neuropraxias and will resolve after the elbow is relocated. Persistent neurologic deficits may require electrodiagnostic testing and possible neurologic decompression if symptoms persist.

Compartment syndrome may occur after a simple elbow dislocation although very rarely. While this is extremely uncommon, awareness of the potential for compartment syndrome is important. Typical history and examination findings including pain out of proportion and with passive stretch of the digits and compression of the forearm compartments should raise awareness for a probable compartment syndrome. Emergent fasciotomies must be done promptly of the forearm and possibly the hand and arm if clinical signs indicate a compartment syndrome even in the presence of intact pulses [23].

Chronic instability after a simple elbow dislocation is uncommon [23]. Symptomatic laxity is an indication for ligament reconstruction and most laxity occurs with failure of the lateral collateral ligament complex resulting in posterolateral rotatory instability [28]. Nonoperative management for posterolateral rotatory instability is not effective and typically requires reconstruction of the lateral ulnar collateral ligament to restore stability. Chronic medial collateral ligament insufficiency is not typical of chronic instability after a simple dislocation. If medial collateral ligament insufficiency is symptomatic in a chronic setting, it is usually a result of chronic global instability requiring both medial and lateral collateral ligament reconstructions simultaneously.

Finally, articular injury may result in late arthrosis affecting the long-term functional outcome of the joint [46]. Articular cartilage may be damaged from the initial injury, even if there is no evidence of fracture or osteochondral injury on radiographs [28]. Josefsson et al. [35] reported radiographic signs of degenerative joint disease in 19 out of 50 patients. These signs included sclerosis, osteophytes, subchondral bone irregularities, and cysts. No joint space narrowing was demonstrated.

## Author's Preferred Treatment

The patient lies supine with the arm across his chest, elbow flexed 90°, and forearm supinated. The physician reducing the elbow stands on the injured side. After applying adequate traction, the arm is held and the olecranon is manipulated into position with the physician's thumb. Next, the elbow is flexed and extended through a full range-of-motion in neutral rotation to assess for stability. If the joint is stable throughout the range-of-motion without any subluxation or crepitus, a posterior splint is applied for comfort until the patient returns to clinic 7 days later. Active elbow mobilization is encouraged as soon as the splint is removed. Nonsteroidal anti-inflammatory drugs are prescribed for 2 weeks for pain relief and to decrease the risk of heterotopic ossification. If the elbow subluxates or dislocates in extension, reassessment in full pronation is performed. If forearm pronation eliminates instability in extension, a hinged brace that allows unlimited flexion and extension and holds the forearm in full pronation is applied. If there is residual instability in full extension or near full extension, an extension block is added. Surgical repair is considered if an extension block of more than 45° is needed.

If a surgical repair is required, a posterior skin incision is preferred and a lateral fasciocutaneous flap is developed. Using a suture anchor, the lateral collateral ligament, together with the capsule and common extensors, is attached to the isometric point on the lateral epicondyle with the elbow in 30° of flexion. The isometric point is approximately 2 mm superior to the center of rotation of the capitellum. Typically, the entire extensor mechanism and the lateral collateral ligament are avulsed and should be repaired as a unit. In general, the ligament should not be dissected out from the overlying common extensor and extensor carpi ulnaris (ECU) but rather a locking Krackow stitch with heavy nonabsorbable high strength suture should be passed through the combined ligament and extensors. Passage of the suture is often aided by creating Kocher's interval between anconeus and ECU. The locking stitch should then be passed through the combined ligament/tendon anterior to the interval. If there is gross instability after lateral collateral ligament repair, then a medial fasciocutaneous flap is elevated and the ulnar nerve is isolated and decompressed in situ. The medial collateral ligament complex and flexor/pronator muscle mass are reattached to the medial epicondyle using suture anchors or bone tunnels. The MCL complex typically resides deep to the humeral head of the flexor carpi ulnaris (FCU) which is typically injured in the setting of a dislocation, as well as the more proximal flexor-pronator mass. With the ulnar nerve decompressed, the location of the humeral head of FCU is easy to identify as it is just anterior to the ulnar nerve. The MCL is typically repaired as a unit with the deep capsule. The common flexor and humeral head of the FCU should then be reattached. The MCL takes origin from the most lateral point of the anterior/inferior aspect of the medial epicondyle. A suture anchor should be placed in this location for ligament repair or a bone tunnel for docking of a locked stitch passed through the ligament. A more posterior/superior anchor can then be placed for flexor/pronator repair. A posterior splint is applied for 10 days to protect the incision, and then the arm is transitioned to a hinged brace with an extension block as needed. The extension block is gradually decreased until full extension is achieved by 3 weeks postoperatively. The brace is removed 4 weeks postoperatively. Before removal of the brace, the patient is allowed to remove the brace only for motion exercises under a therapists' guidance.

## Case Example

A 15-year-old male presented to the emergency department hours after he felt a pop in his left elbow while wrestling. He had a gross deformity about his elbow and the elbow was neurovascularly intact on exam. X-rays revealed a simple elbow dislocation (Fig. 4.7).

The patient was sedated in the emergency department and underwent a closed reduction. He was laid supine with a sheet wrapped around his body. The person responsible for the reduction stood on the patient's left side, while an assistant stood across the bed holding the sheet from under

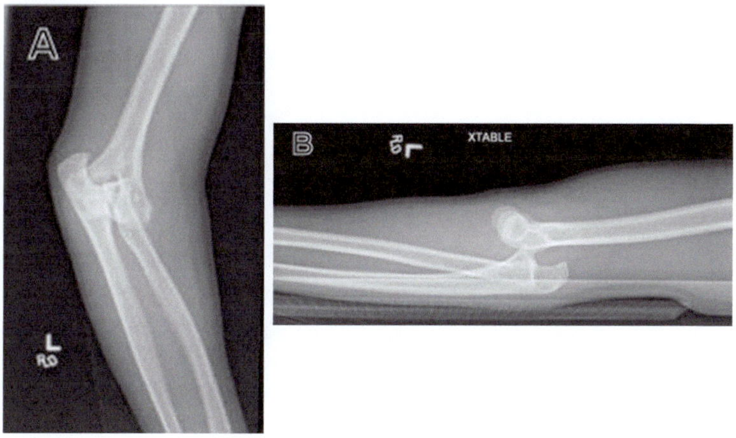


**Fig. 4.7** Pre-reduction radiographs of a simple dislocation. Anterposterior (**a**) and cross table lateral (**b**) view

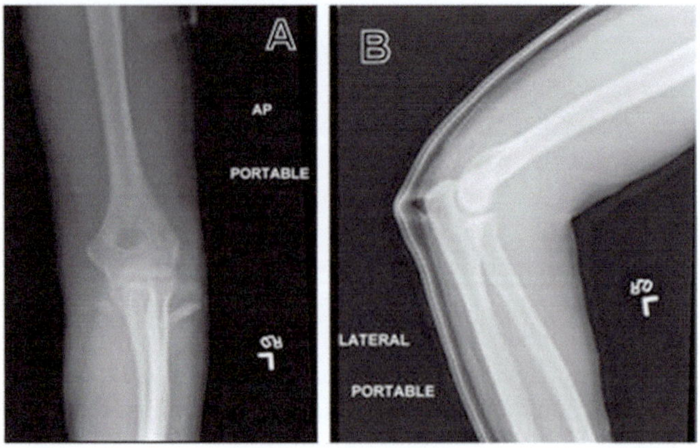


**Fig. 4.8** Post-reduction radiographs of a simple dislocation. Anteroposterior (**a**) and lateral (**b**) view

his left axilla to provide counter-traction. The patient's forearm was fully supinated and axial traction was placed on the proximal forearm with the elbow bent at 90°. The elbow was reduced using a thumb on the tip of the olecranon and coaxing the distal humerus back into the semilunar notch with maintenance of the supination and axial traction of the forearm. His range of motion was tested under fluoroscopy in neutral rotation once he was reduced. The elbow was found to be stable throughout an entire range of motion. He was neurovascularly intact after reduction. Post-reduction radiographs showed a concentrically reduced elbow (Fig. 4.8).

At that time the decision was made to place the patient in a posterior mold splint in 90° of elbow flexion for 7 days. When he returned to clinic 7 days later, the splint was removed and an active range of motion protocol was instituted. The patient did not require formal physical therapy, and he regained nearly full range of motion within 6 weeks, lacking only 5° of extension from his contralateral side. He was able to return to wrestling at 3 months.

**Acknowledgments** We thank Lyn Camire, MA, ELS, of our department for editorial assistance.

## References

1. De Haan J, Schep NWL, Tuinebreijer WE, Patka P, Den Hartog D. Simple elbow dislocations: a systematic review of the literature. Arch Orthop Trauma Surg. 2010;130(2):241–9.
2. Coonrad RW, Roush TF, Major NM, Basamania CJ. The drop sign, a radiographic warning sign of elbow instability. J Shoulder Elbow Surg. 2005;14(3):312–7.
3. Heo YM, Yi JW, Lee JB, Lee DH, Park WK, Kim SJ. Unstable simple elbow dislocation treated with the repair of lateral collateral ligament complex. Clin Orthop Surg. 2015;7(2):241–7.
4. Sheps DM, Hildebrand KA, Boorman RS. Simple dislocations of the elbow: evaluation and treatment. Hand Clin. 2004;20(4):389–404.
5. Stoneback JW, Owens BD, Sykes J, Athwal GS, Pointer L, Wolf JM. Incidence of elbow dislocations in the United States population. J Bone Joint Surg Am. 2012;94(3):240–5.
6. Josefsson PO, Nilsson BE. Incidence of elbow dislocation. Acta Orthop Scand. 1986;57(6):537–8.
7. O'Driscoll SW, Jupiter JB, King GJW, Hotchkiss RN, Morrey BF. The unstable elbow. Instr Course Lect. 2001;50:89–102.
8. O'Driscoll SW, Bell DF, Morrey BF. Posterolateral rotatory instability of the elbow. J Bone Joint Surg Am. 1991;73(3):440–6.
9. Hildebrand KA, Patterson SD, King GJW. Acute elbow dislocations: simple and complex. Orthop Clin North Am. 1999;30(1):63–79.
10. Murthi AM, Keener JD, Armstrong AD, Getz CL. The recurrent unstable elbow: diagnosis and treatment. Instr Course Lect. 2011;60:215–26.
11. Mehlhoff TL, Noble PC, Bennett JB, et al. Simple dislocation of the elbow in the adult. Results after closed treatment. J Bone Joint Surg Am. 1988;70(2):244–9.
12. Cohen MS, Hastings H. Acute elbow dislocation: evaluation and management. J Am Acad Orthop Surg. 1998;6(1):15–23.
13. Sanchez-Sotelo J, O'Driscoll SW, Morrey BF. Medial oblique compression fracture of the coronoid process of the ulna. J Shoulder Elbow Surg. 2005;14(1):60–4.
14. Potter HG, Weiland AJ, Schatz JA, Paletta GA, Hotchkiss RN. Posterolateral rotatory instability of the elbow: usefulness of MR imaging in diagnosis. Radiology. 1997;204(1):185–9.

15. Hotchkiss R. Displaced fractures of the radial head: internal fixation or excision? J Am Acad Orthop Surg. 1997;5(1):1–10.
16. Modi CS, Lawrence E, Lawrence TM. Elbow instability. J Orthop Trauma. 2012;26(5):316–27.
17. McCabe M, Savoie F. Simple elbow dislocations: evaluation, management, and outcomes. Phys Sportsmed. 2012;40(1):62–71.
18. Kuhn MA, Ross G. Acute elbow dislocations. Orthop Clin North Am. 2008;39(2):155–61.
19. O'Driscoll SW, Morrey BF, Korinek S, An KN. Elbow subluxation and dislocation. A spectrum of instability. Clinical orthopaedics and related research. 1992; 186–97.
20. Parvin RW. Closed reduction of common shoulder and elbow dislocations without anesthesia. AMA Arch Surg. 1957;75(6):972–5.
21. Kumar A, Ahmed M. Closed reduction of posterior dislocation of the elbow: a simple technique. J Orthop Trauma. 1999;13(1):58–9.
22. Parsons BO, Ramsey ML. Acute elbow dislocations in athletes. Clin Sports Med. 2010;29:599–609.
23. Hobgood ER, Khan SO, Field LD. Acute dislocations of the adult elbow. Hand Clin. 2008;24(1):1–7.
24. Cohen MS, Hastings H. Rotatory instability of the elbow. J Bone Joint Surg Am. 1997;79-A(2):225–33.
25. Schippinger G, Seibert FJ, Steinböck J, Kucharczyk M. Management of simple elbow dislocations: does the period of immobilization affect the eventual results? Langenbeck's Arch Surg. 1999;384(3):294–7.
26. Maripuri SN, Debnath UK, Rao P, Mohanty K. Simple elbow dislocation among adults: a comparative study of two different methods of treatment. Injury. 2007;38(11):1254–8.
27. Kesmezacar H, Sarikaya IA. The results of conservatively treated simple elbow dislocations. Acta Orthop Traumatol Turc. 2010;44(3):199–205.
28. Ahmed I, Mistry J. The management of acute and chronic elbow instability. Orthop Clin North Am. 2015;46(2):271–80.
29. Josefsson PO, Johnell O, Wendeberg B. Ligamentous injuries in dislocations of the elbow joint. Clin Orthop Relat Res. 1987;221:221–5.
30. Josefsson O, Gentz C-F, Johnell O, Wendeberg B. Surgical versus non-surgical treatment of ligamentous injuries following dislocation of the elbow joint. J Bone Joint Surg Am. 1987;69-A(4):605–8.
31. Fraser GS, Pichora JE, Ferreira LM, Brownhill JR, Johnson JA, King GJW. Lateral collateral ligament repair restores the initial varus stability of the elbow: an in vitro biomechanical study. J Orthop Trauma. 2008;22(9):615–23.
32. Moritomo H, Murase T, Arimitsu S, Oka K, Yoshikawa H, Sugamoto K. The in vivo isometric point of the lateral ligament of the elbow. J Bone Joint Surg Am. 2007;89(9):2011–7.
33. Jeon IH, Kim SY, Kim PT. Primary ligament repair for elbow dislocation. Keio J Med. 2008;57(2): 99–104.
34. Anakwe RE, Middleton SD, Jenkins PJ, McQueen MM, Court-Brown CM. Patient-reported outcomes after simple dislocation of the elbow. J Bone Joint Surg Am. 2011;93(13):1220–6.
35. Josefsson PO, Johnell O, Gentz CF. Long-term sequelae of simple dislocation of the elbow. J Bone Joint Surg Am. 1984;66(6):927–30.
36. Micic I, Kim SY, Park IH, Kim PT, Jeon IH. Surgical management of unstable elbow dislocation without intra-articular fracture. Int Orthop. 2009;33(4): 1141–7.
37. Protzman RR. Dislocation of the elbow joint. J Bone Joint Surg. 1978;60(4):539–41.
38. Royle SG. Posterior dislocation of the elbow. Clin Orthop Relat Res. 1991;269:201–4.
39. Linscheid RL, Wheeler DK. Elbow dislocations. JAMA. 1965;194(11):1171–6.
40. Green DP, McCoy H. Turnbuckle orthotic correction of elbow-flexion contractures after acute injuries. J Bone Joint Surg Am. 1979;61(7):1092–5.
41. Failla JM, Amadio PC, Morrey BF, Beckenbaugh RD. Proximal radioulnar synostosis after repair of distal biceps brachii rupture by the two-incision technique. Report of four cases. Clin Orthop Relat Res. 1990;253:133–6.
42. Morrey BF. Complex instability of the elbow. Instr Course Lect. 1998;47:157–64.
43. Mehta JA, Bain GI. Elbow dislocations in adults and children. Clin Sports Med. 2004;23(4):609–27.
44. Summerfield S, DiGiocanni C, Weiss A-P. Heterotopic ossification of the elbow. J Shoulder Elbow Surg. 1997;6(3):321–32.
45. Akansel G, Dalbayrak S, Yilmaz M, Bekler H, Arslan A. MRI demonstration of intra-articular median nerve entrapment after elbow dislocation. Skeletal Radiol. 2003;32(9):537–41.
46. Dürig M, Müller W, Rüedi TP, Gauer EF. The operative treatment of elbow dislocation in the adult. J Bone Joint Surg Am. 1979;61(2):239–44.

# Management of Terrible Triads

# 5

Dane H. Salazar and Jay D. Keener

## Background

The term "terrible triad of the elbow" was coined by Hotchkiss to describe the constellation of a traumatic elbow dislocation, radial head fracture, and associated coronoid fracture [1]. This dislocation pattern and its associated bony fractures earned this nickname due to their historically poor outcomes and the propensity for early recurrent instability, chronic instability, and posttraumatic arthritis [2–6]. In a description of the historical treatment of patients with elbow dislocations associated with radial head and coronoid fractures treated without a consistent surgical algorithm, 64 % of patients had a "poor" outcome [7]. In a report of the Arbeitsgemeinschaft fur Osteosynthesefragen (AO) experience, Heim and coworkers found that 73 % of patients developed premature arthrosis with residual instability [8]. Recent clinical and biomechanical studies have better defined surgical indications and protocols that have led to improved patient outcomes [9]. Good functional outcome can be achieved if stable, anatomic fixation of all osseous structures that contribute to elbow stability is performed [2, 4, 6, 10, 11]. This allows early motion of the joint at the same time allowing healing of the capsuloligamentous structures. Despite an improved understanding of the pathoanatomy and advances in surgical technique, complications are still frequent and include stiffness, residual instability, and posttraumatic arthrosis [12].

This chapter focuses on the evaluation, treatment options, published outcomes, and complications of terrible triad injuries of the elbow. A systematic approach to the management of this injury complex is provided, with an emphasis on the understanding of the pathoanatomy and current surgical treatments.

## Evaluation

Fracture-dislocations of the elbow are typically acute and traumatic, and thus the patient presentation and history are typically straightforward. The patient presents with a history of trauma, often related to a fall on the outstretched hand. In addition, these injuries may occur due to high-energy trauma and thus a thorough work-up to rule out concomitant musculoskeletal and visceral injuries must be performed. Careful inspection of the soft tissue envelope for open wounds and abrasions should be performed to rule out occult open fractures. In addition to a careful evaluation of the involved elbow, the ipsilateral shoulder and wrist shoulder also be inspected for any signs or symptoms of injury. Other associated

D.H. Salazar, MD • J.D. Keener, MD (✉)
Department of Orthopedic Surgery, Washington University, 660 Euclid Ave. Campus Box 8233, St. Louis, MO 63110, USA
e-mail: salazard@wudosis.wustl.edu; keenerj@wudosis.wustl.edu

© Springer International Publishing Switzerland 2017

R.Z. Tashjian (ed.), *The Unstable Elbow*, DOI 10.1007/978-3-319-46019-2_5

injuries have been reported in 10–15 % of cases, such as distal radius fracture, perilunate dislocations, and shoulder injuries [13]. The distal radioulnar joint and forearm should be specifically evaluated for tenderness or instability as a longitudinal injury of the forearm needs to be ruled out if there is a concomitant radial head fracture.

The documentation of peripheral nerve function and vascular status in the injured extremity, both before and after any attempted closed reduction is critical. Due to pain and swelling from the acute injury, extensive examination of the elbow is often poorly tolerated. It is unusual for a patient to tolerate varus and valgus stress testing to investigate collateral ligament rupture in the acute setting. Nevertheless, the clinician should maintain a high index of suspicion for collateral ligament injury.

Plain radiographs in orthogonal anterior–posterior and true lateral planes should be obtained of the elbow (Fig. 5.1). X-rays should be performed prior to attempted closed reduction. If patients present in clinic from an emergency department or are transferred from an outside facility, cast or splint material can often obscure bony detail. In certain circumstances it may be unclear on X-ray if the fracture fragments come from the radial head or coronoid process. The coronoid fracture is typically distinguished as a triangular fragment anterior to the trochlea in the dislocated elbow and proximally, within the coronoid fossa, after concentric reduction. Frequently computed tomography (CT) scans with reformatted images and three-dimensional reconstructions are needed for better understanding of the fracture patterns and amount of displacement. These images are also useful for preoperative surgical planning (Fig. 5.2).

The individual components of the terrible triad can be individually classified to aid in the evaluation of this injury:

## Fractures of the Radial Head

The radial head is an important secondary stabilizer of the elbow to valgus stress and the radiocapitellar joint accounts for 60 % of load transfer through the elbow joint [14]. Several classification systems exist for fractures of the radial head. The most common cited classification system is that described by Mason [15] and later modified by Johnston [16]. The classification system is purely radiographic and in many cases has proven insufficient to guide clinical treatment. Mason type 1 fractures are nondisplaced fractures of the radial head. Type II fractures are displaced more than 2 mm and involve greater than 30 % of the surface of the head. Type III fractures are described as comminuted fractures often

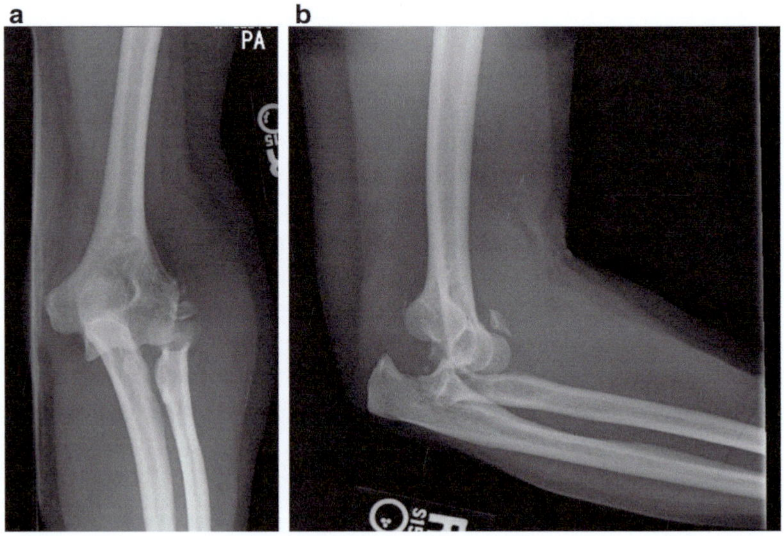


**Fig. 5.1** (**a**) AP and (**b**) Lateral radiographs of a right elbow demonstrating the three components of the terrible triad: posterior dislocation, radial head fracture, and coronoid process fracture

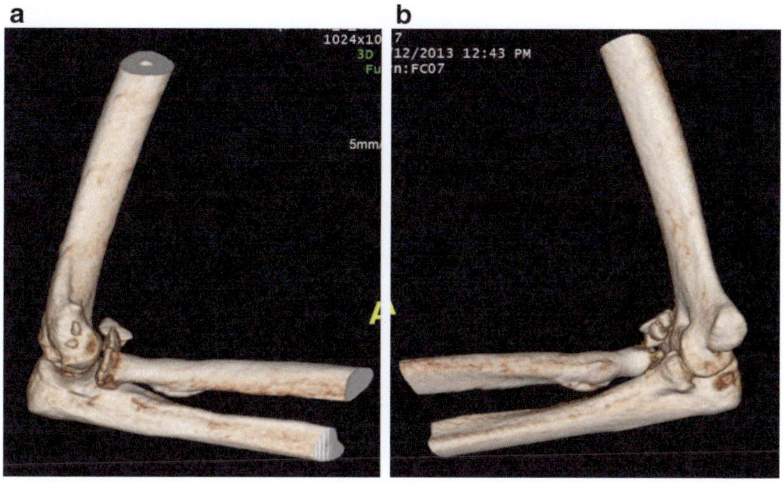

**Fig. 5.2** 3-Dimensional reconstruction CT scan of a right elbow with a terrible triad injury, as viewed (**a**) laterally and (**b**) medially

involving the entire head. Johnston later added the type IV fracture category, which is characterized by a radial head fracture with concurrent ulnohumeral dislocation (Fig. 5.3). This system does not account for associated injuries, which include tears of the interosseous membrane or mechanical blocks to range of motion from osteochondral shear injuries, which often influence both treatment and outcome. The Hotchkiss modification includes clinical examination and provides guidelines for the treatment (Fig. 5.4). In spite of the limitations as a comprehensive classification system, the Mason classification endures as one of the most popular and often cited systems used to describe radial head fractures.

## Fractures of the Coronoid Process

The coronoid process of the ulna serves as a bony anterior buttress, which prevents the posterior displacement of the forearm relative to the humerus. The triceps, brachialis, and biceps muscles have a net resultant posteriorly directed force. Thus when a coronoid fracture reaches a critical threshold and becomes large enough that it no longer acts as a restraint against this posterior force, the elbow will remain subluxed or dislocated, despite an initial reduction of the joint. Coronoid fractures were first classified by Regan

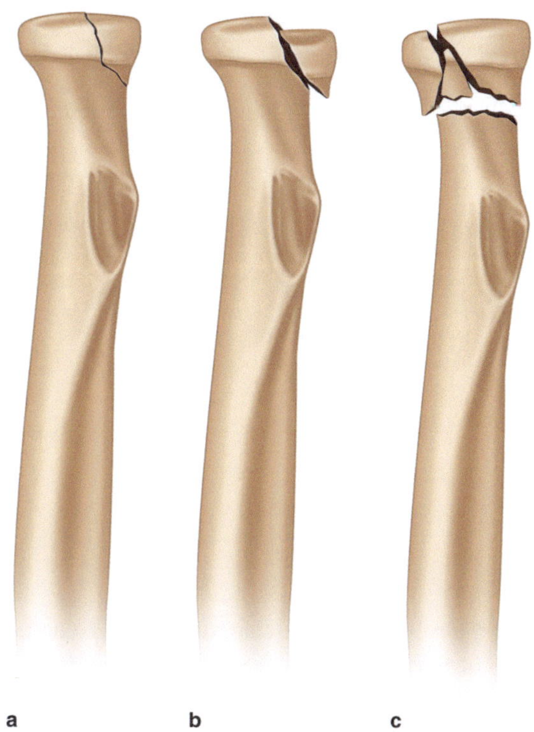

**Fig. 5.3** Mason classification of radial head fractures. (**a**) Type I—Fissures or marginal fractures without displacement; (**b**) Type II—marginal sector fracture with displacement (Segment of the lateral border of the radial head is separated from the other quadrants, is impacted and depressed, or is tilted out of line) (**c**) Type III—Comminuted fractures involving the whole head of the radius

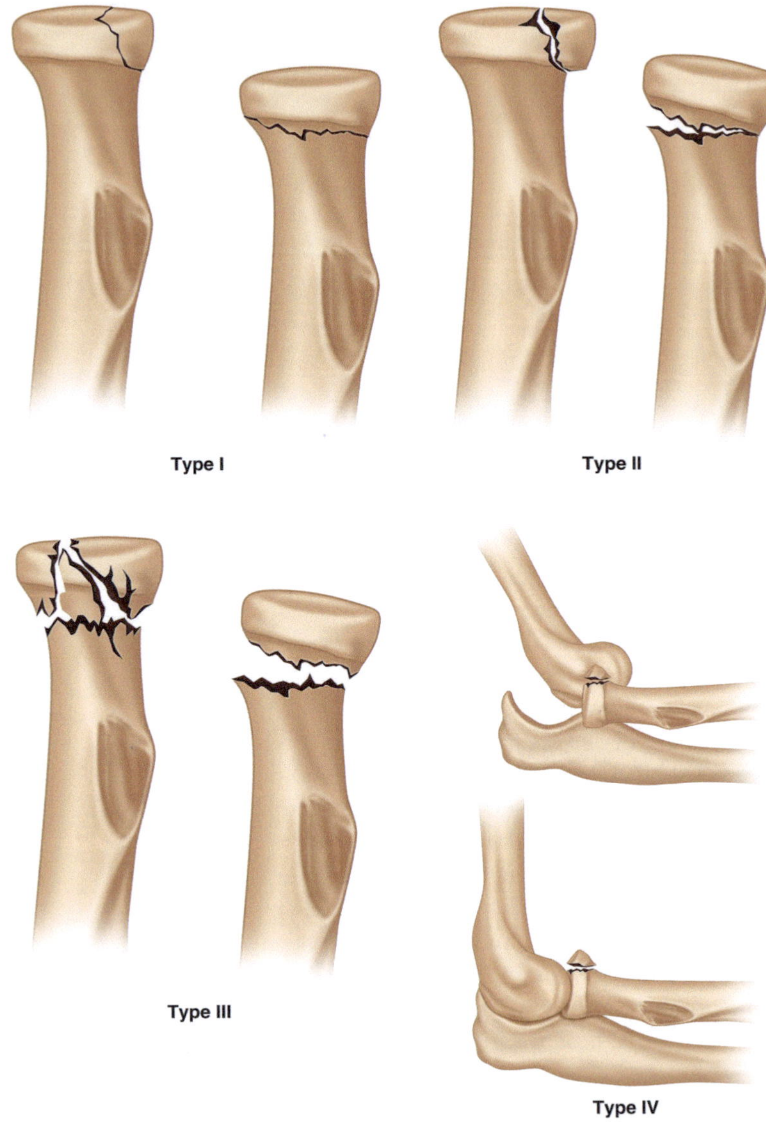


**Fig. 5.4** Hotchkiss modification. Type I—nondisplaced or minimally displaced (<2 mm) fractures of the radial head or neck with no mechanical block, Type II—displaced fractures (>2 mm) that are reparable and may have a mechanical block to motion, Type III—comminuted fractures that are not reparable that require excision or replacement, Type IV—radial head fracture with ipsilateral ulnohumeral dislocation

and Morrey into three categories based on the size of the fragment as seen on a perfect lateral radiograph of the elbow [17, 18]. Type I fractures involve only the tip of the coronoid process, which does not have any soft tissue attachments and thus often does not require fixation. Type II fractures involve less than 50 % of the height of the coronoid process. The brachialis and anterior capsule have attachments attach to this portion of the coronoid [19–21]. Type III fractures involve more than half of the coronoid and render the elbow unstable. Because the anterior band of the ulnar collateral ligament inserts at the base of the coronoid, these fractures cause instability both posteriorly and to valgus stress [22]. A modification of the system later added a "B" to represent the presence and an "A" to indicate the absence of an associated elbow dislocation (Fig. 5.5). This classification system has prognostic implications, as larger fractures were associated with worse outcomes due to greater instability of the elbow joint [17]. This classification system predates the routine use of advanced imaging and does not provide information about the mechanism of injury or the

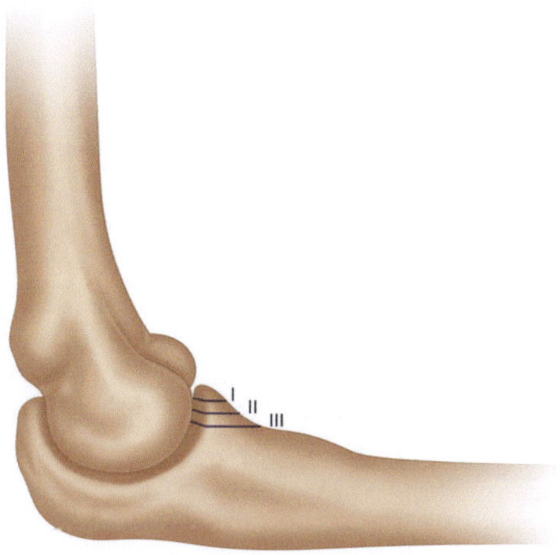


**Fig. 5.5** Regan and Morrey classification of coronoid fractures. Type 1—avulsion of the tip, Type II—fracture involving <50 % of the coronoid process height, Type III—fracture involving >50 % of the coronoid process height

obliquity of the fracture. However due to its simplicity and prognostic utility it remains a useful and popular classification in the management of coronoid fractures.

The availability of CT scans has advanced our ability to accurately delineate the morphology of coronoid fractures. In 2003 a new classification system was proposed by O'Driscoll in order to improve the description of coronoid fracture patterns [23]. This system accounts for the mechanism of injury, provides information regarding associated osseous and soft tissue injuries and ultimately guides treatment. The classification is comprised of three main types: type I is a transverse fracture of the tip of the coronoid process, type II is a fracture of the anteromedial facet and type III is a fracture of the base of the coronoid. These three types are further subdivided based on the severity of involvement (Fig. 5.6).

In the O'Driscoll classification, type I fractures involve the tip of the coronoid process but do not extend medially into the sublime tubercle, anteromedial facet, or distally into the coronoid body. They are transverse in orientation and usually include the insertion of the anterior capsule [24]. These fractures occur due to a shearing mechanism as the coronoid is driven against the distal humerus during an elbow dislocation. Type I fractures are further sub-classified into two types, based on the size of the fractured tip: subtype 1 involve less than 2 mm of bone and subtype 2 fractures involve more than 2 mm of the coronoid tip. Tip fractures are the most commonly encountered pattern in a classic terrible triad injury.

Type II fractures involve the anteromedial aspect of the coronoid process (anteromedial facet) and are associated with a varus and posterormedial mechanism of injury. These fractures are often associated with disruption of the lateral collateral ligament (LCL) and can result in persistent elbow instability leading to rapid posttraumatic arthritis if not recognized and appropriately treated. Not all fractures require surgical repair but identification of this injury pattern is necessary as indications for surgery differ compared to tip fractures. In addition to LCL disruption the medial collateral ligament (MCL) can also be involved in the injury pattern. Anteromedial subtype 1 fractures are located between the tip of the coronoid and the sublime tubercle, with the fracture line exiting medially at the cortex in the anterior half of the sublime tubercle. Laterally, the fracture line exits just medial to the tip of the coronoid. In sub-type 2 fractures the fracture line extends laterally to include the tip of the coronoid process. Sub-type 3 fractures are characterized by having the entire sublime tubercle involved. Type II subtype 3 fractures, by definition, involve the insertion of the anterior bundle of the MCL. Anteromedial facet fractures are most commonly associated with posteromedial rotatory instability of the elbow, not posterolateral rotatory instability seen in terrible triad injuries. In general, these fractures do not typically occur in a classic terrible triad injury although very rarely can be seen.

Basal coronoid fractures (type III) involve the body of the coronoid, indicated by the fracture involving at least 50 % of the height of the coronoid. These fractures are often associated with a less severe soft-tissue injury compared with the tip and anteromedial fracture patterns. The differentiation between basal subtype 1 and subtype 2 fractures is made based on an associated olecranon fracture. Additionally, subtype 1 fractures

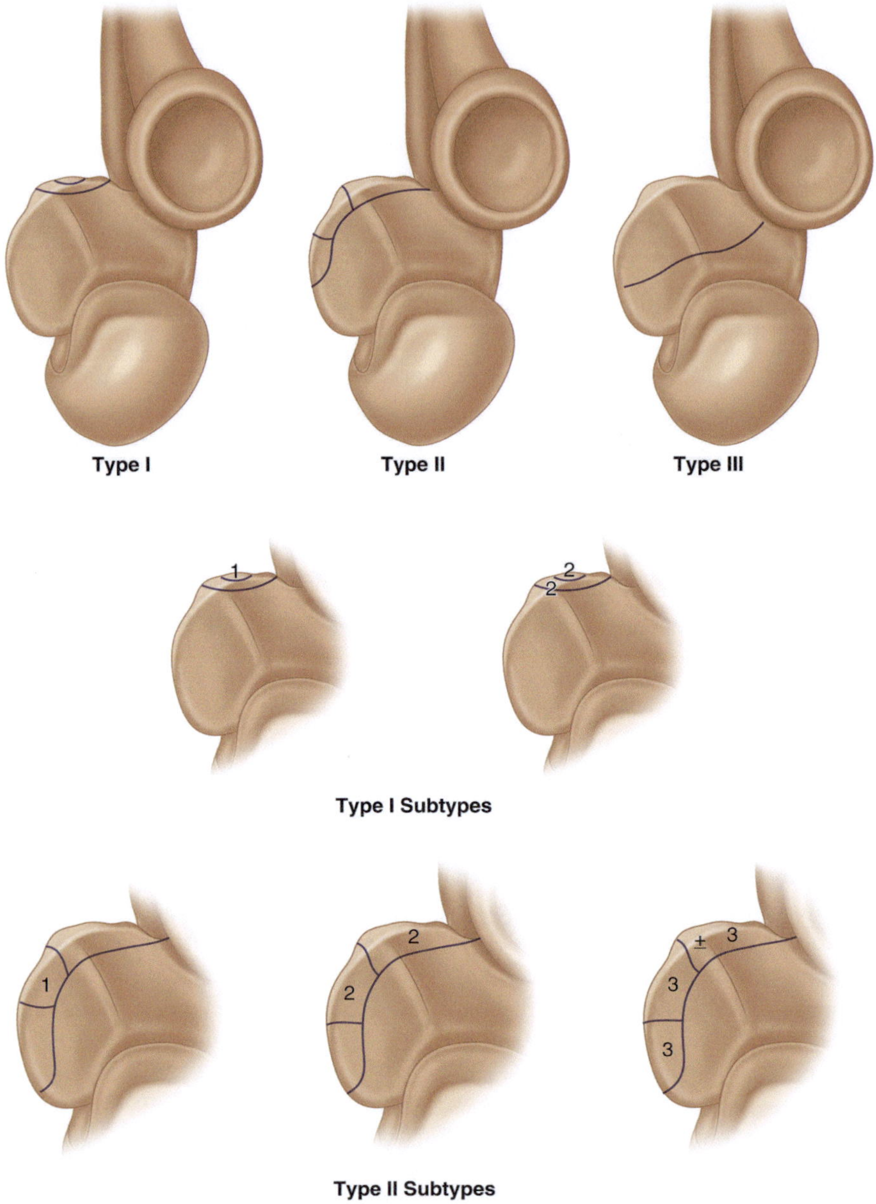


**Fig. 5.6** O'Driscoll classification of coronoid fractures (Type 1 tip fractures: subtype 1— <2 mm, subtype 2— >2 mm; Type 2 anteromedial facet fractures: subtype 1—amteromedial rim, subtype 2—anteromedial rim and tip, subtype 3—anteromedial rim and sublime tubercle $\pm$ tip; Type 3 basal fractures—subtype 1—coronoid body and base, subtype 2—transolecranon basal coronoid fracture)

are typically fragmented, extend into the proximal radioulnar articulation and are often associated with a radial head injury as well. Basal injuries can rarely be seen in terrible triad injuries but more commonly in fracture dislocation patterns involving a fracture of the olecranon process (posterior Monteggia fracture-dislocation).

## Injury to the Lateral Collateral Ligaments

In addition to bony fractures, terrible triad injuries also compromise the lateral ligamentous stabilizers of the elbow. The lateral ligamentous stabilizers include the lateral ulnar collateral (LUCL), the radial collateral (RCL), and the annular ligaments. In 2003 McKee and his coworkers described the pattern of lateral soft-tissue injury in a series of patients with elbow dislocations and fracture dislocations requiring open operative repair [25]. Six injury patterns to the lateral stabilizers were described: (1) proximal avulsion of the lateral ligaments, (2) bony avulsion fracture of the lateral epicondyle, (3) mid-substance rupture of the lateral ligaments, (4) ulnar avulsion of the LUCL at its insertion, (5) ulnar bony avulsion of the LUCL at the supinator crest (cristae supinatoris) and (6) a combination of 2 or more of the described patterns. The most common pattern in their series was proximal avulsion of the lateral ligaments, which was encountered in 52 % of patients (32 of 62 patients). In 41 cases (66 % of patients) a concomitant rupture of the common extensor origin was also discovered [25].

## Treatment Algorithm

Following closed reduction of a complex elbow dislocation, the joint often remains unstable and incongruent. Prolonged immobilization is fraught with complications and can lead to either long-term stiffness or continued instability. Thus most terrible triad injuries are most appropriately managed with surgical fixation except a very isolated group that can be considered for nonoperative management.

A step-wise approach aids in addressing all the critical components of this injury complex if surgical repair is performed. This includes fixation or replacement of the radial head, fixation of the coronoid fragment and repair of the lateral collateral ligament. Once this has been completed, the elbow is assessed for stability to determine the need for adjunctive treatment such repair of the medial collateral ligament or placement of an external fixator.

## Nonoperative Strategies/Therapy Protocols

Initial treatment involves closed reduction and splinting with radiographs to confirm concentric elbow joint reduction. If reduction cannot be obtained or maintained, repeated attempts at closed reduction should not be attempted. Repeated reduction maneuvers are postulated to contribute to the formation of heterotopic ossification about the elbow. Because this injury complex is particularly prone to instability, patients can knowingly or unknowingly dislocate while immobilized in a long arm cast. Even if cast immobilization is successful at maintaining a concentric reduction over time, it precludes early range of motion and leads to contracture. In general, several criteria are required for patients being considered for nonoperative treatment. These include: (1) obtaining and maintaining a concentric reduction of the ulnohumeral and radiocapitellar joints, (2) the reduction must remain stable through a functional arc of motion (within 30° of full extension) and thus allow for early active motion, (3) patients should have small (type I or type II) minimally displaced coronoid fractures, and (4) pronation/supination should be tested to insure the radial head fracture does not cause a mechanical block to motion. Patients should be able to perform supine overhead passive flexion and extension exercises without crepitation or the sensation of instability. Regular weekly surveillance radiographs are required for the first 3–4 weeks to ensure maintenance of a concentric elbow joint.

A recent study reviewed a small series of select patients with terrible triad injuries of the elbow treated nonsurgically utilizing the previously described criteria. The authors reported mean MEPI score of 94 and demonstrated acceptable post injury range of motion (mean flexion 134°, extension 6°, pronation 87° and supination 82°) and strength (strength as mean percentage of the contralateral unaffected elbow: flexion 100 %, extension 89 %, pronation 79 %, and supination 89 %) [26]. 36 % of patients went on to have some radiographic evidence of arthritis and two patients required surgery, one for early recurrent instability and a second for arthroscopic debridement of heterotopic ossification. Overall, these are comparable results to surgically repaired injuries although strict criteria must be used to attempt nonoperative treatment for it to be successful. While a very select group of these injuries can be treated without surgery it is rare and operative fixation is indicated in most cases.

## Surgical Management/Technique-Based/Surgical Pearls

A systematic approach helps to address the critical components of this injury and has been shown to improve clinical outcomes [9]. Traditionally this includes fixation or replacement of the radial head, fixation of the coronoid fragment and repair of the LCL. Once this is completed the elbow is reassessed for stability, to determine the need for repair of the medial collateral ligament and whether an external fixator is required.

### Patient Set-Up and Surgical Approach

Surgery can be performed under regional or general anesthesia. The patient is typically positioned supine using a arm board or "lazy" lateral with the arm brought over the chest. A nonsterile tourniquet can be applied under the final drapes or a sterile tourniquet can be placed depending on the size of the patient's arm. Preoperative imaging and fluoroscopy should be available for use intraoperatively. Two types of incisions may be used, either an extensile posterior skin incision or a lateral skin incision. With the posterior incision full-thickness fasciocutaneous flaps are raised starting on the lateral side. The medial flap is only developed if medial exposure is required for medial collateral ligament repair or ulnar nerve release.

The injury is initially exposed via a lateral arthrotomy. The injured structures are identified from superficial to deep. The deep lateral approach is performed either through Kocher's (Fig. 5.7) or Kaplan's interval or a combination of both. Typically the lateral collateral ligament complex with the common extensor is avulsed off the lateral epicondyle and either the Kaplan or Kocher interval or both can be developed distally to gain access to the radial head and coronoid [25, 27]. Although usually not necessary, releasing a portion of the extensor origin from the lateral supracondylar ride of the humerus can improve lateral exposure. Distally, the annular ligament is incised and later repaired. Deep to the common extensor tendon, the origin of the lateral ligament complex is assessed. Often, the common extensor and the lateral ligament complex are detached as a unit and do not need separation but rather are repaired en mass. Commonly a bare lateral epicondyle is encountered, consistent with a complete proximal avulsion of the LUCL [25]. Next the radial head is assessed. The decision to proceed with either radial head fracture fixation or replacement with arthroplasty is made based on the age of the patient, the degree of comminution and bone quality. If the radial head fracture is deemed repairable attention is turned to fixation of the coronoid process. However, if arthroplasty is planned then a radial neck osteotomy is performed in preparation for the prosthetic implant. The radial neck osteotomy and removal of the remaining head fragments have the benefit of dramatically improving exposure of the fracture bed of the coronoid process from the lateral side.

When the radial head is amenable to fixation, visualization of the coronoid injury can be challenging. Several maneuvers can assist with visualization and exposure from the lateral arthrotomy. The fragments of the radial head, if loose, can be temporarily removed from the wound. Alternatively, the fragments can sometimes be hinged distally on their intact soft tissue attachments. If additional exposure is still required the elbow joint can be subluxed posterolaterally to deliver the coronoid into the field of view. In some cases, a separate medial approach will be needed for adequate exposure and internal fixation of the coronoid fracture. This is more common in cases where the radial head fracture fragments are small and reparable precluding good coronoid exposure and/or the coronoid fracture is large, comminuted, or preferentially involves the anteromedial facet.

### Coronoid Fracture Fixation

Surgical repair and stabilization are carried out from deep to superficial, and the coronoid injury is addressed first. Fixation of the coronoid fracture depends on its size and degree of comminution [21, 22, 24]. Small O'Driscoll type 1

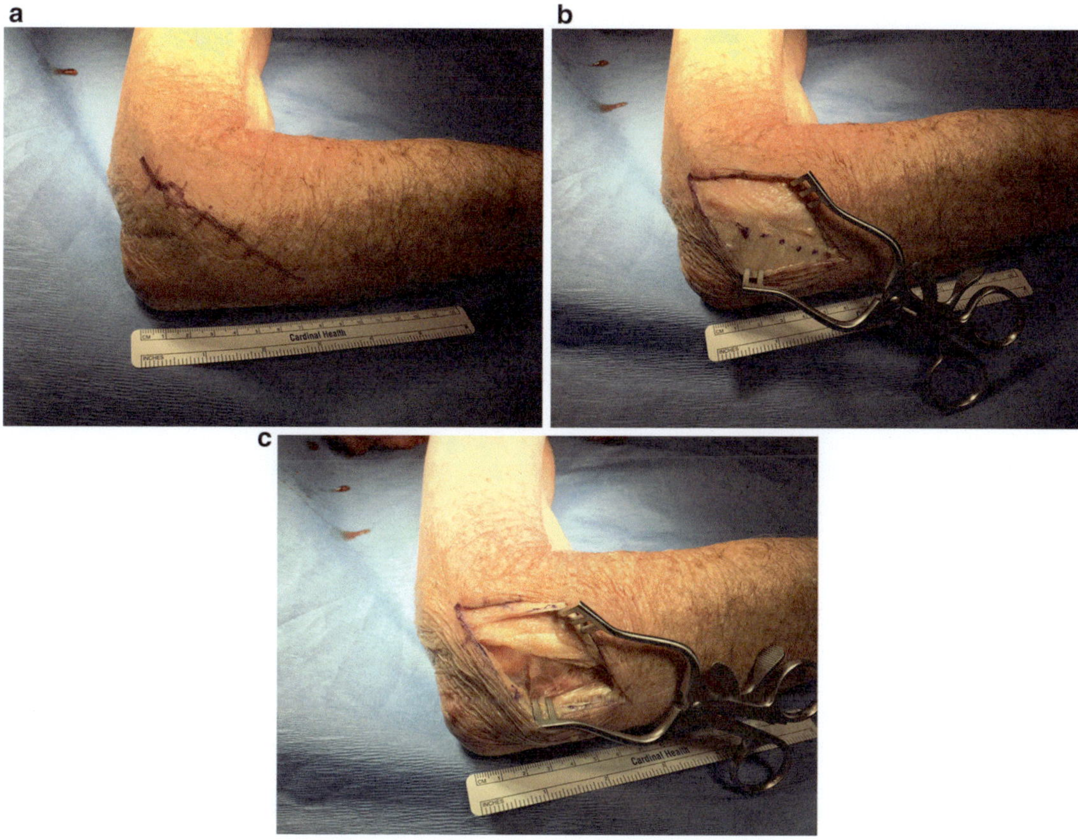

**Fig. 5.7** Posteriolateral approach to the elbow (Kocher) (**a**) Skin incision begins proximal to the lateral epidondyle and is carried distally and obliquely to a point 5 cm from the tip of the olecranon on the ulna. (**b**) In line with its fibers, the interval between the Anconeus (*target sign*) and the Extensor Carpi Ulnaris (*open circle*). (**c**) the Anconeus (*target sign*) is retracted dorsally and the Extensor Carpi Ulnaris (*open circle*) is retracted volarly to reveal the underlying deep structures

fractures can often be ignored as there is minimal bony compromise and the benefits of anterior capsular repair are minimal. If fixation is needed for stability this can be accomplished with sutures passed through drill holes from the dorsal aspect of the proximal ulna into the fracture bed and can be facilitated by utilizing a targeting guide (Fig. 5.8). This device can typically be found in any anterior cruciate ligament (ACL) reconstruction tray. In Type 1 fractures with only a small osseous fragment, sutures provide more reliable fixation than screws.

The requirement for fixation of small coronoid tip fractures remains controversial. Recent research has called into question the need for coronoid fracture fixation [28]. Terada et al. [29] and Josefsson et al. [30] both reported that chronic elbow instability was more common in patients with smaller fractures of the coronoid process. The authors suggested that even small coronoid fractures should be repaired to reconstruct the anterior buttress provided by the anterior capsule. However, a recent biomechanical study suggests that fixation of small type I coronoid tip fractures contributes little to stability in spite of this anterior capsular attachment [31]. Repair of the collateral ligaments was found to be more critical than suture fixation of the coronoid process in the treatment of small type I coronoid fractures [31]. However, because the overwhelming majority of published protocols still support coronoid or anterior capsule fixation, repair of even small coronoid fractures is currently the standard [6, 12, 21, 32].

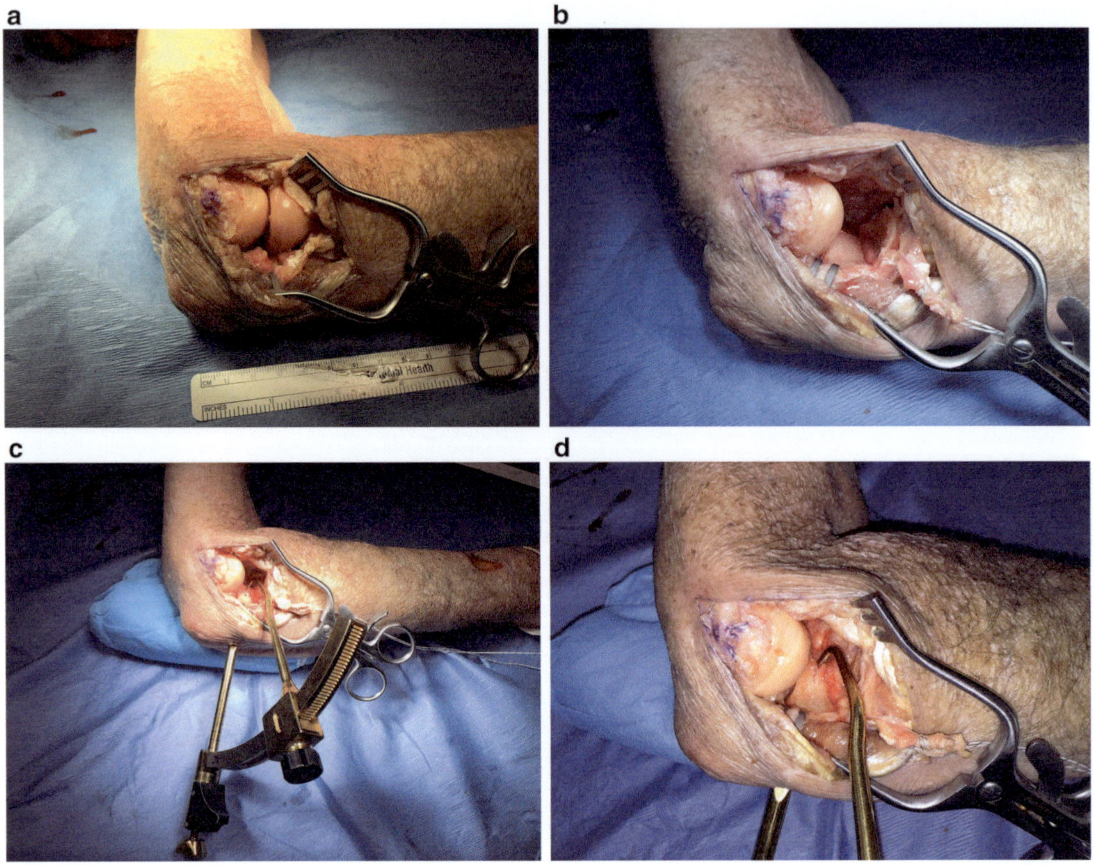

**Fig. 5.8** Coronoid fracture fixed with targeting guide. (**a**) lateral joint exposure (**b**) radial head resection (**c**) targeting guide into the coronoid fracture bed (**d**) drilling transosseous tunnels in the proximal ulna

For larger transverse fragments the suture is passed through drill holes in the fragment and is also passed through the capsule. With larger osseous fragments screw fixation can be performed with a large pointed reduction forceps to hold the fracture reduced while an ACL drill guide is utilized to pass a guide wire from the proximal posterior ulna into the coronoid fragment. A partially threaded cannulated screw can then be advanced over the guide wire and the fracture is compressed. If the size of the coronoid fragment allows, a second screw is placed in the same manner. Anatomic reduction of the fracture is often challenging and is likely unnecessary as long as the anterior buttress and capsular attachments are securely restored [21].

A medial approach offers excellent visualization of the entire coronoid, including the base. Fixation from the medial side can also be achieved with targeted screws into the coronoid through the dorsal surface of the ulna. Larger fracture fragments or fractures with medial comminution can be repaired using fracture specific plates or mini-fragment plates molded to the contour of the medial coronoid. Various medial approaches are available including a split of the flexor pronator, a flexor carpi ulnaris splitting approach through the bed of the ulnar nerve or the Taylor-Scham approach between the ulnar shaft and the ulnar head of the flexor carpi ulnaris. Each of the these approaches has been previously described in Chap. 3.

## Radial Head Fractures

The goals of treatment for the fracture of the radial head are to have a stable construct allowing the radial head to function both as an elbow stabilizer and also permitting early protected mobilization. In general, aggressive operative treatment of radial head injuries restoring the load bearing capacity of the lateral column is preferred in patients with terrible triad injuries. Because the radial head is an important secondary stabilizer, excision in the setting of complex elbow instability is contraindicated acutely [33]. The radial head resists valgus load when the MCL is injured and acts as a buttress to posterior instability with a deficient coronoid [34, 35]. Additionally, it restores the lateral column of the elbow, acting to tension the repaired lateral ligaments resisting varus and posterolateral rotatory instability. Previous studies have demonstrated elbow instability and posttraumatic arthrosis following resection of the radial head in complex elbow dislocations [7]. Therefore, the preferred surgical treatment options in the setting of terrible triad injuries include open reduction and internal fixation (ORIF) or radial head arthroplasty.

The decision between performing open reduction and internal fixation is based upon several factors including fracture location, number of fragments, and comminution. Previous studies have demonstrated inferior outcomes in radial head fractures with greater than three articular fragments treated with open reduction and internal fixation [30]. In a series of 56 radial head fractures treated with ORIF, 13 of the 14 Mason Type III fractures with more than three fragments had unsatisfactory results in contrast to all 15 Mason type II fractures which had satisfactory results [36]. A recent study compared radial head fractures treated with ORIF versus radial head arthroplasty in patients with terrible triad injuries [31]. All patients were managed with a standard algorithm consisting of either repair or replacement of the radial head, repair of the lateral ligaments and repair of the coronoid fracture. The decision to replace or repair the radial head was based on the number of articular fragments; patients with three or less fragments underwent internal fixation. With a minimum of 18 months of follow-up no differences were found in DASH score, Broberg-Morrey index, or in overall range of motion. All patients that underwent arthroplasty at the index procedure had a stable elbow at final follow-up where as 3 or 9 patients in the ORIF group were found to have residual instability. However, 37 % of the patients in the arthroplasty group demonstrated radiographic signs of arthritis compared to none in the ORIF group [37]. Based upon this data, open reduction internal fixation will likely reduce the long-term chance of developing arthritis but should only be considered in patients in whom stable fixation can be achieved with good bone, no comminution, and a limited number of fragments. Otherwise, arthroplasty provides a more reliable outcome in terms of restoring stability.

## Radial Head Fracture Open Reduction and Internal Fixation

Open reduction and internal fixation is reserved for radial head fractures with three or fewer fragments, good bone quality, minimal comminution, and ideally when there is not complete disruption at the radial neck. Advances in contemporary techniques have improved surgical outcomes using internal fixation [36]. Variable pitch headless screws, 1.5 or 2.0 mm cortical mini-fragment screws, pre-contoured radial rim and neck plates, T-plates, mini-condylar plates, and absorbable pins have all been described for the restoration of the fractured radial head and neck.

The articular surface should be reduced under direct visualization using a dental pick or small point-to-point reduction forceps, and should be confirmed with fluoroscopic imaging. Provisional fixation is obtained with small diameter Kirschner wires. Hardware is then placed with the goal of achieving enough stability to allow postoperative functional mobilization (Fig. 5.9). Headless or countersunk screws are utilized to avoid radiocapitellar chondrolysis. Additionally, careful attention to screw lengths will avoid radioulnar joint penetration and avoid painful rotation, diminished range of motion and osteoarthritis. If the fracture pattern involves extension into the radial neck, then operative fixation usually requires the addition of a plate. The nonarticulating portion of the radial head is referred to as the "safe zone" [38–40] which is the preferred region of plate placement. The safe zone corresponds to an approximately 90–110° arc of radial head sur-

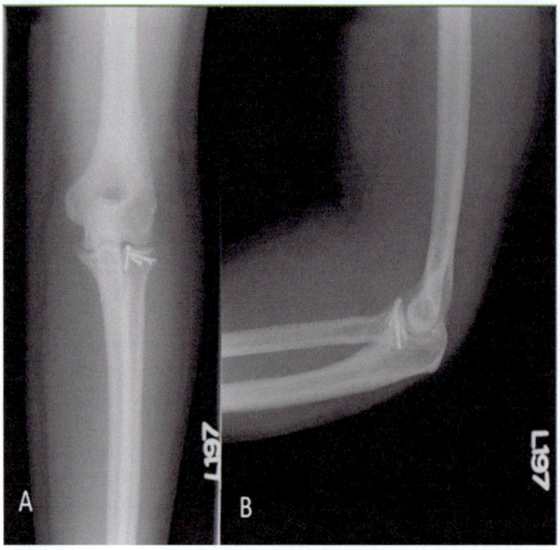


**Fig. 5.9** X-rays of ORIF of the radial head (**a**) Anterior–posterior (**b**) Lateral

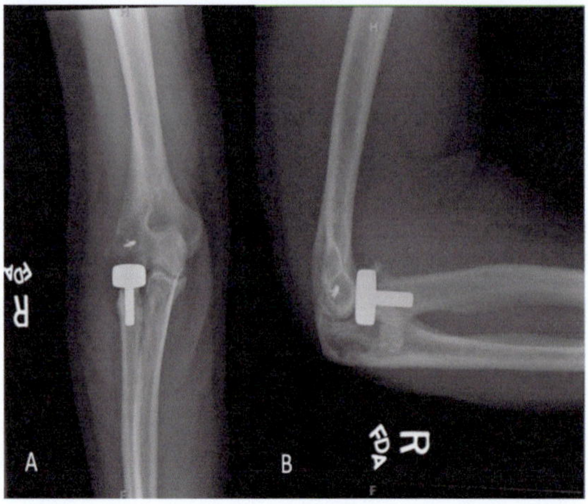


**Fig. 5.10** X-rays of a radial head arthroplasty (**a**) Anterior–posterior (**b**) Lateral

face and is defined as the lateral portion of the radial head/neck that lies between perpendicular axes through the radial styloid and Lister's tubercle [40]. Application of the plate to the radial side of the neck with the forearm in neutral rotation ensures placement in the "safe zone". Care should be taken to avoid plating distally past the bicipital tuberosity as distal dissection places the posterior interosseous nerve at risk for injury.

## Radial Head Arthroplasty

As a result of non-unions and loss of fixation seen with more complex fracture patterns treated with open reduction and internal fixation [36, 41], radial head arthroplasty has become the preferred treatment for acute comminuted fractures (Fig. 5.10). This is particularly relevant in terrible triad injuries where elbow stability is augmented by immediate restoration of lateral column load bearing. The residual head should be resected at the metaphyseal flare to preserve the function of the annular ligament. To provide a stable rim for the prosthesis and aid in accuracy of implant sizing, the maximum amount of radial neck should be preserved.

Optimal sizing of the implant is important in achieving a successful result [42, 43]. Sizing relates to recreation of the normal radial head diameter and radial length. The ideal sized implant should be chosen by comparing the aggregate of the excised fragments of the radial implants to the various radial head size options. In general, downsizing the head diameter slightly is recommended over placing a larger diameter head. If the diameter is too large it will cause undue loading of the margins of the sigmoid notch and potential loss of forearm motion. Reestablishing radial length is critical to normalizing elbow kinematics and stability. That being said an overstuffed radial head will result in pain, diminished range of motion, and capitellar erosion. Under sizing will prevent proper restoration of lateral column loading needed to minimize the risk of persistent instability. Most modern arthroplasty systems are modular allowing for variable head and neck sizing combinations. A trial implant should be inserted to test for stability and motion. To ensure joint congruity and the absence of impingement, the elbow range of motion, both flexion-extension and pronation-supination should be evaluated and documented. To avoid overstuffing, the articular surface of the radial head should lie flush with the proximal aspect of the radioulnar joint at the lesser sigmoid notch just distal to the articular surface of the base of the coronoid. The lateral ulnohumeral joint should be directly visualized to judge for any gapping, as this is the most sensitive intraoperative test for oversizing [42, 43]. Fluoroscopic imaging is then obtained to ensure concentric reduction and appropriate sizing.

## Repair of the Lateral Ligament Complex

In most terrible triad injuries, the lateral ligament complex (LUCL and RCL) and common extensor origin are avulsed from the lateral epicondyle. Multiple successful repair techniques including transosseous tunnels and suture anchors have been described [27]. Typically a running locking suture is passed through the lateral ligaments and the posterolateral joint capsule. The isometric point on the lateral epicondyle is then identified at the center of the arc of the capitellum [44]. The sutures are fixed at the isometric point either through a bone tunnel or anchor. The sutures are tensioned with the elbow concentrically reduced in 90° of flexion and full forearm pronation (Fig. 5.11). After the lateral ligament complex is repaired the common extensor layer is repaired in a side-to-side fashion closing Kocher's and/or Kapan's intervals (Fig. 5.12). Reconstruction of the lateral ligaments is rarely needed in the acute setting although it should be considered when these injuries present in a delayed fashion, beyond 6 or 8 weeks, where the elbow has been subluxated and the tissue quality is compromised.

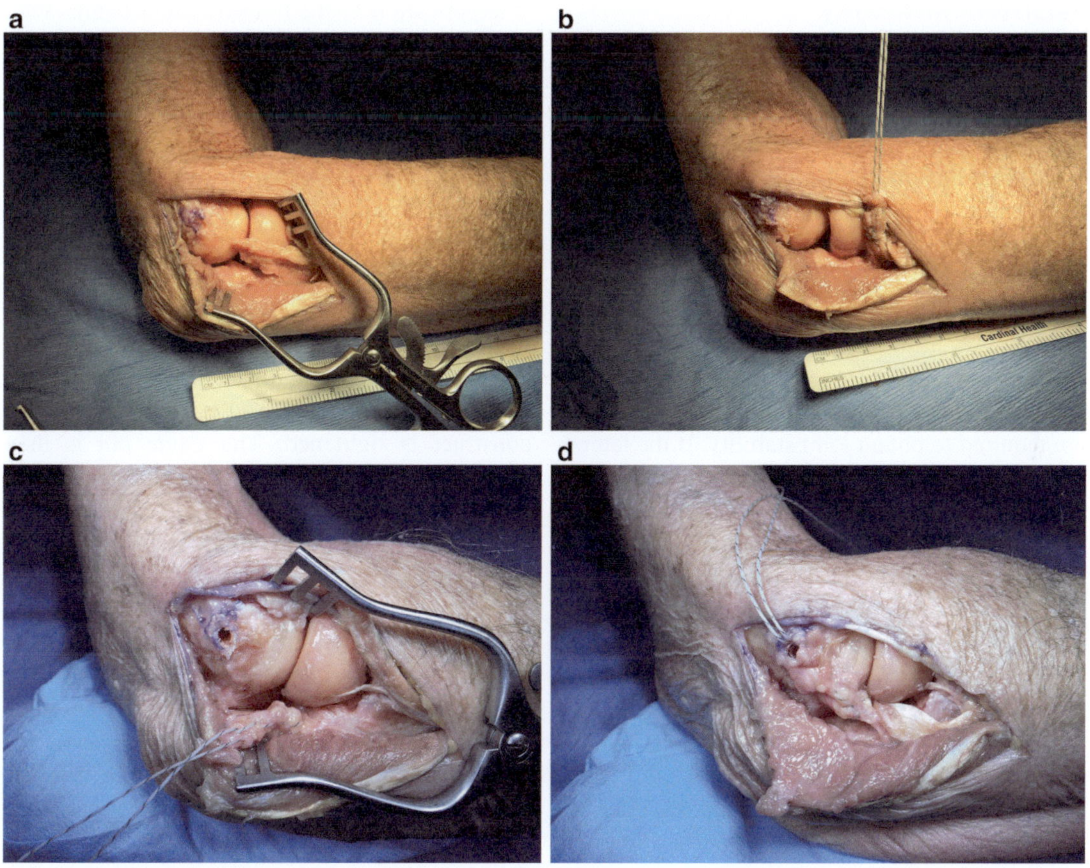

**Fig. 5.11** Lateral collateral ligament repair. (**a**) Demonstrates a lateral ulnar collateral ligament (*black arrow*) avulsed off its origin at the lateral epicondyle (*star*). (**b**) The lateral ulnar collateral ligament (*black arrow*) is prepared using an #2 ultrastrong nonabsorbable suture placed using a running locking technique (Krachow). (**c**) A drill hole is placed for a suture anchor at the isometric point on the lateral epicondyle (*arrow*). (**d**) The lateral collateral ligament tensioned and repaired (*solid black lines*) using an anchor while the elbow is held in approximately 90° of flexion

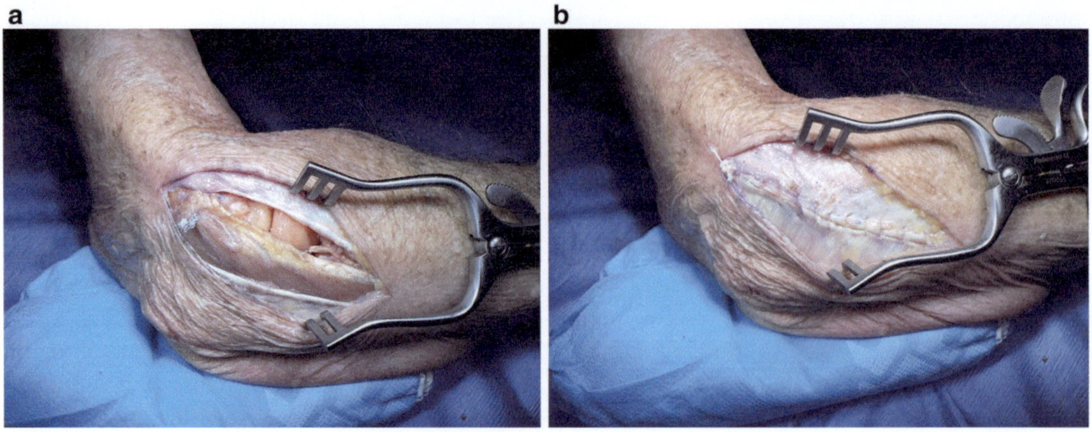


**Fig. 5.12** Repair of the common extensor tendons and fascial closure. (**a**) The anconeus (*target sign*) and common extensor tendon are incorporated into the repair, (**b**) The overlying fascia is repaired

## Persistent Instability

After repair of the coronoid, fixation or replacement of the radial head and repair of the lateral ligaments joint stability should be assessed throughout flexion extension of the elbow in neutral rotation. Ideally the ulnohumeral joint should demonstrate no asymmetric gapping or subluxation out to 30° shy of terminal extension with the forearm in neutral rotation or pronation. On occasion persistent instability that would limit early postoperative range of motion is encountered. In this circumstance further surgical efforts are required to obtain joint stability. If the lateral incision has been utilized, repair of the MCL through a separate medial incision is indicated. If a posterior incision has been utilized the MCL can be repaired by elevating a full-thickness medial flap and performing a deep approach to the MCL just anterior to the ulnar nerve. The ulnar nerve at risk during this approach and it is imperative that the nerve be identified and protected during the MCL repair. If the elbow remains unstable after repair of the MCL then application of a hinged external fixator is the final option to salvage early postoperative range of motion [45–48]. Alternatively placing a static external fixator can be performed to maintain a concentric reduction of the joint for 3–4 weeks and then removed to allow graduated range of motion.

Application of the hinged fixator begins with the insertion of a center axis guide pin through the center of elbow rotation aided by fluoroscopic guidance. This pin can be placed either from the lateral or medial side of the joint. After verifying on orthogonal views that the pin is through the center of rotation, the elbow is held reduced while the frame is assembled around it. Two pins are inserted into the humerus above the elbow through small open incision to ensure the radial nerve and its branches are protected. Two pins are placed into the ulna at its subcutaneous border. The pins are affixed to the hinge and the construct is tightened. The guide pin is then removed. Next the elbow is taken through a functional range of motion from 30 to 130° to confirm that the joint remains reduced.

## Alternative Surgical Protocols

Other operative treatments include "internal" hinged fixation, and static external fixators for persistent instability of complex fracture dislocations. Although effective in select situations these methods all have drawbacks. Orbay et al. published results on the use of an internal stabilizer fashioned from a Steinmann pin to manage complex fracture-dislocations of the elbow [49]. Their technique utilizes a bent Steinmann pin introduced through the axis of ulnohumeral

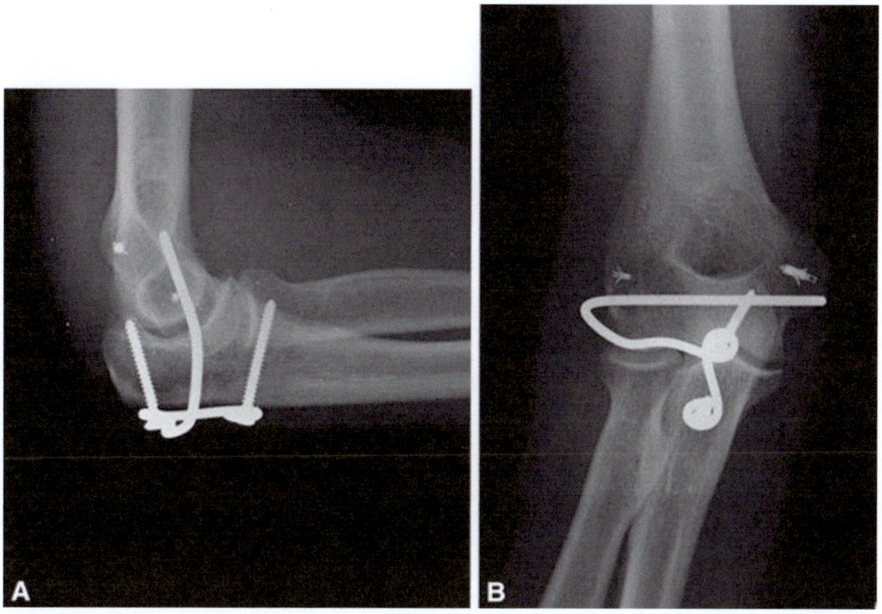


**Fig. 5.13** Internal elbow hinge (**a**) Anterior–posterior (**b**) Lateral (Courtesy of Jorge Orbay, MD Miami Hand & Upper Extremity Institute)

rotation and fixed to the proximal ulnar shaft (Fig. 5.13). They reported on a series of ten patients treated with their device, which acts as an internal hinged fixator. Mean range of motion at latest follow-up was flexion 134°, extension −19°, pronation 75°, and supination 64°. All elbows were clinically and radiographically stable. Complications resulting in additional procedures occurred in four patients. They concluded that their device allowed early postoperative range of motion of the elbow in patients that demonstrated persistent elbow instability without out the need to place a device that requires transcutaneous pins [49].

In some patients the ligamentous and bony disruption of the elbow does not allow application of a hinged external fixation device, in these cases static external fixation may be utilized to obtain and maintain joint stability. Range of motion may be started after removal of the static fixator. Eventual secondary procedures such as capsular releases may be necessary to reach maximum range of motion. Both static and hinged external fixators neutralize forces across the injured segment until the joint has healed enough to accept those forces.

Although not widely utilized, several centers have successfully treated terrible triad elbow injuries with a protocol that involves placing a single 4.5 mm large fragment cortical transarticular screw from the medial proximal ulna into the lateral distal humerus for persistent instability (Fig. 5.14). This screw is placed utilizing fluoroscopic guidance in the operating room and the patient is placed into a long arm cast for complete joint immobilization. After 3–4 weeks, the patient is taken back to the operating room where the transarticular screw is removed and the joint is check for stability. If the elbow remains concentrically reduced through a functional arc of motion then a hinged elbow brace is applied and a range of motion protocol is begun. If any concerns for instability remain, the patient is placed back into a long arm cast and followed up in clinic in 2–3 weeks at which point the motion protocol is begun. Caution should be utilized when incorporating these alternative surgical techniques into the operative treatment of terrible triad injuries as future research is still required to guide the surgical indications for their use and to elucidate the appropriate patient or injury characteristics that may require them.

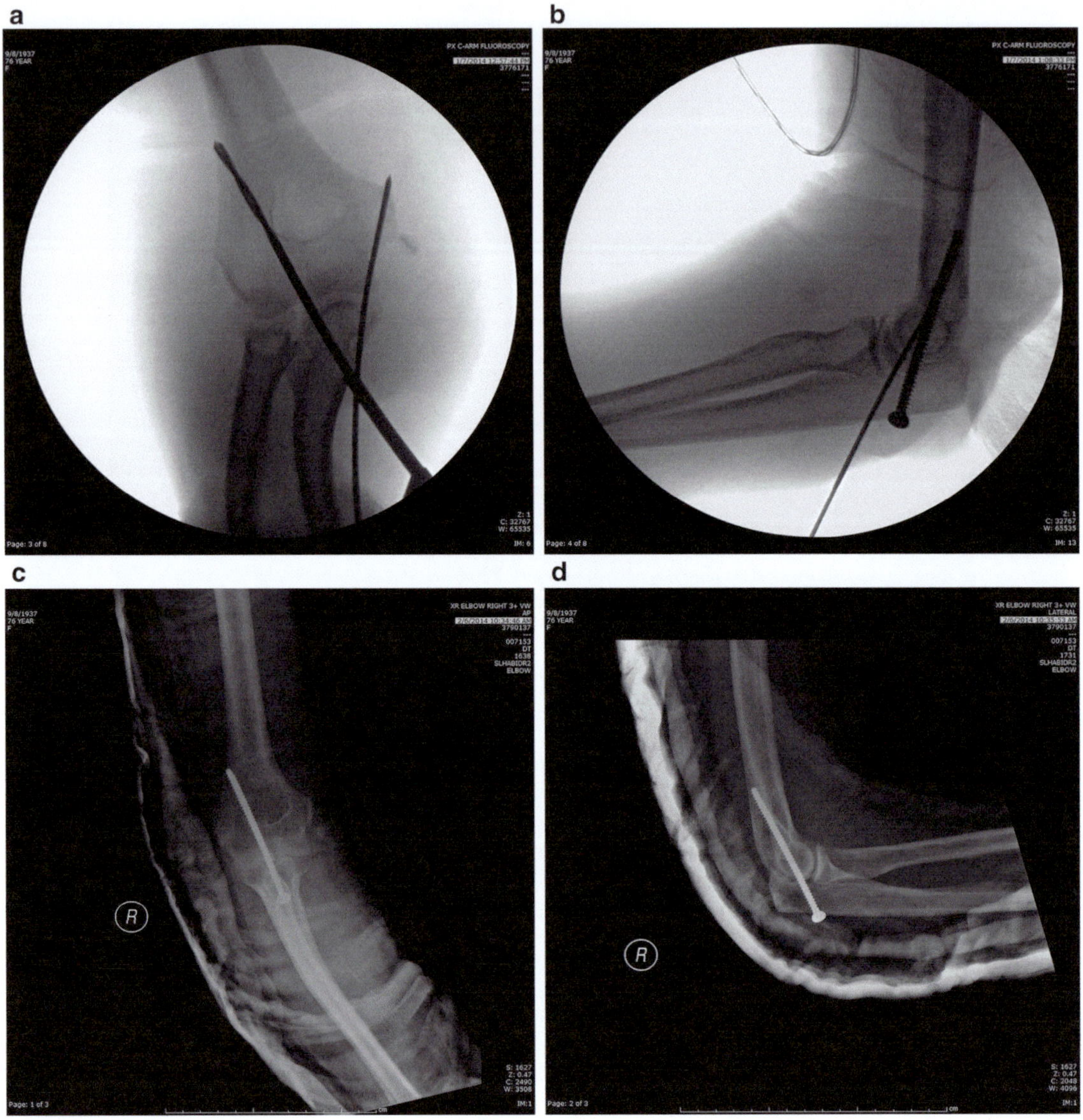

**Fig. 5.14** Trans-articular screw (**a**) Fluoroscopic intraoperative anterior–posterior (**b**) Fluoroscopic intraoperative lateral (**c**) Postoperative anterior–posterior radiograph (**d**) Postoperative lateral radiograph

## Published Outcomes/Complications

### Outcomes

A retrospective review of 36 consecutive patients with an elbow dislocation and an associated fracture of both the radial head and the coronoid documented the outcomes of a standardized surgical protocol utilizing current surgical techniques [9, 50]. The authors surgical protocol included fixation or replacement of the radial head, fixation of the coronoid fracture if possible, repair of associated capsular and lateral ligamentous injuries, and in selected cases repair of the medial collateral ligament and/or adjuvant-hinged external fixation. Patients were evaluated both radiographically and with a clinical examination at the time of the latest follow-up. At a mean of 34 months postoperatively, the flexion-extension arc of the elbow averaged 112°±11° and forearm rotation averaged 136°±16°. The mean Mayo Elbow Performance Score was 88 points (range, 45–100 points) and corresponded to 15 excellent results, 13 good results, seven fair results, and one poor result. Concentric stability was restored to 34 elbows. Eight patients had complications requiring a reoperation: two developed a synostosis; one developed recurrent instability; four required hardware removal and elbow release; and one developed a wound infection. They concluded that a standardized systematic surgical protocol for terrible triad fracture-dislocations of the elbow restored sufficient elbow stability to allow early motion postoperatively and reasonable functional outcomes.

Another retrospective study reported on the results of all patients aged 18 years or older whom underwent surgical treatment for "terrible triad" elbow fracture dislocation at one institution over a 7 year period [10]. Surgical treatment involved fixation or replacement of the radial head, repair of the anterior capsule or coronoid fracture in most cases, and repair of the lateral collateral ligament. Outcomes included grip strength, range of motion, Disabilities of the Arm, Shoulder, and Hand (DASH) questionnaire score, and a visual analog score for pain as well as radiographic assessment. Eleven patients were presented; seven patients had suture fixation of the coronoid fragment and anterior capsule, two had screw fixation of the coronoid, and two had no repair of the coronoid. The radial head was replaced in nine patients and repaired in one, and a fracture fragment was excised in another. The average follow-up for the cohort was 38 months. The average arc of motion of the injured elbow was 112° and that of the contralateral elbow was 142°. The average DASH score was 19.7 (scale, 0–100), with the mean visual analog pain score being 2.2 (scale, 0–10). No patients had recurrent elbow instability. Three patients underwent further surgical procedures, all for loss of motion. The authors concluded that a systematic approach to the fixation of "terrible triad" elbow fracture dislocations provides predictable elbow stability and functional range of motion in the medium term.

In a retrospective series over a 5 year period, a single surgeon reported on 22 patients with the terrible triad injury complex of the elbow [52]. Operative treatment consisted of open reduction internal fixation (ORIF) or prosthetic replacement of all fractures of the radial head and coronoid and reattachment of the origin of the lateral collateral ligament (LCL) complex to the lateral epicondyle. The MCL was not repaired in any of the 22 patients. Postoperatively one patient had instability that was attributed to noncompliance and required revision surgery. At an average of 32 months after injury, patients had an average of 117° ulnohumeral motion and 137° forearm rotation, and 17 of 22 patients (77 %) had good or excellent results. This author concluded that MCL repair is unnecessary in the treatment of dislocation of the elbow with associated intra-articular fractures provided that the articular fractures and the LCL are repaired or reconstructed.

In a multicenter study of patients with terrible triad injuries, Pierrart et al. reported on a series of 18 patients treated operatively [11]. At an average follow up of 31.5 months postoperatively, the mean MEPS score value was 78 (25–100) and corresponded to three excellent results, ten good results, three fair results, and two poor results. Five early and three late complications were reported. The authors recommended that the goals of surgery should be: to restore stability by preserving the radial head whenever possible through repair or replacing it with a prosthesis, by repairing the lateral collateral ligament and performing fixation of the coronoid fracture. If the elbow remains persistently unstable, options include repair of the medial collateral ligament or application of a hinged fixator.

Finally, recent research has challenged the concept that coronoid process fractures in the setting of the terrible triad injury require operative fixation [28]. In a small series of 14 patients that were treated for acute terrible triad injuries (two Regan-Morrey type I and 12 Regan-Morrey type II coronoid fractures) with a surgical protocol that included radial head repair or prosthetic replacement and repair of the LCL only. No coronoid fracture fixation was performed if intraoperative fluoroscopy confirmed stability throughout a full arc of motion after radial head repair or replacement and LCL repair. Repair of the medial collateral ligament or application of external fixation was not performed in any case. At a minimum follow-up of 2 years the mean arc of ulnohumeral motion at final follow-up was 123° (range, 75–140°) and mean forearm rotation was 145° (range, 70–170°). The mean Broberg and Morrey score was 90 and the average DASH score was 14. Radiographs revealed mild arthritic changes in one patient. One patient developed radiographically apparent but asymptomatic HO and none of the patients demonstrated instability postoperatively [28]. These results should be interpreted with caution. Future research is required to corroborate their findings, which demonstrate that terrible triad injuries with type I and II coronoid process fractures could be treated without fixation of coronoid fractures when repair or replacement of the radial head fracture and repair of the LUCL complex sufficiently restores intraoperative stability of the elbow through a functional range of motion underflouroscopy.

## Complications

Complications are frequently encountered following treatment for terrible triad injuries. The frequency of complications is related to the severity of the injury. Common complications are instability/subluxation, malunion, nonunion, stiffness, heterotopic ossification, infection, and ulnar neuropathy [9, 24, 51–53].

In rare circumstances instability persists following repair of the osseous and ligamentous structures in a terrible triad injury. In two recent series of elbows treated with a modern surgical algorithm for terrible triad persistent postoperative instability ranged from 0 to 15% [10, 54]. Persistent instability is likely due to unrecognized/unaddressed medial collateral ligament injury, unreconstructable coronoid fracures, chronic dislocations, or failure of repair. In patients in whom the distal humerus is subluxated over the coronoid base, there may be impaction or attritional bone loss, making simple repair of the coronoid insufficient. In these cases, coronoid reconstruction with bone bone graft can be considered; both radial head and olecranon autografts have been described [55, 56].

Loosening or failure of radial head implants has been reported, although newer designs offer much more modularity, thereby allowing for more accurate implant sizing, which may lead to improved results [57, 58]. The major issue with radial head arthroplasty is overstuffing the radiocapitellar joint [42, 43]. This can lead to abnormal radiocapitellar joint pressures causing pain, loss of flexion, capitellar erosion, and subluxation of the ulnohumeral joint. The native radial head should be used as a template whenever possible. If the native radial head falls between sizes, the implant with the smaller diameter or length should be selected. Intraoperatively the proximal portion of the radial head implant should be flush with the proximal aspect of the lesser sigmoid notch.

Posttraumatic stiffness is a common complication after treatment of terrible triad injuries of the elbow. The best treatment is prevention, such that at the time of index surgery, the elbow should be rendered sufficiently stable to allow early ROM. Should stiffness occur, the first line of treatment is nonsurgical, with passive stretching and static progressive splinting. Stiffness that is recalcitrant to nonoperative treatment may be treated surgically with open or arthroscopic capsular release. If heterotopic ossification is associated with stiffness, an open surgical approach is commonly required. Ring et al. [59] reported good results with open capsular excision in 46 patients with posttraumatic stiffness. At a mean follow-up of 48 months, there was restoration of a functional arc of motion of nearly 100°. Heterotopic ossification that becomes clinically significant is relatively uncommon and the use of prophylactic measures for heterotopic ossification is controversial. Some authors recommend prophylactic measures only for those patients with a concomitant head injury, burns, or those who have failed initial surgical treatment.

Posttraumatic arthritis can occur because of chondral damage at the time of injury as well as because of residual elbow instability or articular incongruity [7, 45]. The primary rationale for operative treatment is to restore stability to the elbow because early subluxation of the joint will usually lead to rapid posttraumatic arthrosis of the ulnohumeral joint. Treatment options include debridement, radial head excision, radial head arthroplasty, and total elbow arthroplasty depending on the severity of the joint destruction.

As with any surgical procedure, infection remains a potential complication after surgical fixation of elbow injuries. Surgical site infections around the elbow should be treated in the same way as any infection that occurs around a joint. If the infection is thought to be superficial, oral or intravenous antibiotics may be used. In deep infections serial surgical débridement with a course intravenous organism specific antibiotics are indicated.

A systematic review of 16 studies, involving 312 patients with terrible triad fracture dislocations treated with surgery demonstrated Mayo elbow performance scores ranging from 78 to 95. Mean DASH scores ranged from 9 to 31. The proportion of patients who required reoperation due to complications ranged from 0 to 54.5 % (overall70/312 [22.4 %]). Most of these complications were related to hardware fixation problems, joint stiffness, joint instability, and ulnar neuropathy. The two most common complications that did not require reoperation were heterotopic ossification (39/312 [12.5 %] patients) and arthrosis (35/312 [11.2 %] patients).

## Conclusions

Terrible triad injuries of the elbow remain challenging to treat and require careful examination of the injured limb and accurate assessment of the imaging to determine the extent of the bony and ligamentous injury. In most cases prompt surgical attention with a systematic approach to restore or replace bony anatomy and provide joint stability is indicated. Restoration of elbow stability that allows for early range of motion is felt to be a key factor in successful outcome.

## References


1. Rockwood CA, Green DP, Bucholz RW, et al. Rockwood and Green's fractures in adults. 4th ed. Philadelphia, PA: Lippincott-Raven; 1996.
2. Tashjian RZ, Katarincic JA. Complex elbow instability. J Am Acad Orthop Surg. 2006;14(5):278–86.
3. Giannicola G, Sacchetti FM, Greco A, Cinotti G, Postacchini F. Management of complex elbow instability. Musculoskelet Surg. 2010;94 Suppl 1:S25–36.
4. Bohn K, Ipaktchi K, Livermore M, Cao J, Banegas R. Current treatment concepts for "terrible triad" injuries of the elbow. Orthopedics. 2014;37(12):831–7. Johnson DL, editor, SLACK Incorporated.
5. Xiao K, Zhang J, Li T, Dong Y-L, Weng X-S. Anatomy, definition, and treatment of the "terrible triad of the elbow" and contemplation of the rationality of this designation. Orthop Surg. 2015;7(1):13–8.
6. Chen NC, Ring D. Terrible triad injuries of the elbow. J Hand Surg Am. 2015;40(11):2297–303.
7. Ring D, Jupiter JB, Zilberfarb J. Posterior dislocation of the elbow with fractures of the radial head and coronoid. J Bone Joint Surg. 2002;84-A(4):547–51.
8. Heim U. Combined fractures of the radius and the ulna at the elbow level in the adult. Analysis of 120 cases after more than 1 year. Rev Chir Orthop Reparatrice Appar Mot. 1998;84(2):142–53.
9. Pugh DMW, Wild LM, Schemitsch EH, King GJW, McKee MD. Standard surgical protocol to treat elbow dislocations with radial head and coronoid fractures. J Bone Joint Surg. 2004;86-A(6):1122–30.
10. Fitzgibbons PG, Louie D, Dyer GSM, Blazar P, Earp B. Functional outcomes after fixation of "terrible triad" elbow fracture dislocations. Orthopedics. 2014;37(4):e373–6.
11. Pierrart J, Bégué T, Mansat P. GEEC. Terrible triad of the elbow: treatment protocol and outcome in a series of eighteen cases. Injury. 2015;46 Suppl 1:S8–12.
12. Mathew PK, Athwal GS, King GJW. Terrible triad injury of the elbow: current concepts. J Am Acad Orthop Surg. 2009;17(3):137–51.
13. Neviaser JS, Wickstrom JK. Dislocation of the elbow: a retrospective study of 115 patients. South Med J. 1977;70(2):172–3.
14. Morrey BF, Tanaka S, An KN. Valgus stability of the elbow. A definition of primary and secondary constraints. Clin Orthop Relat Res. 1991;(265):187–95.
15. MASON ML. Some observations on fractures of the head of the radius with a review of one hundred cases. Br J Surg. 1954;42(172):123–32.
16. Johnston GW. A follow-up of one hundred cases of fracture of the head of the radius with a review of the literature. Ulster Med J. 1962;31(1):51–6.
17. Regan W, Morrey B. Fractures of the coronoid process of the ulna. J Bone Joint Surg Am. 1989; 71(9):1348–54.
18. Regan W, Morrey BF. Classification and treatment of coronoid process fractures. Orthopedics. 1992;15(7): 845–8.

19. Doornberg JN, van Duijn J, Ring D. Coronoid fracture height in terrible-triad injuries. J Hand Surg Am. 2006;31(5):794–7.
20. Budoff JE. Coronoid fractures. J Hand Surg Am. 2012;37(11):2418–23.
21. Ring D, Horst TA. Coronoid fractures. J Orthop Trauma. 2015;29(10):437–40.
22. Doornberg JN, Ring D. Coronoid fracture patterns. J Hand Surg Am. 2006;31(1):45–52.
23. O'driscoll SW, Jupiter JB, Cohen MS, Ring D, McKee MD. Difficult elbow fractures: pearls and pitfalls. Instr Course Lect. 2003;52:113–34.
24. Ring D. Fractures of the coronoid process of the ulna. J Hand Surg Am. 2006;31(10):1679–89.
25. McKee MD, Schemitsch EH, Sala MJ, O'driscoll SW. The pathoanatomy of lateral ligamentous disruption in complex elbow instability. J Shoulder Elbow Surg. 2003;12(4):391–6.
26. Chan K, MacDermid JC, Faber KJ, King GJW, Athwal GS. Can we treat select terrible triad injuries nonoperatively? Clin Orthop Relat Res. 2014; 472(7):2092–9.
27. Cohen MS. Lateral collateral ligament instability of the elbow. Hand Clin. 2008;24(1):69–77.
28. Papatheodorou LK, Rubright JH, Heim KA, Weiser RW, Sotereanos DG. Terrible triad injuries of the elbow: does the coronoid always need to be fixed? Clin Orthop Relat Res. 2014;472(7):2084–91.
29. Terada N, Yamada H, Seki T, Urabe T, Takayama S. The importance of reducing small fractures of the coronoid process in the treatment of unstable elbow dislocation. J Shoulder Elbow Surg. 2000;9(4): 344–6.
30. Josefsson PO, Gentz CF, Johnell O, Wendeberg B. Dislocations of the elbow and intraarticular fractures. Clin Orthop Relat Res. 1989;(246):126–30.
31. Beingessner DM, Stacpoole RA, Dunning CE, Johnson JA, King GJW. The effect of suture fixation of type I coronoid fractures on the kinematics and stability of the elbow with and without medial collateral ligament repair. J Shoulder Elbow Surg. 2007;16(2):213–7.
32. Zeiders GJ, Patel MK. Management of unstable elbows following complex fracture-dislocations--the "terrible triad" injury. J Bone Joint Surg Am. 2008;90 Suppl 4:75–84.
33. Beingessner DM, Dunning CE, Gordon KD, Johnson JA, King GJW. The effect of radial head excision and arthroplasty on elbow kinematics and stability. J Bone Joint Surg. 2004;86-A(8):1730–9.
34. Jensen SL, Olsen BS, Tyrdal S, Søjbjerg JO, Sneppen O. Elbow joint laxity after experimental radial head excision and lateral collateral ligament rupture: efficacy of prosthetic replacement and ligament repair. J Shoulder Elbow Surg. 2005;14(1):78–84.
35. Deutch SR, Jensen SL, Tyrdal S, Olsen BS, Sneppen O. Elbow joint stability following experimental osteoligamentous injury and reconstruction. J Shoulder Elbow Surg. 2003;12(5):466–71.
36. Ring D. Open reduction and internal fixation of fractures of the radial head. Hand Clin. 2004;20(4): 415–27. vi.
37. Watters TS, Garrigues GE, Ring D, Ruch DS. Fixation versus replacement of radial head in terrible triad: is there a difference in elbow stability and prognosis? Clin Orthop Relat Res. 2014;472(7):2128–35.
38. Witt J. Toward safe exposure of the proximal part of the radius: landmarks and measurements. J Bone Joint Surg. 2001;83-A(10):1589–90.
39. Diliberti T, Botte MJ, Abrams RA. Anatomical considerations regarding the posterior interosseous nerve during posterolateral approaches to the proximal part of the radius. J Bone Joint Surg Am. 2000;82(6): 809–13.
40. Caputo AE, Mazzocca AD, Santoro VM. The nonarticulating portion of the radial head: anatomic and clinical correlations for internal fixation. J Hand Surg Am. 1998;23(6):1082–90.
41. Ikeda M, Sugiyama K, Kang C, Takagaki T, Oka Y. Comminuted fractures of the radial head. Comparison of resection and internal fixation. J Bone Joint Surg Am. 2005;87(1):76–84.
42. Frank SG, Grewal R, Johnson J, Faber KJ, King GJW, Athwal GS. Determination of correct implant size in radial head arthroplasty to avoid overlengthening. J Bone Joint Surg Am. 2009;91(7):1738–46.
43. Athwal GS, Frank SG, Grewal R, Faber KJ, Johnson J, King GJW. Determination of correct implant size in radial head arthroplasty to avoid overlengthening: surgical technique. J Bone Joint Surg Am. 2010;92(Suppl 1, Pt 2):250–7.
44. Cohen MS, Bruno RJ. The collateral ligaments of the elbow: anatomy and clinical correlation. Clin Orthop Relat Res. 2001;(383):123–30.
45. McKee MD, Bowden SH, King GJ, Patterson SD, Jupiter JB, Bamberger HB, et al. Management of recurrent, complex instability of the elbow with a hinged external fixator. J Bone Joint Surg Br. 1998;80(6):1031–6.
46. Ruch DS, Triepel CR. Hinged elbow fixation for recurrent instability following fracture dislocation. Injury. 2001;32 Suppl 4:SD70–8.
47. Jupiter JB, Ring D. Treatment of unreduced elbow dislocations with hinged external fixation. J Bone Joint Surg. 2002;84A(9):1630–5.
48. Tan V, Daluiski A, Capo J, Hotchkiss R. Hinged elbow external fixators: indications and uses. J Am Acad Orthop Surg. 2005;13(8):503–14.
49. Orbay JL, Mijares MR. The management of elbow instability using an internal joint stabilizer: preliminary results. Clin Orthop Relat Res. 2014;472(7):2049–60.
50. McKee MD, Pugh DMW, Wild LM, Schemitsch EH, King GJW. Standard surgical protocol to treat elbow dislocations with radial head and coronoid fractures. Surgical technique. J Bone Joint Surg Am. 2005; 87(Suppl 1, Pt 1):22–32.
51. Forthman C, Henket M, Ring DC. Elbow dislocation with intra-articular fracture: the results of operative

treatment without repair of the medial collateral ligament. J Hand Surg Am. 2007;32(8):1200–9.
52. O'Driscoll SW, Morrey BF, Korinek S, An KN. Elbow subluxation and dislocation. A spectrum of instability. Clin Orthop Relat Res. 1992;(280):186–97.
53. Pugh DMW, McKee MD. The "terrible triad" of the elbow. Tech Hand Up Extrem Surg. 2002;6(1):21–9.
54. Giannicola G, Calella P, Piccioli A, Scacchi M, Gumina S. Terrible triad of the elbow: is it still a troublesome injury? Injury. 2015;46 Suppl 8:S68–76.
55. Moritomo H, Tada K, Yoshida T, Kawatsu N. Reconstruction of the coronoid for chronic dislocation of the elbow. Use of a graft from the olecranon in two cases. J Bone Joint Surg Br. 1998;80(3):490–2.
56. Papandrea RF, Morrey BF, O'driscoll SW. Reconstruction for persistent instability of the elbow after coronoid fracture-dislocation. J Shoulder Elbow Surg. 2007;16(1):68–77.
57. Knight DJ, Rymaszewski LA, Amis AA, Miller JH. Primary replacement of the fractured radial head with a metal prosthesis. J Bone Joint Surg Br. 1993;75(4):572–6.
58. Duckworth AD, Wickramasinghe NR, Clement ND, Court-Brown CM, McQueen MM. Radial head replacement for acute complex fractures: what are the rate and risks factors for revision or removal? Clin Orthop Relat Res. 2014;472(7):2136–43.
59. Ring D, Adey L, Zurakowski D, Jupiter JB. Elbow capsulectomy for posttraumatic elbow stiffness. J Hand Surg Am. 2006;31(8):1264–71.

# Varus Posteromedial Rotatory Instability

# 6

Kevin Chan and George S. Athwal

## Introduction

Traumatic complex elbow instability can be a difficult problem to manage for orthopedic surgeons. Inadequate treatment can lead to long-term disability, instability, pain, and posttraumatic arthritis. Recognition of patterns of injury can help to predict associated injuries, guide treatment, and restore a functional elbow. This chapter will discuss the management of anteromedial coronoid fractures and associated varus posteromedial rotatory elbow instability (PMRI).

The exact incidence of anteromedial coronoid fractures is unknown, although they are decidedly less common than other patterns of complex elbow instability such as the terrible triad injury. Their recognition began with the realization that not all coronoid fractures occurred in the coronal plane with a varying amount of height involvement [1]. The increasing understanding of elbow instability has led to improved treatment concepts for anteromedial coronoid fractures.

K. Chan, MD, MSc, FRCSC
G.S. Athwal, MD, FRCSC (✉)
Division of Orthopedic, Department of Surgery, Roth McFarlane Hand & Upper Limb Centre, Western University, 268 Grosvenor St, London, ON, Canada, N6A 4L6
e-mail: chank85@gmail.com; gsathwal@hotmail.com

## Anatomy of Elbow Stability

The primary stabilizers of the elbow are classically thought to be the ulnotrochlear articulation, medial collateral ligament (MCL), and lateral collateral ligament (LCL). Of these, the coronoid, anterior band of the MCL, and the lateral ulnar collateral ligament (LUCL) are believed to be the most important [2, 3]. The radial head acts as a secondary stabilizer [4]. The anterior and posterior capsule and muscles that cross the joint also enhance overall elbow stability.

The coronoid forms the anterior part of the trochlear notch in the proximal ulna. It provides an important anterior buttress to resist posterior ulnohumeral displacement [2, 5]. Together with the radial head, the coronoid also provides posterolateral rotatory stability [6]. Recognition of the anteromedial facet of the coronoid has been relatively recent and it has been [7] described as the region located between the coronoid tip and sublime tubercle. A quantitative three-dimensional CT study found that on average, 58 % of the anteromedial facet is unsupported by the proximal ulnar meta-diaphysis [8]. This suggests that it is a separate osseous process that can be prone to fracture, which is thought to occur from a varus posteromedial rotatory mechanism [7]. The anteromedial coronoid is fractured by a shearing mechanism from contact with the medial trochlea [7]. Associated injuries include a LCL disruption

© Springer International Publishing Switzerland 2017

R.Z. Tashjian (ed.), *The Unstable Elbow*, DOI 10.1007/978-3-319-46019-2_6

and possibly, a radial head fracture [7]. The posterior band of the MCL can also be disrupted by the injury mechanism as well [7].

## Initial Evaluation

A standard, thorough history and physical examination should be conducted for all complex elbow injuries. Clarification of the mechanism of injury may help to predict the pathology and guide treatment. An understanding of the patient's medical, functional, and occupational status may affect treatment decisions. Routine examination of neurovascular structures and the joints above and below the elbow should be done to rule out associated injuries. Particular attention to ulnar nerve function is important, since it can be susceptible to compressive neuropathy due to its proximity to the posterior band of the MCL, which is thought to be disrupted from the fracture mechanism [7]. Although an associated elbow dislocation is uncommon with an anteromedial coronoid fracture, if present, a closed reduction under sedation should be promptly performed.

A specific physical examination of patients with anteromedial coronoid fractures is currently not well defined. It is worth remembering that one of the goals when examining these patients is to identify those with significant elbow instability, specifically the PMRI pattern, who would benefit from surgical stabilization. While gross instability seen statically on plain radiographs is relatively easy to identify, the ability to document more subtle elbow instability is a much more difficult task. In the acute setting, physical examination of the elbow is limited by pain. When this occurs, some authors believe that an examination under anesthesia is more reliable [9]. Rhyou et al. [10] retrospectively reviewed their results using the size of the anteromedial coronoid fracture and varus stress testing under fluoroscopy to guide treatment. If fragments were ≤5 mm and there was no instability detected with varus stress testing, then conservative management was recommended. Rhyou et al. [10] reported good results after a mean follow-up of 37 months with an average Disabilities of the Arm, Shoulder, and Hand (DASH) score of 6. However, limitations of stress testing include variability in the amount of force applied by the treating orthopedic surgeon. In the authors' opinion, given adequate muscle relaxation and pain relief, most patients would likely demonstrate varus posteromedial elbow instability; but, similar to the management of an acute simple dislocation of the elbow, nonoperative treatment can be successful even though there is demonstrable instability detected under anesthesia [11].

Another difficulty encountered when treating patients with anteromedial coronoid fractures is the lack of a universally accepted physical examination maneuver to detect PMRI. In the more common instability pattern, that is the valgus posterolateral rotatory instability, several examination techniques are described and well accepted, including the pivot shift test [12], chair sign [13], and pushup sign [13]. However, there is a paucity of validated physical exam tests for PMRI in the orthopedic literature. In the senior author's experience, the most useful test is the gravity varus stress test (Fig. 6.1). This coincides with the opinion of Ramirez et al. [9]. The patient is asked to place the shoulder in 90° abduction with the forearm in neutral rotation. The test is considered positive if the patient experiences instability or crepitation, while the elbow is actively moved from flexion to extension. Additionally, the treating physician may palpate for ulnohumeral subluxation with hyperpronation of the forearm, termed the hyperpronation test. The hyperpronation test is usually conducted with the patient comfortably seated. The examiner passively places the elbow at 90° of flexion and then passively hyperpronates the patient's forearm. This hyperpronation imparts a medial rotatory force to the ulnohumeral joint. In cases of medial sided insufficiency, the examiner may visualize or palpate posteromedial rotatory ulnohumeral subluxation. Currently, the authors use the gravity varus stress test and the hyperpronation test as part of their criteria for treating certain anteromedial coronoid fractures nonoperatively [14]. In the published nonoperative series after a mean follow-up of 50 months, there were no complications identified, including recurrent instability or

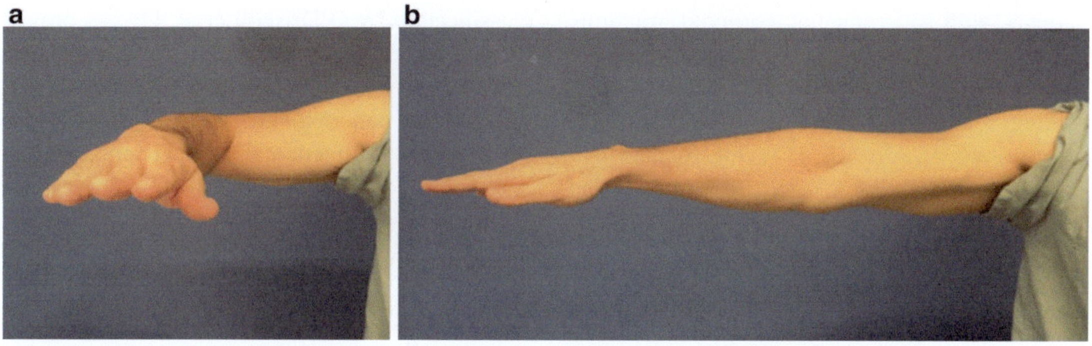

**Fig. 6.1** Gravity varus stress test for posteromedial rotatory instability. The patient is asked to place the shoulder in 90° abduction with the forearm in neutral rotation. The test is positive when the patient experiences instability or crepitations while the elbow is actively moved from flexion (**a**) to extension (**b**)

delayed surgical intervention. Further studies are required to validate a physical examination test to detect PMRI in cases of anteromedial coronoid fractures.

## Imaging Studies

Standard anteroposterior (AP) and lateral radiographic views of the affected elbow are the mainstay initial diagnostic tools for patients with suspected anteromedial coronoid fractures. It is important to maintain a high index of suspicion, since abnormal findings on plain radiographs can be subtle. On the AP view, there can be decreased medial ulnohumeral joint space with resultant asymmetry of the ulnohumeral joint [1]. Occasionally, the elbow may be aligned in varus if the fracture is substantially displaced, and the radiocapitellar joint space may be widened due to disruption of the LCL [1]. Sanchez-Sotelo et al. [1] also described the double crescent sign, which is thought to be pathognomonic for anteromedial coronoid fractures (Fig. 6.2). On the lateral view, the displaced anteromedial coronoid fragment leads to a double subchondral density with subsequent loss of parallelism between the medial aspect of the coronoid and the opposing distal humeral articular surface [1]. Oblique views of the elbow may assist with recognition of these fractures as well [9].

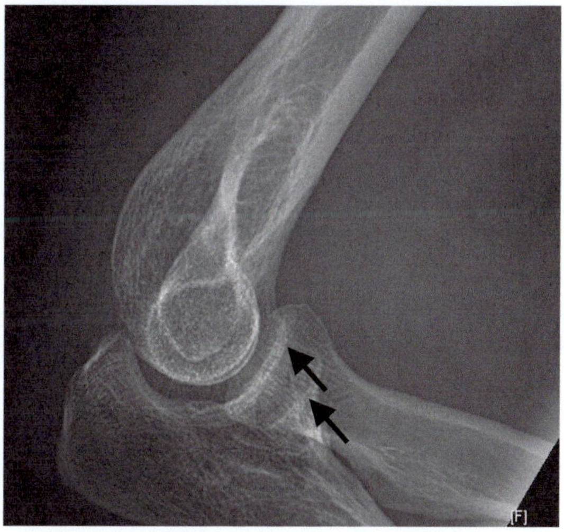

**Fig. 6.2** The "double crescent" sign (*arrows*) representing a displaced anteromedial coronoid fracture

All patients with suspected coronoid fractures should undergo computed tomography (CT) scans of the affected elbow, preferably with three-dimensional reconstructions, if available. This will confirm the diagnosis and aid in recognition of the type of coronoid fracture. CT scans are also needed to measure the size and displacement of the fracture fragments. The information obtained from CT scans is invaluable and helps to guide treatment recommendations.

Magnetic resonance imaging (MRI) of the affected elbow is generally not required when managing patients with anteromedial coronoid fractures. Rhyou et al. [10] investigated their patients with MRI scans and confirmed that the LCL is invariably injured to some degree in patients with anteromedial coronoid fractures. However, the information obtained from the MRI studies did not affect treatment decision, confirming that this imaging modality is usually unnecessary.

## Classification

Regan and Morrey [15] provided the initial classification of coronoid fractures, which were based on the size of the fracture fragment as seen on lateral radiographic views. In this classification, type 1 represented tip avulsion fractures, type 2 involved up to 50 % of the coronoid, and type 3 involved greater than 50 % of the coronoid. The recognition that some coronoid fractures were not oriented in the transverse plane necessitated a more comprehensive classification. O'Driscoll et al. [7] proposed their classification of coronoid fractures, which accounted for the anatomic location and the amount of coronoid injured (Fig. 6.3). In this classification, O'Driscoll et al. [7] observed three types of coronoid fractures: tip, anteromedial, and basal. The anteromedial coronoid fractures are further grouped as subtype 1 (anteromedial rim), subtype 2 (rim + tip), and subtype 3 (rim + sublime tubercle). The current classification by O'Driscoll et al. [7] has proven to be more clinically relevant, since it takes into consideration the mechanism of injury and specific fracture patterns. Thus, it ultimately provides guidance for treatment and surgical approach.

## Treatment Principles

In general, the goals of treatment of traumatic complex elbow instability are to restore a stable trochlear notch and maintain proper joint alignment while the collateral ligaments heal [16]. Nonoperative treatment can be considered if these goals can be satisfied with brief immobilization of the elbow. Otherwise, surgery is required to prevent elbow instability and posttraumatic arthrosis.

## Nonoperative Treatment

Our understanding of anteromedial coronoid fractures has evolved over time. Initial concerns with persistent elbow instability, joint incongruity, and rapid development of arthritis led many authors to suggest surgical intervention for most of these fractures [1, 7]. In fact, Doornberg and

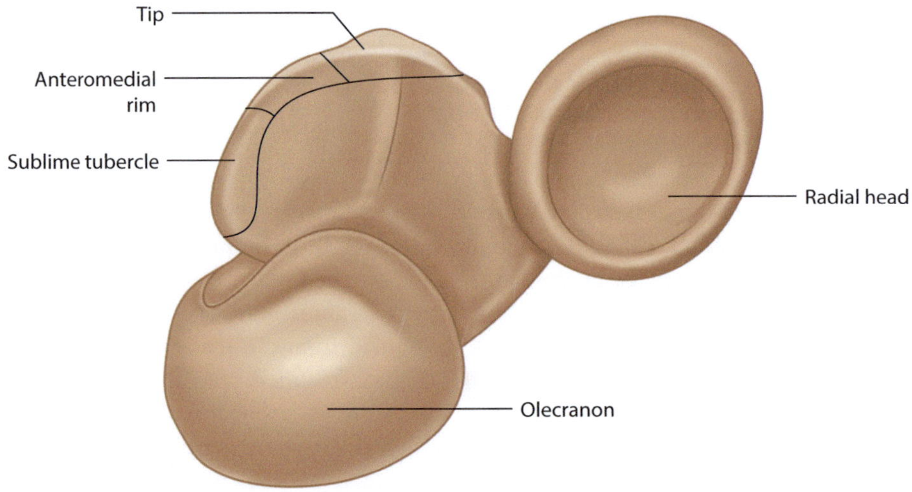


**Fig. 6.3** O'Driscoll classification of coronoid fractures, consisting of type 1 (tip), type 2 (anteromedial), and type 3 (basal). In this figure, the anteromedial subtype fractures are demonstrated, including subtype 1 (rim), subtype 2 (rim + tip), and subtype 3 (rim + sublime tubercle)

Ring [17] identified six patients with varus malalignment of the elbow and attributed it to lack of fixation in four and loss of fixation in two patients. However, more recent opinions indicate that certain anteromedial coronoid fractures can be managed nonoperatively if they are small, minimally displaced, and not associated with static elbow subluxation [16]. Moon et al. [18] followed three patients with minimally displaced anteromedial coronoid fractures (two subtype 2, one subtype 3) treated nonoperatively and found excellent results without complications. Similarly, van der Werf et al. [19] retrospectively reviewed the results of six patients who elected to have nonoperative treatment for their anteromedial coronoid fractures (all subtype 2) after elbow subluxation had been ruled out. Only three patients had medium-term follow-up (two at 3 years and one at 7 years). Of these, all patients had regained full elbow motion and there were no radiographic signs of arthrosis. Rhyou et al. [10] also managed one patient with an anteromedial coronoid subtype 2 fracture nonoperatively after CT imaging demonstrated that the fragment was <5 mm and a varus stress test showed no instability. After 4 years' follow-up, the patient had regained full range of motion.

Although current studies demonstrate that select anteromedial coronoid fractures can be treated nonoperatively, the exact indications remain controversial. Moon et al. [18] and van der Werf et al. [19] did not report on the sizes of the fracture fragments or the amount of displacement accepted. In a biomechanical study, Pollock et al. [20] demonstrated that the size of the fractured anteromedial coronoid and the status of the LCL had effects on elbow stability, particularly in varus stress. They concluded that small subtype 1 fractures (approximately less than 5 mm) might be treated conservatively if rehabilitation allows the LCL to heal. This was tested on cadavers with an intact MCL. As Pollock et al. [20] noted, examination of both collateral ligaments remains important before applying their criteria.

In a clinical study, the current authors have also attempted to clarify the indications for nonoperative management [14]. Patients were treated conservatively if they met the following criteria, including a congruent elbow joint seen radiographically, and a stable arc of active elbow motion to a minimum of 30° of extension to allow early motion within the first 10–14 days. Between 2006 and 2012, ten suitable patients were included in the study. After a mean follow-up of 50 months, the authors reported an average motion of $137 \pm 8°$ of flexion, $2 \pm 5°$ of extension, $88 \pm 5°$ of pronation, and $86 \pm 10°$ of supination. All fractures had united and there were no cases requiring delayed surgical intervention for recurrent instability. This study included nine anteromedial coronoid subtype 2 fractures and one subtype 3 fracture. The mean fragment size was $5 \pm 1$ mm (range: 2–7 mm) with a mean displacement of $3 \pm 2$ mm for the subtype 2 injuries. The subtype 3 fracture was 9 mm in size with 1 mm of maximal articular gap. Thus, the authors concluded that small, minimally displaced subtype 2 fractures, particularly when $\leq 5$ mm in size, could be treated conservatively. While some subtype 3 fractures may be amendable to nonoperative management, these injuries require caution, since they lack both the medial and lateral restraints against instability. If patients elect nonoperative management, it is imperative that the treating physician ensures that the fracture is truly undisplaced or minimally displaced on CT scans. Additionally, it is important that the patients are compliant with rehabilitation and serial clinical and radiographic follow-ups are done to monitor for complications such as instability.

Appropriate anteromedial coronoid fractures treated nonoperatively are referred to physiotherapy early within 10–14 days after injury. Supine positioning with overhead active and active-assisted flexion/extension exercises with the forearm in neutral are initiated. Forearm rotation exercises are allowed at 90° flexion. A resting elbow splint at 90° flexion is used between exercises for approximately 6 weeks. Shoulder abduction is avoided to minimize varus stress on the elbows. Strengthening is added when sufficient healing has progressed, typically around 6–8 weeks after injury.

## Operative Treatment

The surgical strategy to treating anteromedial coronoid fractures remains controversial. Park et al. [21] approached these fractures differently depending on the subtype according to O'Driscoll's classification [7]. They repaired the LCL only if the fracture was small (subtype 1), whereas larger fractures (subtype 2 and 3) underwent open reduction internal fixation (ORIF) using a buttress plate and LCL repair. The MCL was repaired last if there was residual elbow instability. Similarly, Rhyou et al. [10] fixed the LCL only if the fracture was small (≤5 mm) and the elbow demonstrated instability with varus stress testing. Still, other authors advocate suture fixation through capsular attachments if the fracture is too small for plates and/or screws [9, 16].

Although high-level evidence is lacking, this surgical strategy satisfies the principles of restoring stability to the elbow to promote early range of motion. It is analogous to the surgical treatment of "terrible triad" fracture-dislocations of the elbow [22, 23]. Patients are typically positioned supine with the arm resting on an arm table. Depending on surgeon preference, initial exposure is obtained through either a posterior skin incision or through separate medial and lateral incisions. The anteromedial coronoid fracture is exposed using a medial deep approach (see Fig. 6.4). In a cadaveric study, Huh et al. [24] demonstrated improved exposure using an FCU-splitting approach compared to a flexor-pronator split. However, Ring and Doornberg [25] recommend the use of a flexor-pronator split for smaller anteromedial coronoid fractures that remain anterior to the sublime tubercle. Larger fractures that extend into the base of the coronoid can also be approached by elevating the entire flexor-pronator mass from a dorsal to volar direction [25, 26]. The integrity of the MCL is then assessed, but not repaired until after the anteromedial coronoid and LCL are addressed. The fracture is evaluated, reduced, and fixed using preferably a buttress plate and/or screws (see Fig. 6.5). To reduce the fracture, the authors typically use K-wires directed anterior to posterior to provide temporary fixation. Then, it is the authors' preference to apply an anterior plate 2 or 2.5 mm T or Y plate that is contoured intraoperatively. Conversely, commercially available precontoured plates for the coronoid are available. When applying the plate, care must be taken to direct the screws dorsally or dorsoradially. If directing the screws dorsoradially, the lesser sigmoid notch must be avoided. Intraoperatively, fluoroscopic views of the ulnohumeral, radiocapitellar, and lesser sigmoid notch must be obtained to ensure all hardware is extra-articular. Once secure fixation is obtained of the fracture, the medial collateral ligament is repaired, followed by the lateral collateral ligament using suture anchors or transosseous tunnels (see Fig. 6.6).

Alternatively, in cases with a larger anteromedial facet fracture without comminution where solid bony stability can be obtained with ORIF, repair of the LCL is not absolutely necessary. In these cases, after obtaining bony stability and intraoperative fluoroscopy confirms a reduced joint, the elbow can be rehabilitated as a simple elbow dislocation with a protocol that protects the lateral sided ligamentous injury.

In larger highly comminuted anteromedial facet fractures, where rigid bony stability cannot be obtained with ORIF and lateral ligament repair only is insufficient to maintain a congruent elbow reduction, a static or dynamic external fixator is indicated. It is the authors' preference to apply a static large fragment external fixator with two pins directed posterior to anterior in the humerus (trans-triceps) and two pins directed posterior to anterior in the ulna. Typically, the fixator is removed at 4–6 weeks (see Fig. 6.7).

Postoperatively, patients may be immobilized in a splint for 1–2 weeks. Elbow range of motion is initiated after the first postoperative visit. Shoulder abduction is avoided to minimize varus stress on the elbow. Strengthening exercises may be started once satisfactory healing has occurred, typically around 6 weeks.

Park et al. [21] reviewed 19 patients treated operatively with their surgical protocol. After a mean follow-up of 31 months, the mean arc of flexion and extension was 128°. Functional scores were categorized as excellent in four patients, good in six patients, and fair in one patient according to the Mayo Elbow Performance Score. There were no reported complications

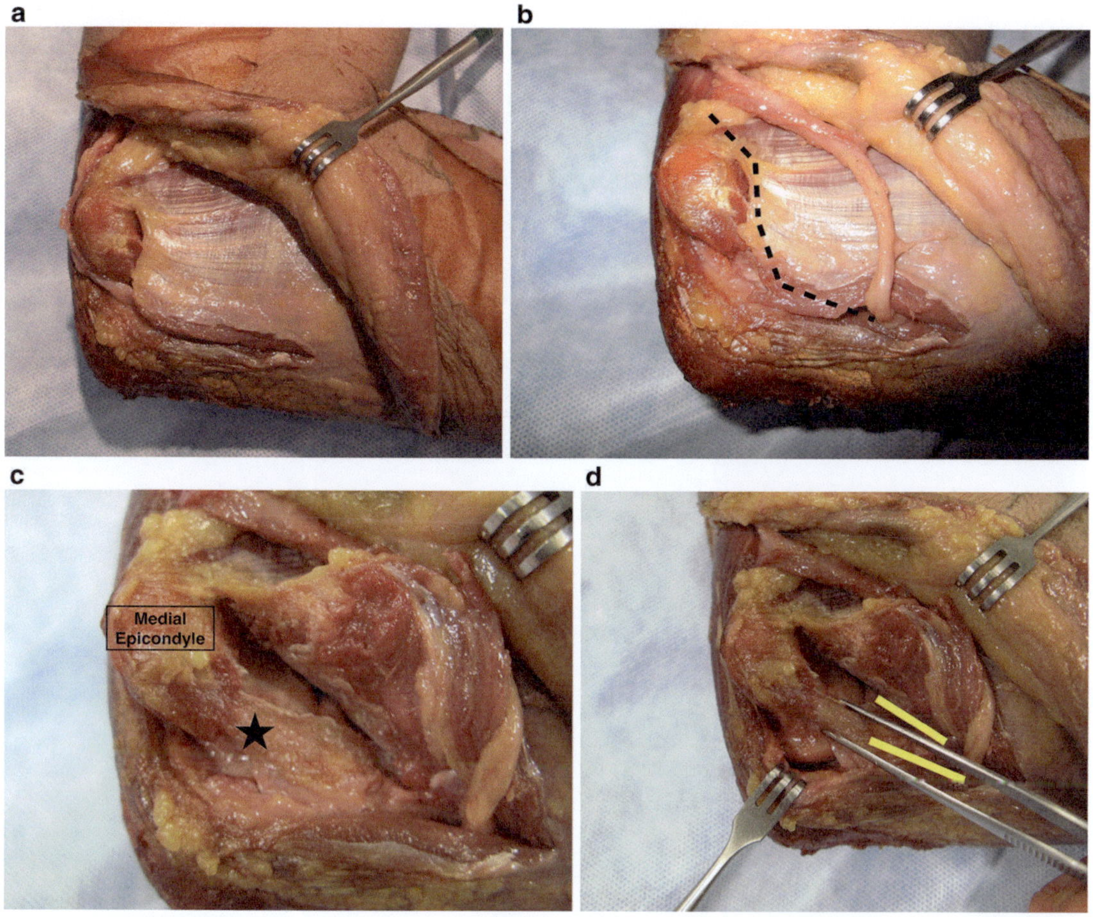


**Fig. 6.4** Exposure of an anteromedial coronoid fracture. A left cadaveric elbow specimen is shown with the hand directed distally toward the right. A posterior skin incision with elevation of a medial flap has been completed (**a**). The ulnar nerve is identified and exposed up to the two heads of flexor carpi ulnaris. The ulnar nerve is elevated and transposed anteriorly (**b**). The flexor pronator mass is then released along the *dashed line* and a flap elevated distally (**b**). The anterior bundle of the medial collateral ligament (*black star*) is protected (**c**). Once the coronoid is exposed, plates may be applied over the sublime tubercle and/or on the anterior aspect of the coronoid (*yellow lines* represent plate locations) (**d**). Release of the ulnar head of the flexor carpi ulnaris from the proximal ulna and distally along the ulna shaft as well as the flexor pronator mass as shown will allow maximal exposure of the proximal ulna for plate application (Taylor-Scham approach)

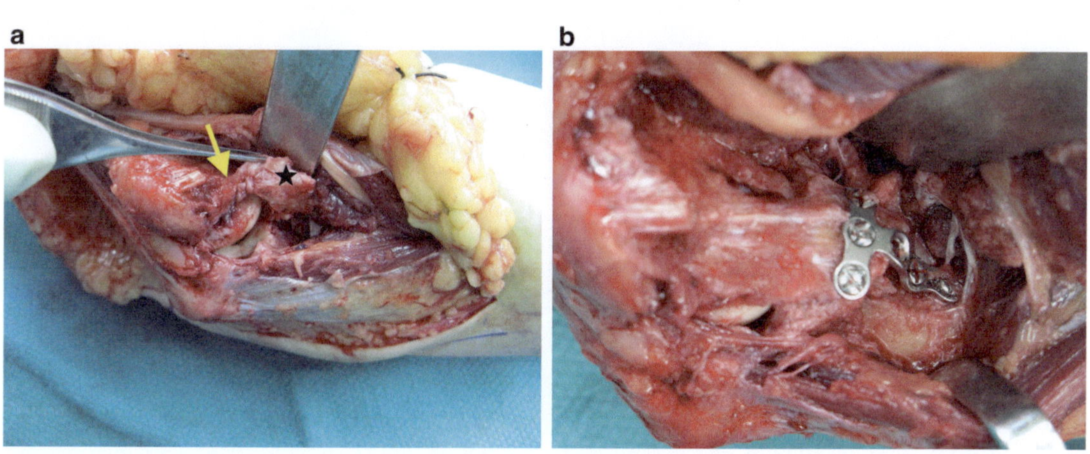


**Fig. 6.5** An anteromedial facet fracture (**a**) involving the sublime tubercle (*black star*). The anterior bundle of the medial collateral ligament maintains its attachment on the sublime tubercle (*yellow arrow*). Open reduction and internal fixation of the facture is accomplished with a 2.0 mm plate placed over the sublime tubercle (**b**)

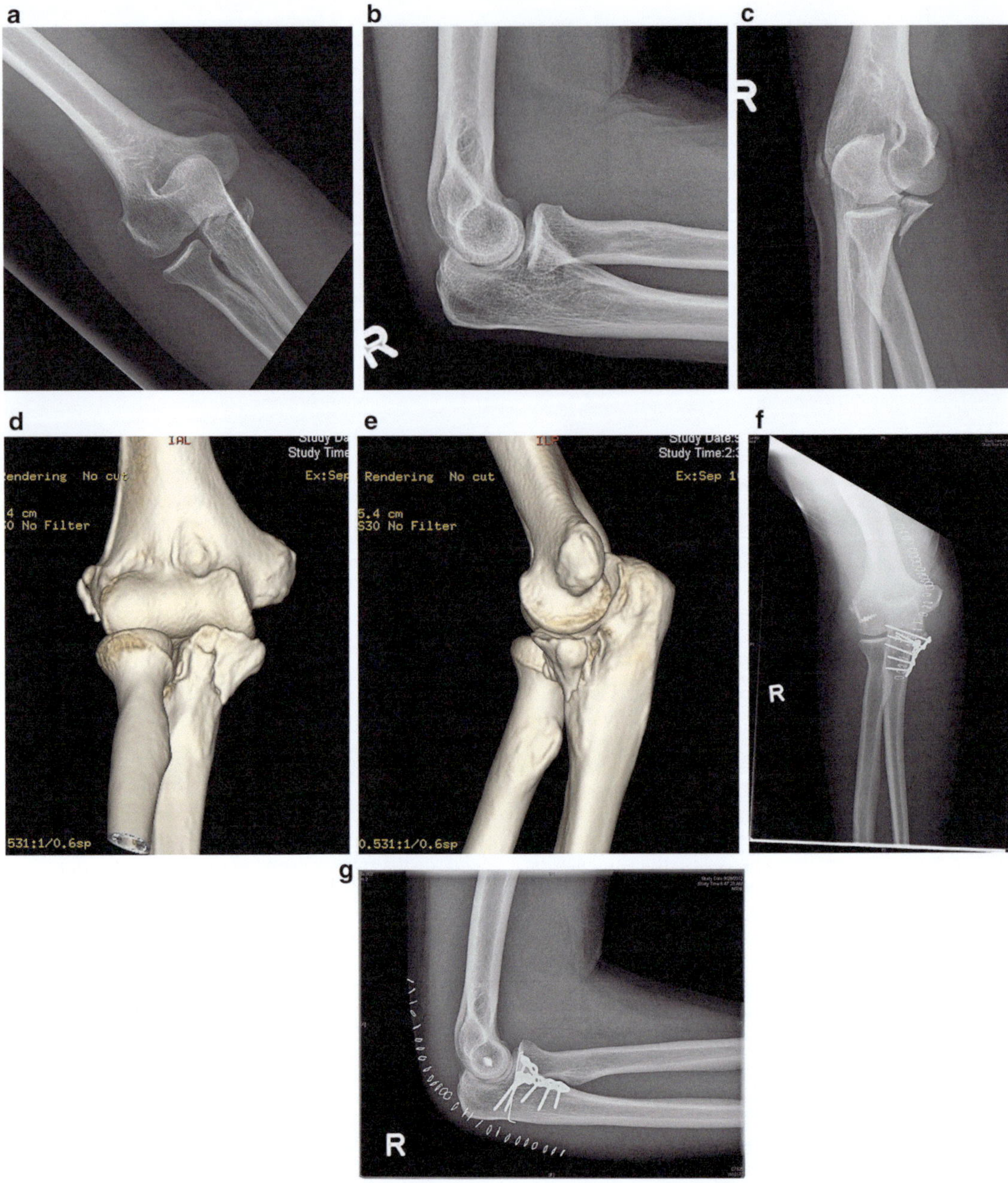


**Fig. 6.6** AP, lateral, and oblique radiographs of an anteromedial facet subtype 3 fracture demonstrating static rotational instability in extension (**a–c**). A 3D CT scan demonstrates involvement of the sublime tubercle with mild comminution of the coronoid tip (**d**, **e**). Postoperative radiographs (**f**, **g**) demonstrate double plate fixation of the coronoid with suture anchor repair of the lateral collateral ligament

requiring additional treatment. Two patients developed heterotopic ossification, one patient had mild joint incongruity, and one patient had persistent mild symptoms of ulnar neuropathy. Rhyou et al. [10] also reported the results of their surgical algorithm in 17 patients. After a mean follow-up of 37 months, they demonstrated an average MEPS of 98, corresponding to an excellent

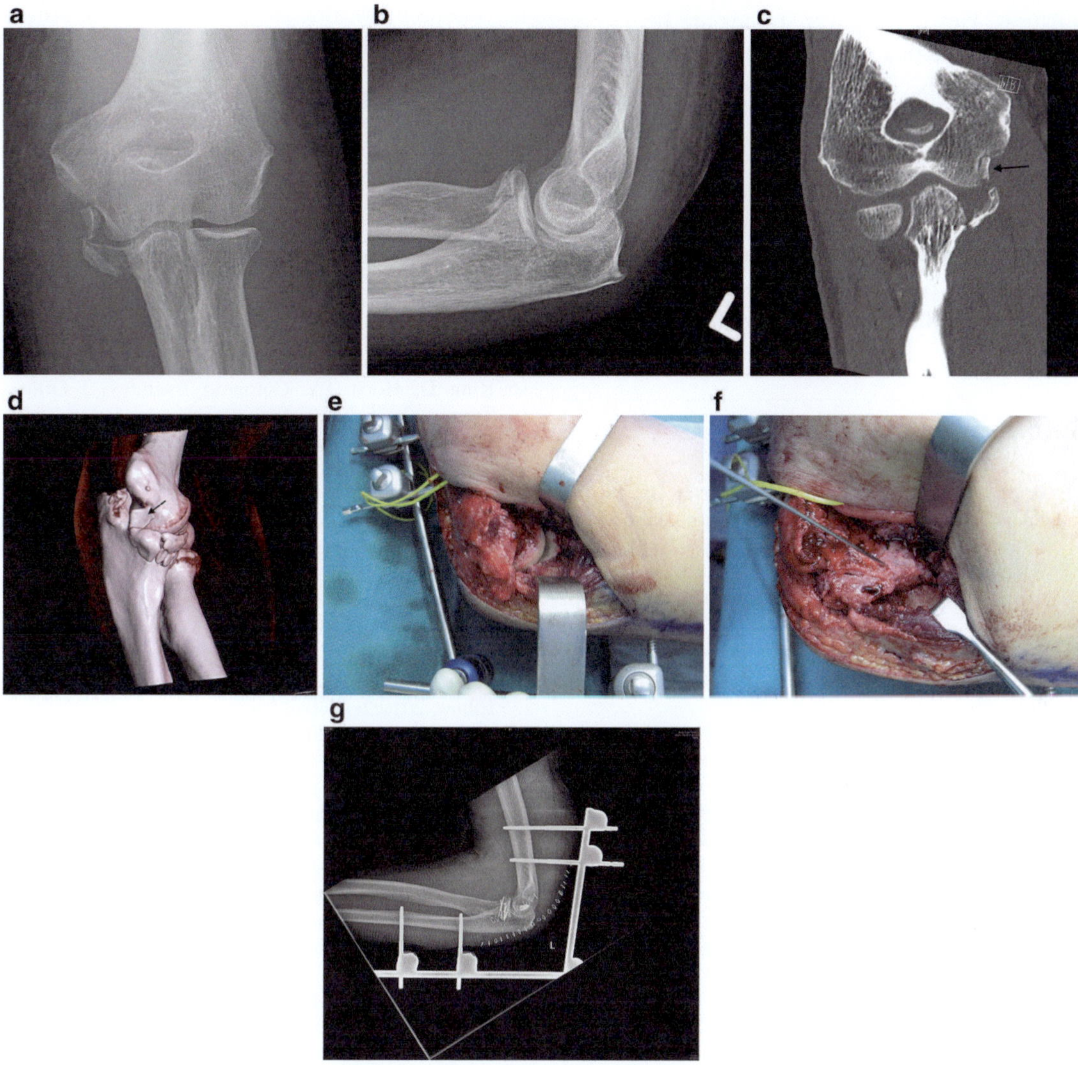

**Fig. 6.7** Anteroposterior and lateral radiographs demonstrate a severely comminuted anteromedial coronoid fracture (**a**, **b**). Coronal CT (**c**) and 3D reconstructions (**d**) demonstrate the degree of comminution and the extruded osteochondral fragment (*black arrow*). Due to the degree of comminution, the patient underwent open reduction and internal fixation with screws and thread wires with application of a static external fixator to neutralize joint forces and to protect the fixation (**e**, **f**). Postoperative radiographs demonstrate satisfactory reduction of the fracture fragments (**g**)

outcome. Doornberg and Ring [17] reviewed 17 patients and reported a mean arc of flexion and extension of 116° and a mean arc of forearm rotation of 153°. Complications involving the 12 patients whose initial surgery was performed at their institution included one deep infection and one recurrent elbow dislocation with wound separation.

## Conclusion

Anteromedial coronoid fractures are thought to occur from a varus posteromedial rotatory mechanism of injury. Initial reports of elbow instability and the development of arthrosis led many authors to recommend internal fixation of these fractures. However, newer studies are beginning to demonstrate that select anteromedial coronoid fractures can be successfully treated nonoperatively. Most fractures, however, that demonstrate static instability or are displaced, are preferentially managed with open reduction and internal fixation with or without ligament repair. Further studies are still needed to clarify methods to detect varus posteromedial instability and the optimal rehabilitation after these fractures.

## References


1. Sanchez-Sotelo J, O'Driscoll SW, Morrey BF. Medial oblique compression fracture of the coronoid process of the ulna. J Shoulder Elbow Surg. 2005;14(1):60–4.
2. Morrey BF, An KN. Stability of the elbow: osseous constraints. J Shoulder Elbow Surg. 2005;14(1 Suppl S):174s–8.
3. Safran MR, Baillargeon D. Soft-tissue stabilizers of the elbow. J Shoulder Elbow Surg. 2005;14(1 Suppl S): 179s–85.
4. Morrey BF, Tanaka S, An KN. Valgus stability of the elbow. A definition of primary and secondary constraints. Clin Orthop Relat Res. 1991; (265):187–95.
5. Closkey RF, Goode JR, Kirschenbaum D, Cody RP. The role of the coronoid process in elbow stability. A biomechanical analysis of axial loading. J Bone Joint Surg Am. 2000;82A(12):1749–53.
6. Schneeberger AG, Sadowski MM, Jacob HA. Coronoid process and radial head as posterolateral rotatory stabilizers of the elbow. J Bone Joint Surg Am. 2004;86A(5):975–82.
7. O'Driscoll SW, Jupiter JB, Cohen MS, Ring D, McKee MD. Difficult elbow fractures: pearls and pitfalls. Instr Course Lect. 2003;52:113–34.
8. Doornberg JN, de Jong IM, Lindenhovius AL, Ring D. The anteromedial facet of the coronoid process of the ulna. J Shoulder Elbow Surg. 2007;16(5):667–70.
9. Ramirez MA, Stein JA, Murthi AM. Varus Posteromedial Instability. Hand Clin. 2015;31(4): 557–63.
10. Rhyou IH, Kim KC, Lee JH, Kim SY. Strategic approach to O'Driscoll type 2 anteromedial coronoid facet fracture. J Shoulder Elbow Surg. 2014;23(7): 924–32.
11. Anakwe RE, Middleton SD, Jenkins PJ, McQueen MM, Court-Brown CM. Patient-reported outcomes after simple dislocation of the elbow. J Bone Joint Surg Am. 2011;93(13):1220–6.
12. O'Driscoll SW, Bell DF, Morrey BF. Posterolateral rotatory instability of the elbow. J Bone Joint Surg Am. 1991;73(3):440–6.
13. Regan W, Lapner PC. Prospective evaluation of two diagnostic apprehension signs for posterolateral instability of the elbow. J Shoulder Elbow Surg. 2006;15(3):344–6.
14. Chan K, Faber KJ, King GJ, Athwal GS. Selected Anteromedial Coronoid Fractures can be Treated Non-Operatively. J Shoulder Elbow Surg. 2016; doi: 10.1016/j.jse.2016.02.025.
15. Regan W, Morrey B. Fractures of the coronoid process of the ulna. J Bone Joint Surg Am. 1989;71(9): 1348–54.
16. Ring D, Horst TA. Coronoid fractures. J Orthop Trauma. 2015;29(10):437–40.
17. Doornberg JN, Ring DC. Fracture of the anteromedial facet of the coronoid process. J Bone Joint Surg Am. 2006;88(10):2216–24.
18. Moon JG, Bither N, Jeon YJ, Oh SM. Non surgically managed anteromedial coronoid fractures in posteromedial rotatory instability: three cases with 2 years follow-up. Arch Orthop Trauma Surg. 2013;133(12):1665–8.
19. Van Der Werf HJ, Guitton TG, Ring D. Non-operatively treated fractures of the anteromedial facet of the coronoid process: a report of six cases. Shoulder Elbow. 2010;2(1):40–2.
20. Pollock JW, Brownhill J, Ferreira L, McDonald CP, Johnson J, King G. The effect of anteromedial facet fractures of the coronoid and lateral collateral ligament injury on elbow stability and kinematics. J Bone Joint Surg Am. 2009;91(6):1448–58.
21. Park SM, Lee JS, Jung JY, Kim JY, Song KS. How should anteromedial coronoid facet fracture be managed? A surgical strategy based on O'Driscoll classification and ligament injury. J Shoulder Elbow Surg. 2015;24(1):74–82.
22. Pugh DM, Wild LM, Schemitsch EH, King GJ, McKee MD. Standard surgical protocol to treat elbow dislocations with radial head and coronoid fractures. J Bone Joint Surg Am. 2004;86A(6):1122–30.
23. McKee MD, Pugh DM, Wild LM, Schemitsch EH, King GJ. Standard surgical protocol to treat elbow dislocations with radial head and coronoid fractures. Surgical technique. J Bone Joint Surg Am. 2005;87(Suppl 1, Pt 1):22–32.
24. Huh J, Krueger CA, Medvecky MJ, Hsu JR. Medial elbow exposure for coronoid fractures: FCU-split versus over-the-top. J Orthop Trauma. 2013;27(12):730–4.
25. Ring D, Doornberg JN. Fracture of the anteromedial facet of the coronoid process. Surgical technique. J Bone Joint Surg Am. 2007;89(Suppl 2, Pt 2):267–83.
26. Taylor TK, Scham SM. A posteromedial approach to the proximal end of the ulna for the internal fixation of olecranon fractures. J Trauma. 1969;9(7):594–602.

# Posterior Monteggia Fracture-Dislocations

## 7

Justin C. Wong, Joseph A. Abboud, and Charles L. Getz

## Background

### Historical Perspective

Classically, *Monteggia fractures* have been described as diaphyseal ulnar fractures associated with radial head dislocation. In 1814, Monteggia described two clinical cases of a proximal-third diaphyseal ulna fracture associated with anterior dislocation of the radial head and highlighted the residual radial head instability after closed management of the injuries. Further classification and description of Monteggia fractures was refined by Bado, in 1967, who recognized that radial head instability may occur anteriorly, posteriorly, or laterally and that the associated ulna fracture may occur at the diaphysis or more proximally and with or without an associated radial shaft fracture [1]. Whereas the anterior variant of Monteggia injuries is more common among the pediatric population, the posterior Monteggia is more common among adults [2–4]. Historically, outcomes of Monteggia fractures were inconsistent and often poor [5–9]. Although treatment of these injuries remains a challenge, advances in imaging techniques, a greater understanding of the anatomy and stabilizers of the elbow and enhanced methods of internal fixation have led to improved outcomes [10–14].

J.C. Wong, MD (✉)
Department of Orthopedic Surgery, Thomas Jefferson University Hospital, 1020 Walnut Street, Rm 516 College Building, Philadelphia, PA 19107, USA
e-mail: jcwong330@gmail.com

J.A. Abboud, MD
Department of Orthopedic Surgery, The Rothman Institute, Thomas Jefferson University, 925 Chestnut St, 5th Floor, Philadelphia, PA 19107, USA
e-mail: Joseph.Abboud@RothmanInstitute.com

C.L. Getz, MD
Department of Orthopedic Surgery, The Rothman Institute, Thomas Jefferson University Hospital, 925 Chestnut Street, Philadelphia, PA 19107, USA
e-mail: Charlie.getz@rothmaninstitute.com

### Elbow Anatomy and Stability

The elbow is a complex joint with three articulations (ulnohumeral, radiocapitellar, and proximal radioulnar) that permit stable range of motion of the forearm through flexion-extension and pronation-supination (Fig. 7.1). Stability of the elbow is dependent upon the highly congruous articular surfaces as well as medial and lateral ligamentous structures [15–17]. The trochlear notch formed between the coronoid and olecranon processes provides a nearly 180° arc of articulation with the distal humerus but has a transverse bare-spot devoid of articular cartilage at its lowest point. In profile, the coronoid projects higher than the olecranon, such that a line drawn from the tips of the coronoid and olecranon

© Springer International Publishing Switzerland 2017
R.Z. Tashjian (ed.), *The Unstable Elbow*, DOI 10.1007/978-3-319-46019-2_7

processes, should form a 30° angle with a line drawn along the axis of the ulna. The sublime tubercle on the medial aspect of the coronoid serves as the insertion site of the medial collateral ligament, which provides primary stability against valgus-forces throughout the range of elbow motion [15–18]. The radial head, which articulates with the capitellum and the proximal ulna, is a secondary stabilizer to valgus forces. The lateral ulnar collateral ligament complex is composed of the radial collateral ligament, lateral ulnar collateral ligament, and the annular ligament (Fig. 7.2). The annular ligament encircles the radial head with an origin and insertion on the proximal ulna and provides stability to the proximal radio-ulnar joint. The radial collateral ligament provides restraint against varus forces and originates on the lateral epicondyle and has a broad insertion along the annular ligament [15, 19]. The lateral ulnar collateral ligament takes origin off of the lateral epicondyle and traverses the posterior half of the radial head before inserting on the crista supinatoris of the proximal ulna providing restraint against posterolateral rotatory instability.

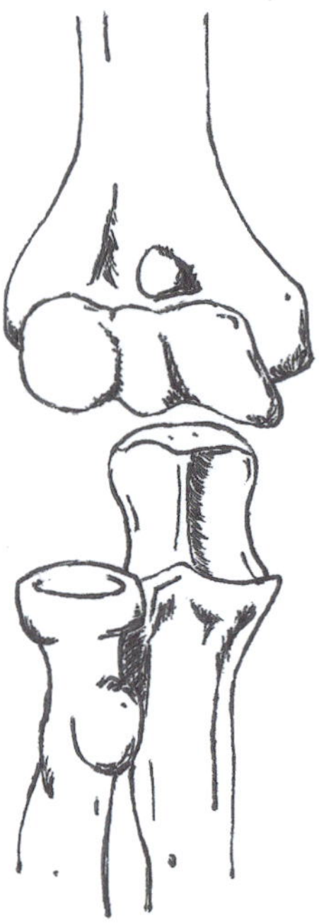

**Fig. 7.1** Bony anatomy of elbow joint. Anterior view of distal humerus and proximal radius and ulna demonstrate highly congruous joint surfaces (From Wong JC, Getz CL, Abboud JA. Adult Monteggia and Olecranon Fracture Dislocations of the Elbow. *Hand Clin*. 2015;31(4):565–80)

The relative contributions of the bony and ligamentous structures to elbow stability have been studied biomechanically [20–25]. Whereas elbow stability may be maintained with isolated fractures of the coronoid up to 50 % of the coronoid height, smaller coronoid fractures in conjunction with ligamentous or radial head injury can lead to joint instability [23–27]. These studies help to underscore the complementary nature of the bony and ligamentous stabilizers of the elbow. When treating complex elbow dislocations such as the

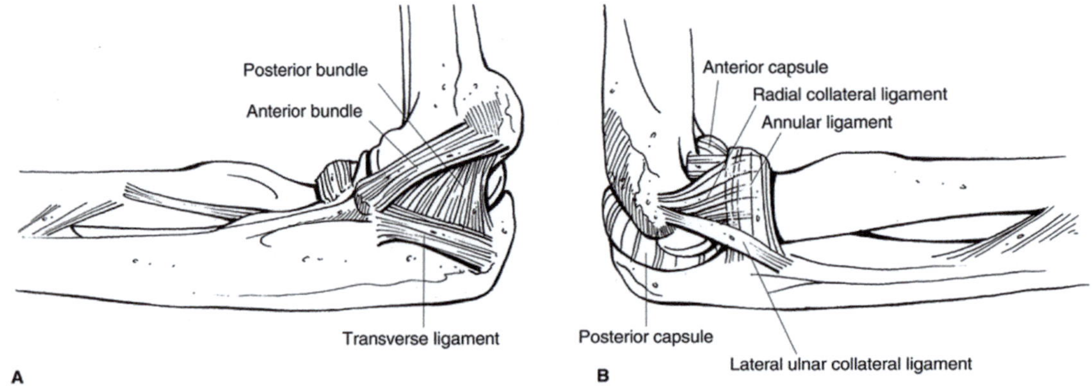


**Fig. 7.2** Elbow ligamentous anatomy. Structure of the medial collateral ligament complex (**a**) and the lateral collateral ligament complex (**b**) (From Tashjian RZ, Katarinic JA. Complex elbow instability. *J Am Acad Orthop Surg*. 2006;14(5):278–86)

posterior Monteggia fracture-dislocation, it is critical to identify and manage all of the bony or ligamentous stabilizers of the elbow so that joint stability may be restored and early range of motion may be performed to optimize outcomes.

## Classification of Injury Pattern

Bado described a four-category classification of Monteggia fractures based upon the direction of radial head displacement and whether or not an associated fracture of the radial diaphysis was present (Fig. 7.3).

- In Type I fractures, there is apex anterior angulation of the ulnar fracture and anterior dislocation of the radial head.
- Type II fractures demonstrate apex posterior ulnar fracture with posterior or posterolateral dislocation of the radial head.
- Type III fractures demonstrate metphyseal ulnar fractures with lateral radial head dislocation.
- Type IV fractures concomitant radial and ulnar diaphyseal fracture in conjunction with anterior radial head dislocation.

A more simplified approach has been proposed to classify adult Monteggia fractures as occurring either anteriolateral (Bado Type I, III, and IV) or posterior (Bado Type II) [28]. The anterolateral Monteggia injuries in adults occur predominantly through the ulnar diaphysis with anterolateral radial head dislocation, but importantly do not have any element of ulnohumeral

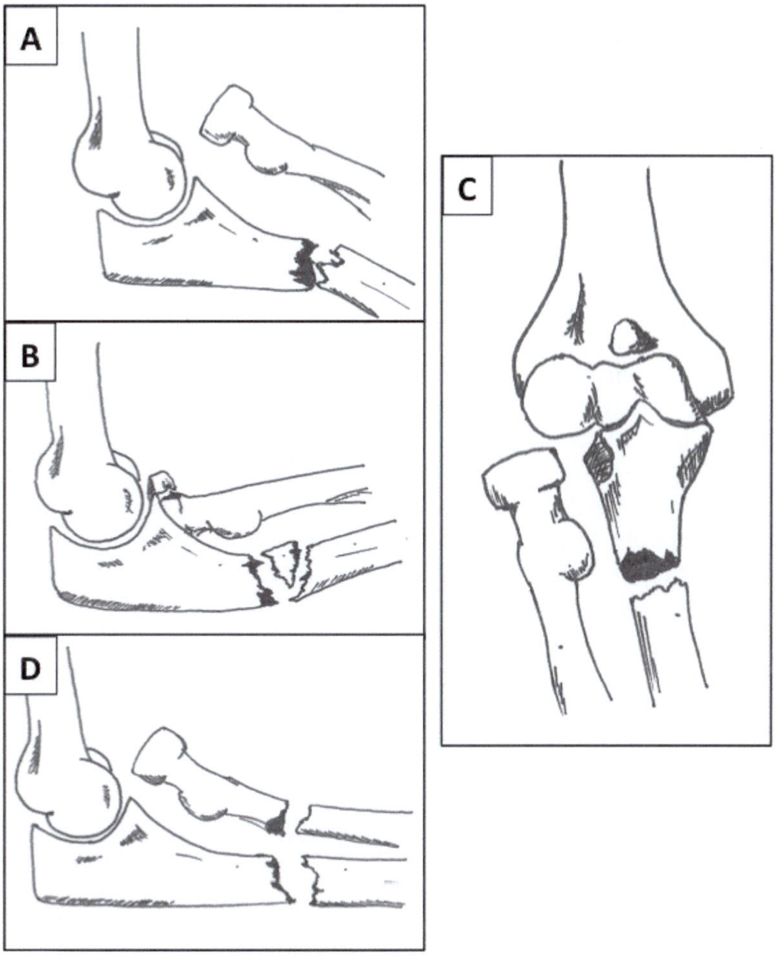


**Fig. 7.3** Bado classification of monteggia fractures. (**a**) Type I—Anterior Monteggia, (**b**) Type II—Posterior Monteggia, (**c**) Type III—Lateral Monteggia, (**d**) Type IV—Monteggia fracture with diaphyseal radial shaft fracture (From Wong JC, Getz CL, Abboud JA. Adult Monteggia and Olecranon Fracture Dislocations of the Elbow. *Hand Clin*. 2015;31(4):565–80)

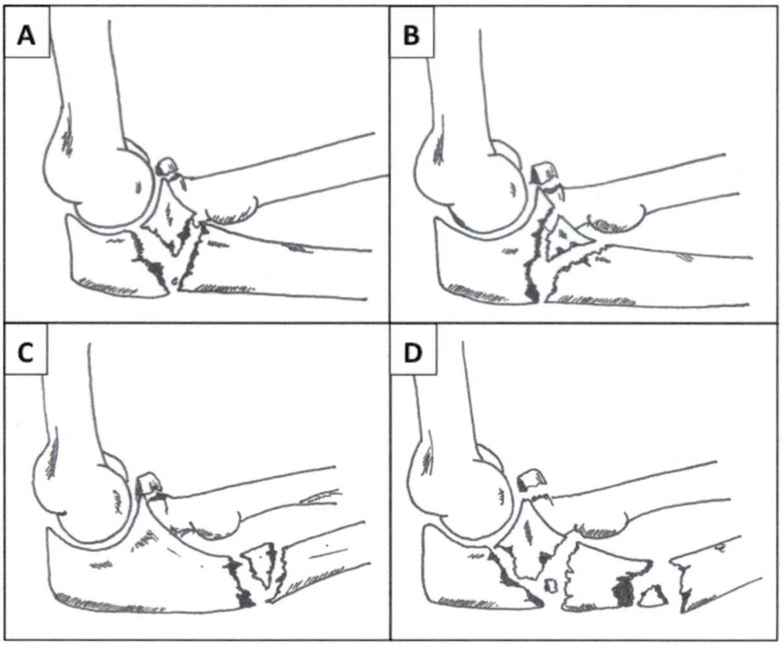


**Fig. 7.4** Jupiter sub-classification of posterior monteggia fractures. (**a**) IIA—the ulnar fracture involves the distal olecranon and coronoid process, (**b**) IIB—the ulnar fracture is at the metaphyseal-diaphyseal junction distal to the coronoid, (**c**) IIC—the ulnar fracture is diaphyseal, (**d**) IID—ulnar fracture extends along proximal third to half of the ulna (From Wong JC, Getz CL, Abboud JA. Adult Monteggia and Olecranon Fracture Dislocations of the Elbow. *Hand Clin.* 2015;31(4):565–80)

instability. Treatment of anterolateral Monteggia injuries is directed at restoration of ulnar length and alignment to indirectly achieve radial head reduction. It is rarely necessary that the proximal radiocapitellar joint be opened to achieve radial head reduction, but may be necessary in some cases as a result of annular ligament interposition [11, 28]. In contrast, the posterior Monteggia injury has been shown to have more concomitant injuries involving either the radial head, coronoid process, or lateral ulnar collateral ligament complex, which sometimes results in ulnohumeral instability [10, 12, 29]. Posterior Monteggia fractures (Bado Type II) are further subclassified based upon the location of the ulnar fracture in relation to the coronoid process, with the IIA and IIB subtypes being the most common [10, 12] (Fig. 7.4). In particular, when the fracture involves the coronoid process (IIA, IID), the fragment is often a large anterior quadrangular or triangular fragment that requires anatomic reduction to restore ulnohumeral joint stability.

- Type IIA—fracture of proximal ulna involving the coronoid process
- Type IIB—fracture occurring distal to the coronoid process at the junction of the ulnar metaphysis and diaphysis
- Type IIC—fracture along the ulnar diaphysis
- Type IID—severely comminuted fracture of ulna extending from olecranon to ulnar diaphysis

## Evaluation

The posterior Monteggia fracture occurs most commonly in elderly females with underlying osteoporotic bone as a result of low-energy ground level fall [10, 12]. Although these injuries may occur in isolation, patients have been observed to have concomitant skeletal, thoracoabdominal, or head trauma in up to 30% of cases [10, 12]. This is a reminder that initial evaluation of any trauma patient should begin according to the Advanced Trauma Life Support protocol. Once deemed stable, a more thorough evaluation of the extremity can begin. While posterior Monteggia lesions are most often closed injuries, attention should be paid to the soft-tissue envelope to look for potential open injury. Concomitant injury proximally, distally, or in the contralateral extremity is not uncommon and should be thoroughly assessed. Vascular injury is rare in Monteggia fracture dislocations, but injury to the posterior interosseous nerve or ulnar nerve has been reported although nerve exploration is not usually required and spontaneous resolution is often observed [12]. Although rare, compartment syndrome has been reported [11].

Standard anterior-posterior, lateral, and oblique radiographs of the elbow and forearm should be obtained to evaluate the osseous injuries. As previously mentioned, if the ulnar fracture involves the coronoid process the fracture fragment is often large and represents a significant loss to intrinsic ulnohumeral stability, which may result in ulnohumeral subluxation/dislocation. Associated radial head fractures are common and are thought to occur through a shearing mechanism as the radial head dislocates posterolaterally across the capitellum [9, 10, 29]. If standard radiographs are unable to provide a clear picture of the spectrum of injury, then cross-sectional imaging such as computed tomography should be obtained.

Initial management of these injuries should include well-padded splinting of the elbow in a comfortable position. Due to the inherent instability of these injuries, closed reduction is unlikely to be successful and excessive manipulation of the elbow/forearm should be avoided. Ideally, definitive surgical management of these injuries should occur as soon as the patient is medically stable for surgery.

## Treatment Algorithm

The goals of treatment include (1) a stable elbow joint including radiocapitellar as well as ulnohumeral joint and (2) stable internal fixation of the ulna fracture to permit early range of motion. The treatment algorithm may be broken down into the individual components of the injury pattern. The radial head dislocation is often reduced indirectly when ulnar length and alignment has been restored. When the ulnar fracture is at the level of the coronoid it is imperative that the coronoid fracture fragment be incorporated into the fixation construct and that an anatomic reconstruction of the trochlear notch be achieved.

Radial head fractures may be seen in 35–100 % of posterior Monteggia injuries and are commonly Mason type II or III [8–11, 30, 31]. Type II radial head fractures should undergo open reduction and internal fixation. Historically, type III radial head fractures were either fixed or excised and outcome measures did not appear to demonstrate significant complication resulting from radial head excision [10–12]. However, since these injuries may also occur in conjunction with lateral ulnar collateral ligament injury it may be prudent for the surgeon to consider metallic radial head replacement as opposed to excision for type III injuries to minimize the chance of persistent instability. Lateral ulnar collateral ligament repair may also be necessary if intraoperative assessment demonstrates residual ulnohumeral instability despite stable anatomic fixation of the coronoid, olecranon, and radial head [29].

## Nonoperative Strategies

While Monteggia injuries in children can be treated nonoperatively with closed reduction and casting, there is little role for nonoperative management of Monteggia injuries in adults. Although it may be possible to perform closed reduction of the ulna and radial head in simple ulna fracture patterns, loss of reduction is common and stable internal fixation of the ulna is recommended [10].

## Surgical Management and Techniques

These injuries are approached through the posterior approach to the elbow with an extension along the subcutaneous border of the ulna. If the ulnar fracture is proximal, access to the radial head can often be obtained through the fracture bed. Alternatively, for diaphyseal ulnar fractures, access to the radial head can be obtained through a separate lateral incision or through elevation of the posterolateral skin flap. For fractures at the ulnar metaphysis and more proximally, the ideal fixation construct involves a 3.5 mm dynamic compression plate or a limited contact dynamic compression plate placed along the dorsal cortex of the ulna and contoured around the olecranon so that the proximal screws are orthogonal to the more distal screws [11–14, 32]. Constructs with tension band wiring, tubular, or semi-tubular plates provide inadequate fixation and are at risk for loss of fixation [32]. Similarly, for fractures proximal to the metaphysis, medial or lateral placement of the plate may only permit one to two screws to be engaged in the proximal olecranon fragment [11, 32]. True diaphyseal ulna fractures may be fixed with the plate placed volarly or dorsally to minimize hardware prominence and the need for late hardware removal.

Typically, reduction of the radial head is achieved by restoring length and alignment of the ulna fracture. The injury may be fixed step-wise either from proximal-to-distal or distal-to-proximal [14, 29, 33]. Ring and Jupiter have advocated the use of a distractor to allow for indirect reduction of the ulnar fracture fragments in cases with severe comminution along the trochlear notch [29]. The first step involves placement of a smooth 0.062 Kirschner wire through the olecranon fragment and into the distal humerus. Distraction is then achieved between the K-wire and a second wire or pin that is placed in the distal ulna away from the fracture and out of the way of the intended are of definitive fixation. The distal humerus can be utilized as a template to reconstruct the ulnar trochlea.

Alternatively, Beingessner et al. have proposed a stepwise approach from distal-to-proximal for the extensively comminuted Type IID posterior Monteggia injuries, but their principles may be applicable to all posterior Monteggia fractures and ensure that the surgeon has addressed all of the bony and ligamentous contributions to elbow and forearm stability [14]. If the radial head is fractured and accessible through the ulnar fracture plane, then the first step should be reduction and fixation of the radial head or prosthetic replacement if the surgeon feels it cannot be fixed. Radial head fractures with more than three articular fragments may be better served with prosthetic replacement—internal fixation of more comminuted radial head fractures commonly results in radial head malunion and loss of forearm rotation [34]. After the radial head has been addressed, a combination of lag screws and mini-fragment plates can be utilized to reconstruct the ulnar shaft from distal-to-proximal. If the radial head cannot be accessed through the ulna fracture, the ulna should be repaired and then the radial head addressed through a lateral approach (Kocher, Kaplan or EDC split—see Chap. 3). The reduction of the coronoid fragment can be obtained through one of the ulnar fracture planes. Smaller coronoid fragments may require transosseous suture fixation whereas larger coronoid fragments may potentially be captured with screws. The most proximal portion of the ulna fracture (olecranon) is addressed last with provisional reduction of the olecranon to the distal ulna with pointed reduction clamps and placement of a contoured 3.5-mm compression plate along the dorsal cortex of the ulna. After the osseous structures are stabilized, attention should be paid to potential injury of the medial or lateral ulnar collateral ligaments—with lateral ulnar collateral ligament injuries being more common as a result of the posterior dislocation of the radial head.

When the fracture involves the trochlear notch (Types IIA and IID) it is imperative that the relative relationship of the coronoid and olecranon processes be reconstructed. It is important to remember that there is a naturally occurring bare spot devoid of articular cartilage at the low point of the trochlear notch. Overall, restoration of the relative alignment of the coronoid and olecranon processes to one another may be more important than residual articular incongruity from fracture comminution [35]. Shortening of the olecranon should be avoided if there are comminuted areas of the articular surface at the level of the greater sigmoid notch. The dorsal aspect of the olecranon should be used as the key for olecranon length. Excessive shortening will result in anterior and posterior impingement with flexion and extension restricting motion. Fluoroscopy should be utilized throughout the case to ensure that the ulna is being reconstructed anatomically and that screw tips do not penetrate articular surfaces. The elbow should be put through a gentle range of motion to ensure unrestricted motion and joint stability. If radiocapitellar instability persists then attention should be paid to ensure that appropriate length and alignment of the ulna has been restored. A hinged external fixator to complement internal fixation may be used at the discretion of the surgeon [36]. Our preference is to always check radiocapitellar and ulnohumeral alignment using intraoperative fluoroscopy after fixation is achieved but prior to wound closure. The elbow joint is placed through a flexion-extension arc with the forearm in pronated, neutral, and supinated positions. With the elbow in full extension and forearm in full supination, we carefully scrutinize the lateral view looking for any malalignment of the radiocapitellar joint that would suggest lateral ulnar collateral ligament injury.

Postoperative management for these complex elbow injuries is dictated by multiple factors, including (1) stability of fracture fixation achieved intraoperatively, (2) stability of elbow joint, (3) condition of soft-tissue envelope, and (4) presence or absence of concomitant injury. For the majority of patients, restoration of anatomic bone alignment with stable internal fixation results in a stable elbow joint, which will permit early motion of the elbow. Postoperatively, patients are placed in a well-padded anterior splint with the elbow held in 15–30° of flexion. The anterior placement of the splint limits the pressure over the posterior incision. The splint is maintained for 2 days then removed and the skin incision is assessed. If wound healing allows, the patient is transitioned into a soft dressing and gentle active-assisted range of motion is initiated. The elbow is protected in a sling when exercises are not being performed. If necessary, the splint is continued up to 2 weeks to limit elbow motion and permit wound healing. Serial follow-up is obtained at 2 weeks, then monthly until radiographic union. Passive range of motion and use of nighttime static flexion or static extension splints to help with terminal flexion or extension, are initiated at 6 weeks if necessary. Strengthening is initiated at 2 months if bony healing and elbow range of motion permits.

## Published Outcomes/Complications

Historically, the outcomes of Monteggia fractures have been poor due to inadequate means of obtaining and maintaining ulnar and radial head reduction [5–9]. Improvements in methods of internal fixation combined with a better understanding of the components of the injury pattern as it relates to elbow stability have allowed surgeons to achieve better outcomes than their predecessors [11–14] (Table 7.1). In general, posterior Monteggia fractures that are associated with coronoid or radial head involvement tend to have worse outcomes [10–12].

Ring et al. reported on one of the largest series of Monteggia fractures in adults treated with modern internal fixation devices [11]. The authors were able to compare results of posterior and anterior Monteggia injuries [11]. Although 83 % of the study population eventually had satisfactory outcome, reoperations and complications were high. In particular, they noted a 50 % unsatisfactory result after index operation in posterior Monteggia injuries with associated radial head fracture. Overall, nine (24 %) of their patients required reoperation within 3 months, 16 % of whom were for loss of ulna fixation and 8 % for secondary radial head resection. The method of fracture fixation was variable in their study and ranged from tension-band wiring to fixation with plates placed along the medial, lateral, or dorsal cortex of the ulna. Loss of fracture fixation was highest in injuries treated with tension-band wiring or plate fixation placed on the medial or lateral cortex of the ulna and lowest in patients treated with 3.5 mm contoured plates along the dorsal ulna. The authors highlighted several points about treatment: (1) posterior Monteggia injuries commonly happen in older females with osteoporotic bone and require stout fixation, (2) contoured plates placed along the dorsal ulna allow for improved fixation in the proximal ulna with more screws overall and more screws oriented perpendicular to one another when compared with medial or lateral plate placement, (3) coronoid involvement necessitates stable reconstruction of the trochlear notch, and (4) radial head fractures increase the likelihood of an unsatisfactory result.

Similarly, Konrad et al. reported long-term outcomes in a series of Monteggia fractures in adults and confirmed that radial head fractures, fractures involving the coronoid and posterior

**Table 7.1** Outcomes of posterior monteggia fracture dislocation

| Publication | Ring et al. JBJS 1998 | Konrad et al. JBJS Br 2007 | Beingessner et al. JOT 2011 | Doornberg et al. CORR 2004 |
|---|---|---|---|---|
| Patients | 38[a] | 37[a] | 16 | 16[a] |
| Follow-up | 6.5 years (2–14) | 8 years (5–11) | 37 weeks (9–82) | 6 years (3–10) |
| Age | 58 years (27–88) | 43 years (21–72) | – | 53 years (21–82) |
| Gender | 15 male, 23 female | 18 male, 9 female | – | 8 male, 8 female |
| Injury characteristics | | | | |
| Open fracture | 3 (8 %)—2 type I, 1 type IIA | 4 (11 %)—unspecified | 5 (6 %) | 1 (6 %) |
| Radial head fracture | 26 (68 %)—7 type 2, 19 type 3 | 11 (30 %)—unspecified | 15 (94 %)—unspecified | 13 (81 %)—3 type 2, 10 type 3 |
| Coronoid fracture | 10 (26 %) | 11 (30 %) | 14 (88 %)—5 type 1, 1 type 2, 8 type 3 | 16 (100 %)—1 type 2, 15 type 3 |
| LUCL involvement | – | – | 2 required repair | 2 required repair |
| Neurologic injury | 0 (0 %) | 3[a] | 0 | 1 (6 %)—brachial plexus palsy |
| Other injuries | 3—distal radius fx<br>1—floating elbow<br>1—proximal humerus fx<br>1—shoulder dislocation<br>2—compartment syndrome | – | 1/3—unspecified | 2 (12 %)—distal radius fx<br>1 (6 %)—shoulder dislocation |
| Method of fixation | 3—tension band wiring<br>1—Steinmann pin<br>17—3.5 mm DCP<br>10—3.5 mm LC-DCP<br>2—3.5 mm recon plate<br>4—semitubular plate | 11—tension band wiring<br>26—3.5 mm DCP or LC-DCP | 16—3.5 LC-DCP with mini-fragment plate supplemental fixation | 11—3.5 mm LC-DCP<br>2—3.5 mm DCP<br>1—3.5 mm recon plate<br>1—tension band wiring |
| Avg. Arc ROM (extension-flexion) | 112 (range: 65–140) | 103 (range: 50–130) | 101 | 95 (50–125) |
| Avg. Arc ROM (pronation-supination) | 126 (range: 0–160) | 128 (range: 100–180) | 139 | 115 (0–170) |
| Broberg-Morrey score | Excellent—14 (37 %)<br>Good—18 (47 %)<br>Fair—1 (3 %)<br>Poor—5 (13 %) | Excellent—8 (30 %)<br>Good—9 (33 %)<br>Fair—6 (22 %)<br>Poor—4 (15 %) | – | Excellent—5 (31 %)<br>Good—7 (44 %)<br>Fair—1 |
| ASES | – | – | – | 78 (28.5–100) |
| DASH score | – | 22 (0–70) | – | – |
| Reoperation | 9 (24 %)—6 (16 %) loss of fixation, 3 (8 %) for secondary radial head resection | 12 patients of entire study group (26 %)—6 nonunion, 2 infection, 2 radial head loss of fixation, 2 synostosis | 1 (6 %)—removal of hardware | – |
| Arthrosis | 3 (8 %) | – | 0 (0 %) | 9 (56 %) |
| Other complications | 2 (5 %)—synostosis<br>1 (3 %)—PLRI | 5 (14 %)—heterotopic ossification<br>2 (5 %)—synostosis | 3 (19 %)—heterotopic ossification<br>1 (6 %)—radial head malunion<br>1 (6 %)—late median and radial nerve compression | 3 (18 %)—synostosis |

*LC* limited contact, *DCP* dynamic compression plate, *PLRI* posterolateral rotatory instability
[a]Part of larger study

Monteggia fracture patterns portended worse outcomes as compared with anterior Monteggia injuries [12]. Reoperation (26 %) was common and was performed for either: ulnar nonunion (13 %), infection (4 %), radial head malunion (4 %), and synostosis resection (4 %). Although 30 % of the ulna fractures were treated with tension band wiring, the authors noted that this technique was only utilized in simple fracture patterns without significant comminution. They also commented that using a dorsal countoured plate provides improved fracture stability.

Beingessner et al. described their recommended surgical technique and outcomes of treating the posterior Monteggia injuries with comminution extending from the ulna diaphysis to the olecranon (Jupiter IID) [14]. The methods of ulna fixation were more uniform and employed a combination of mini-fragment plates to reconstruct the ulna in a step-wise fashion in conjunction with a long 3.5 mm plate placed along the dorsal ulna and contoured around the olecranon. They experienced no incidence of loss of fixation of the ulna in their patients and the reoperation rate was low (6 %).

Utilizing the Broberg-Morrey scale for outcomes, good to excellent outcomes may be achievable in 63–84 % of patients when utilizing contemporary means of internal fixation [11–13, 37]. The average flexion-extension arc of motion achievable ranges between 95 and 112° and the average pronation-supination arc of motion ranges between 115 and 128° [11–14]. The observed rate of ulnohumeral arthrosis ranges from 0 to 56 % and is dependent upon whether the fracture extends proximally to involve the coronoid and trochlear notch as well as length of follow-up in the reported studies [11–14]. Proximal radioulnar joint synostosis and heterotopic ossification range from 5 to 19 % of cases and correlate with poorer patient outcomes [11–14].

Reoperation rates range from 6 to 26 % and may be attributable to loss of ulna fixation, ulna nonunion, radial head malunion or loss of fixation, infection, synostosis or heterotopic ossification removal and symptomatic hardware [11–14]. The most commonly reported reasons for reoperation were related to either loss of ulna fixation or secondary procedures for radial head fracture, highlighting the importance in achieving stable anatomic reconstruction of the ulna and in choosing the optimal initial management of any associated radial head fracture [11–14]. Most of the secondary procedures performed on the radial head were due to loss of fixation or malunion of comminuted Mason Type III fractures treated with open reduction and internal fixation. In most cases, the secondary treatment for these complications involved radial head resection to improve forearm pronation-supination. However, in the acute setting radial head arthroplasty may be preferable to radial head resection due to the secondary stabilizing effect of the radial head on elbow stability [19–22, 38].

Ring et al. reported on outcomes of revision surgery for loss of alignment of 17 posterior Monteggia fractures [32]. The initial loss of alignment in this series of patients was often due to technical errors in methods of fixation (i.e., utilizing tension-band wires or intramedullary screws or with plates being placed either medial or lateral) or failure to address all components of the injury pattern (i.e., coronoid fractures, lateral ulnar collateral ligament injuries). The fractures were revised with 3.5-mm contoured plates placed along the dorsal ulna cortex and a variety of procedures to address the radial head, lateral ulnar collateral ligament, or heterotopic ossification. Lateral ulnar collateral ligament repair was required in four (24 %) of patients and hinged external fixation was utilized in five (29 %) to protect the internal fixation or address residual ulnohumeral instability. Overall, 82 % of their patients achieved a good or excellent result according to the Broberg-Morrey system and flexion-extension arc of motion improved from 58° (range: 30–90) to 108° (range: 75–135), while pronation-supination arc of motion improved from 42° (range: 0–110) to 134° (range: 40–150).

## Case Examples

### Case 1

A 46-year-old female sustained a posterior Monteggia fracture at the level of the ulnar metaphysis (Jupiter IIB) with associated comminuted

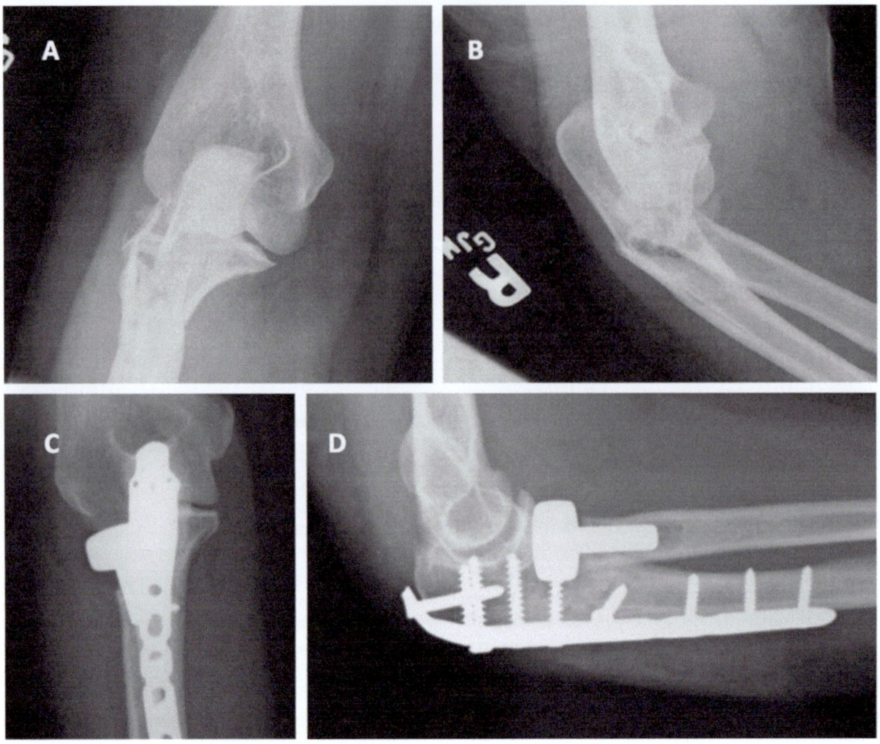


**Fig. 7.5** Posterior Monteggia with radial head fracture. Anteroposerior (**a**) and Lateral (**b**) radiographic views demonstrate posterior Monteggia at metaphyseal level (Jupiter IIB) with associated comminuted radial head fracture. Postoperative Anteroposterior (**c**) and Lateral (**d**) radiographic views after stable fixation with posteriorly placed and contoured plate and metallic radial head arthroplasty (From Wong JC, Getz CL, Abboud JA. Adult Monteggia and Olecranon Fracture Dislocations of the Elbow. *Hand Clin*. 2015;31(4):565–80)

radial head fracture (Fig. 7.5a, b). Surgery was performed through posterior approach to elbow. The fracture site and soft-tissue disruption allowed access to perform radial head arthroplasty. After radial head arthroplasty was performed, the proximal ulna was reconstructed with a combination of inter-fragmentary screw and posteriorly applied pre-contoured 3.5 mm olecranon plate (Fig. 7.5c, d). At final follow-up the patient regained full range of motion in flexion-extension and pronation-supination, comparable to her uninjured elbow. She had no further reoperations.

## Case 2

A 55-year-old male sustained a posterior Monteggia fracture with involvement of the coronoid and extension toward ulnar diaphysis (Jupiter IID) and associated radial head fracture (Fig. 7.6a, b). Fracture fixation was performed through posterior approach. The ulnar nerve was identified and protected for subcutaneous transposition at the end of the case. Wide medial and lateral skin flaps permitted access to either side of the joint. A Kocher approach to the radial head also permitted assessment of lateral ulnar collateral ligament integrity. The radial head fracture fragment could not be fixed with screws so fixation was achieved with K-wires. In this case, the lateral ulnar collateral ligament did not require repair; however if necessary the lateral ulnar collateral ligament can be repaired with a suture anchor placed at the isometric point on the lateral epicondyle. Proximal ulna was reconstructed with a combination of inter-fragmentary screws and posteriorly applied 3.5 mm plate. As is characteristic of Jupiter Type IID Monteggia

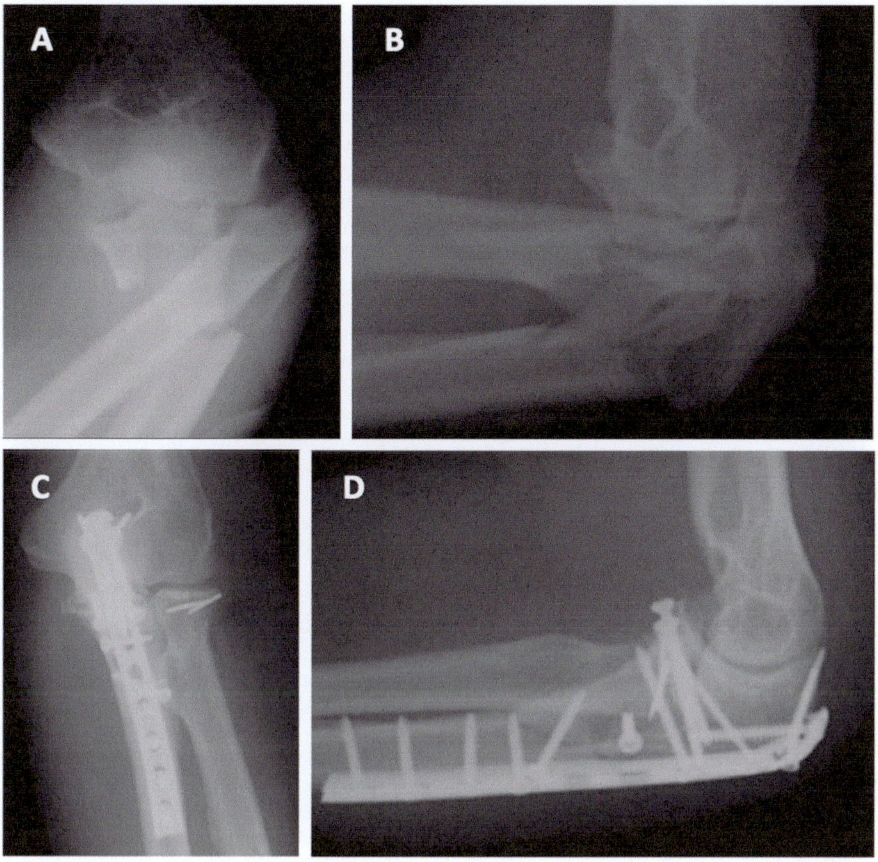


**Fig. 7.6** Posterior Monteggia with coronoid involvement. Anteroposterior (**a**) and Lateral (**b**) radiographic views demonstrate a posterior Monteggia fracture with characteristic large anterior quadrangular ulnar fragment extending into the coronoid process as well as radial head fracture. Anteroposterior (**c**) and Lateral (**d**) radiographs after anatomic reduction and fixation of the ulna with posterior placed plate and screws. Supplemental fixation of the large anterior ulna fragment with anterior-to-posterior directed screws. The radial head fragment is fixed with k-wires (From Wong JC, Getz CL, Abboud JA. Adult Monteggia and Olecranon Fracture Dislocations of the Elbow. *Hand Clin*. 2015;31(4):565–80)

fractures, the coronoid fracture fragment extended into the ulnar shaft. In this case, adequate fracture reduction and fixation could not be achieved indirectly so the decision was made to gain direct visualization of that fragment through a medial approach. The medial skin flap was elevated to allow flexor-pronator elevation and the coronoid fragment was fixed with anterior-to-posterior inter-fragmentary screws (Fig. 7.6c, d). In complex fractures of the proximal ulna associated with coranoid process fractures that require fixation, the Taylor-Scham approach offers an extensile approach allowing access to all components of the injury (see Chap. 3). At final follow-up the patient regained 5–100° of motion in extension-flexion and near-full pronation-supination.

## Summary

Posterior Monteggia fractures are complex injuries that occur more commonly in adults and often times in older females with osteoporotic bone. Associated injuries such as radial head fracture, coronoid fracture, lateral ulnar collateral ligament injury, and ulnohumeral instability are common and must be addressed. Good outcomes can be achieved if the surgeon recognizes the pattern of injury and the influence that the each of the associated injuries has on elbow stability. The most stable method of fixation of the ulna involves a 3.5-mm plate placed along the dorsal cortex and contoured around the olecranon. When the fracture extends proximally into the coronoid or olecranon, then stable reconstruction of the trochlear notch is required. Concomitant radial head fractures may be managed in a variety of ways depending upon fracture displacement and comminution. For comminuted radial head fractures, strong consideration should be given toward radial head arthroplasty as opposed to repairing or resecting the radial head. Lateral ulnar collateral ligament injuries may require repair if ulnohumeral stability persists despite anatomic ulna and radial head reconstruction. Complications like stiffness, posttraumatic arthrosis, heterotopic ossification, and synostosis are common and may require subsequent procedures to address.

## References


1. Bado JL. The Monteggia lesion. Clin Orthop Relat Res. 1967;50:71–86.
2. Ring D, Waters PM. Operative fixation of Monteggia fractures in children. J Bone Joint Surg Br. 1996; 78(5):734–9.
3. Ring D, Jupiter JB, Waters PM. Monteggia fractures in children and adults. J Am Acad Orthop Surg. 1998;6:215–24.
4. Guitton TG, Ring D, Kloen P. Long-term evaluation of surgically treated anterior Monteggia fractures in skeletally mature patients. J Hand Surg Am. 2009;34(9):1618–24.
5. Watson-Jones R. Fractures and joint injuries. 3rd ed. Baltimore, MD: Williams and Wilkins; 1943. p. 520–35.
6. Speed JS, Boyd HB. Treatment of fractures of the ulna with dislocation of the head of the radius (Monteggia fracture). J Am Med Assoc. 1940;115:1699–705.
7. Bruce HE, Harvey Jr JP, Wilson Jr JC. Monteggia fractures. J Bone Joint Surg. 1974;56-A:1563–76.
8. Pavel A, Pitman JM, Lance EM, Wade PA. The posterior Monteggia fracture. A clinical study. J Trauma. 1965;5:185–99.
9. Penrose JH. The Monteggia fracture with posterior dislocation of the radial head. J Bone Joint Surg Br. 1951;33:65–73.
10. Jupiter JB, Leibovic SJ, Ribbans W, Wilk RM. The posterior Monteggia lesion. J Orthop Trauma. 1991;5(4):395–402.
11. Ring D, Jupiter JB, Simpson NS. Monteggia fractures in adults. J Bone Joint Surg Am. 1998;80(12): 1733–44.
12. Konrad GG, Kundel K, Kreuz PC, Oberst M, Sudkaamp NP. Monteggia fractures in adults: long-term results and prognostic factors. J Bone Joint Surg Br. 2007;89(3):354–60.
13. Doornberg J, Ring D, Jupiter JB. Effective treatment of fracture-dislocations of the olecranon requires a stable trochlear notch. Clin Orthop Relat Res. 2004;429:292–300.
14. Beingessner DM, Nork SE, Agel J, Viskontas D. A fragment-specific approach to Type IID Monteggia elbow fracture-dislocations. J Orthop Trauma. 2011;25(7):414–9.
15. Regan WD, Korinek SL, Morrey BF, An KN. Biomechanical study of ligaments around the elbow joint. Clin Orthop Relat Res. 1991;271:170–9.
16. Regan W, Morrey B. Fractures of the coronoid process of the ulna. J Bone Joint Surg Am. 1989;71(9):1348–54.
17. Wilkins KE, Morrey BF, Jobe FW, Kvitne RS, Coonrad RW, Figgie 3rd HE, Jupiter JB, Inglis AE, Wright 2nd PE, Burns EB, et al. The elbow. Instr Course Lect. 1991;40:1–87.
18. Tashijian RZ, Katarinic JA. Complex elbow instability. J Am Acad Orthop Surg. 2006;14(5):278–86.
19. King GJ, Morrey BF, An KN. Stabilizers of the elbow. J Shoulder Elbow Surg. 1993;2(3):165–74.
20. Beingessner DM, Dunning CE, Gordon KD, Johnson JA, King GJ. The effect of radial head fracture size on elbow kinematics and stability. J Orthop Res. 2005;23(1):210–7.
21. Beingessner DM, Dunning CE, Gordon KD, Johnson JA, King GJ. The effect of radial head excision on elbow kinematics and stability. J Bone Joint Surg Am. 2004;86-A(8):1730–9.
22. Johnson JA, Beingessner DM, Gordon KD, Dunning CE, Stacpoole RA, King GJ. Kinematics and stability of the fractured and implant-reconstructed radial head. J Shoulder Elbow Surg. 2005;14(1 Suppl S):195S–201.
23. Closkey RF, Goode JR, Kirschenbaum D, Cody RP. The role of the coronoid process in elbow stability. A biomechanical analysis of axial loading. J Bone Joint Surg Am. 2000;82-A(12):1749–53.
24. Deutch SR, Jensen SL, Tyrdal S, Olsen BS, Sneppen O. Elbow joint stability following experimental osteoligamentous injury and reconstruction. J Shoulder Elbow Surg. 2003;12(5):466–71.
25. Jeon IH, Sanchez-Sotelo J, Zhao K, An KN, Morrey BM. The contribution of the coronoid and radial head to the stability of the elbow. J Bone Joint Surg Br. 2012;94(1):86–92.
26. Schneeberger AG, Sadowski MM, Jacob HA. Coronoid process and radial head as posterolateral rotatory stabilizers of the elbow. J Bone Joint Surg Am. 2004;86-A(5):975–82.
27. Hull JR, Owen JR, Fern SE, Wayne JS, Boardman 3rd ND. Role of the coronoid process in varus

osteoarticular stability of the elbow. J Shoulder Elbow Surg. 2005;14(4):441–6.
28. Ring D. Monteggia fractures. Orthop Clin North Am. 2013;44(1):59–66.
29. Ring D, Jupiter JB. Fracture-dislocation of the elbow. J Bone Joint Surg Am. 1998;80(4):566–80.
30. Mason ML. Some observations on fractures of the head of the radius with a review of one hundred cases. Br J Surg. 1954;42:123–32.
31. Hotchkiss RN. Displaced fractures of the radial head: internal fixation or excision? J Am Acad Orthop Surg. 1997;5(1):1–10.
32. Ring D, Tavakolian J, Kloen P, Helfet D, Jupiter JB. Loss of alignment after surgical treatment of posterior Monteggia fractures: salvage with dorsal contoured plating. J Hand Surg Am. 2004;29(4):694–702.
33. Athwal GS, Ramsey ML, Steinmann SP, Wolf JM. Fractures and dislocations of the elbow: a return to the basics. Instr Course Lect. 2011;60:199–214.
34. Ring D, Quintero J, Jupiter JB. Open reduction and internal fixation of fractures of the radial head. J Bone Joint Surg Am. 2002;84A(10):1811–5.
35. Ring D, Jupiter JB, Sanders RW, Mast J, Simpson NS. Transolecranon fracture-dislocation of the elbow. J Orthop Trauma. 1997;11(8):545–50.
36. Ring D, Hannouche D, Jupiter JB. Surgical treatment of persistent dislocation or subluxation of the ulnohumeral joint after fracture-dislocation of the elbow. J Hand Surg Am. 2004;29(3):470–80.
37. Broberg MA, Morrey BF. Results of treatment of fracture-dislocations of the elbow. Clin Orthop Relat Res. 1987;216:109–19.
38. Harrington IJ, Sekyi-Out A, Barrington TW, Evans DC, Tuli V. The functional outcome with metallic radial head implants in the treatment of unstable elbow fractures: a long-term review. J Trauma. 2001;50(1):46–52.

# 8 Transolecranon Fracture-Dislocations

Nicholas M. Capito, E. Scott Paxton, and Andrew Green

## Background

Due to the congruent osteoarticular anatomy and ligamentous support, the elbow is an inherently stable joint. Nevertheless, instability injuries, which range from simple dislocations to a host of complex fracture-dislocations, exist and can present treatment challenges. Transolecranon fracture-dislocations are a unique injury that combines a fracture of the olecranon with anterior dislocation of the elbow. "Trans-olecranal fractures" were first described by Biga and Thomine in 1974 [1]. They identified two subtypes based on the ulna fracture: Type I (simple) and Type II (comminuted). In contrast to Monteggia injuries, the proximal radioulnar articulation is not disrupted in transolecranon fracture-dislocations. In transolecranon fracture-dislocations, the radius and ulna shafts translate together anteriorly with anterior dislocation of the radiocapitellar joint.

The proximal ulna has four bony component parts including the olecranon, coronoid process, greater sigmoid notch, and the ulnar shaft. The greater sigmoid notch surrounds almost 180° of the trochlea and contributes to anterior-posterior, varus-valgus, and rotational stability. Disruption of these osseous components contributes to elbow instability and joint incongruity. Complex elbow injuries can be difficult to treat and may have a substantial effect on functional outcome. Recent advances in musculoskeletal imaging and fracture fixation implants have enhanced our ability to treat these complex injuries.

## Evaluation

Transolecranon fracture-dislocations usually occur as the result of an axial load to the dorsal aspect of the proximal forearm while the elbow is in a mid-flexion position. This mechanism drives the distal humerus into the greater sigmoid notch causing a proximal ulna fracture, while also displacing the forearm anteriorly causing an anterior dislocation of the radiocapitellar joint. Similar to many other fractures, there is a bimodal distribution of patients; young adults who sustain higher energy trauma and elderly patients with

N.M. Capito, MD
Champion Orthopedics, Augusta, GA, USA
e-mail: ncaps4@gmail.com

E.S. Paxton, MD
Department of Orthopedic Surgery, Warren Alpert Medical School, Brown University, 2 Dudley St., Suite 200, Providence, RI 02905, USA
e-mail: escottpaxton@gmail.com

A. Green, MD (✉)
Division of Shoulder and Elbow Surgery, Department of Orthopedic Surgery, Warren Alpert Medical School, Brown University, 2 Dudley St., Suite 200, Providence, RI 02905, USA
e-mail: agshoulder@aol.com

© Springer International Publishing Switzerland 2017
R.Z. Tashjian (ed.), *The Unstable Elbow*, DOI 10.1007/978-3-319-46019-2_8

poor bone quality who are typically injured in lower energy level falls.

It is important to recognize the differences between transolecranon fracture-dislocations, isolated olecranon fractures, and Monteggia injuries. Monteggia injuries are also fracture-dislocations of the forearm, but unlike transolecranon fracture-dislocations, the defining lesion is a dislocation of the proximal radioulnar joint. Monteggia's original description was of a proximal one-third ulnar shaft fracture with anterior dislocation of the radial head [2]. Bado further subclassified Monteggia injuries according to the direction of the radial head dislocation. Bado Type I Monteggia injuries involve an anterior dislocation of the radial head, but in contrast to transolecranon injuries, the ulna fracture is diaphyseal and the proximal radioulnar joint is disrupted. Ring et al. [3] reported that the unique characteristic of transolecranon fracture-dislocations is the sparing of ligamentous structures. They wrote that the proximal radioulnar joint remains intact in transolecranon fracture-dislocations, as well as both the lateral collateral ligament (LCL) and medial collateral ligament (MCL) complexes [4–7]. Understanding the extent of injury to the bone and soft tissue structures within each of these types of elbow injuries allows one to most successfully treat and rehabilitate the injured patient.

Depending upon the mechanism of injury and quality of bone, the proximal ulna fracture can vary from a relatively simple and transverse olecranon fracture to complex and comminuted fractures that involve the greater sigmoid notch proximally, as well as the coronoid process and the remainder of the proximal ulna [4]. Most coronoid fractures associated with these injuries involve large Regan and Morrey type 3 fragments [5, 8]. It is the complexity of the proximal ulna fracture that dictates the specific fixation techniques required for surgical repair.

Due to the degree of injury and deformity at the elbow, patients sustaining transolecranon fracture-dislocations most commonly present to an emergency care facility. A complete medical evaluation and physical exam is necessary to rule out other injuries. It is important to understand the patient's general health, activity level, daily requirements, and outcome expectations, because these all play an important role in the management and outcome of these injuries.

High-energy mechanisms of injury should raise concern for other visceral and musculoskeletal injuries. The injured upper extremity is evaluated for concomitant ipsilateral injuries that may be less obvious. The condition of the surrounding soft tissue envelope must be assessed and the extent of forearm compartment swelling considered and monitored as necessary. Posterior abrasions are not uncommon and may necessitate either emergent or delayed surgical treatment. Open fractures must also be identified and appropriately treated. The neurologic examination assesses all major peripheral nerves about the elbow and considers other concomitant upper extremity injuries. Anterior displacement of the forearm can cause considerable stretch to the median, ulnar, and radial nerves. Distal pulses and perfusion of the hand are also routinely assessed.

The initial imaging studies should include AP and lateral plain radiographs of the injured elbow joint. Additional plain radiographs of the forearm and wrist are necessary to rule out and assess associated injuries. More distal concomitant diaphyseal ulna fractures can occur and may be missed on isolated elbow radiographs. Simple fractures do not typically require additional imaging. In cases of comminuted and complex injuries, a commuted tomography (CT) scan can provide more detailed definition of the fracture anatomy of the proximal ulna and aid in surgical planning. Lastly, traction radiographs, which are most easily obtained in the operating room with the patient under anesthesia, can also be helpful in understanding the fracture morphology.

## Treatment Algorithm

Transolecranon fracture-dislocations are inherently unstable and almost always require surgical fixation to restore functional anatomy. After the initial evaluation, it is reasonable to attempt a closed reduction, especially if there is marked displacement or the skin is threatened.

Unfortunately, in most cases the ulna fracture is unstable and a closed reduction cannot be maintained. The elbow is splinted in less than 90° of flexion to protect the skin and soft tissues and to minimize further injury prior to surgery.

Definitive nonoperative treatment can be considered in the rare cases of successful closed reduction or in patients with comorbidities, psychosocial or medical, that preclude surgical management.

## Surgical Management

The goal of operative management of complex elbow fractures is to achieve stable, rigid anatomic fixation that allows early elbow motion [9]. Urgent surgery should be considered to minimize the risk of further neurovascular injury that can result from the elbow dislocation and emergent surgery should be carried out in cases of open fractures.

General anesthesia with or without regional anesthesia can be used.

Patient positioning must provide unimpeded access to the injured anatomy to facilitate surgical exposure and fixation. Because a posterior approach is typically used the patient can be placed prone, in the lateral decubitus position, or supine with the injured arm brought across the chest. In the latter, it is helpful to place padding behind the trunk to slightly elevate the affected side so that the forearm and hand are in a dependent position. When the arm is brought across the chest, it can be held in place by clamping it securely to the drapes, held by an assistant, or held in place with a sterile articulating arm holder. It is also important to position the patient so that intraoperative fluoroscopic images can be easily obtained. A tourniquet is placed on the upper arm and used to maintain a bloodless surgical field. The tourniquet time should be limited to a maximum of 2 h.

A posterior incision provides direct access to the ulna fracture site. The skin and soft tissue are incised directly down to the ulna to maintain full-thickness flaps. Careful soft tissue dissection is performed to provide adequate exposure for fracture reduction and fixation while protecting the soft tissue envelope, minimizing devascularization of fracture fragments, and preserving intact ligamentous structures. The distal humerus can usually be visualized through the ulna fracture. Dissection on the medial aspect of the proximal ulna needs to be careful to avoid injuring the ulnar nerve. The ulnar nerve does not necessarily need to be transposed in these injuries but should be identified and protected throughout the case often with in situ decompression. Periosteal elevation that is limited to expose the fracture edges in simpler olecranon fractures may be all that is needed. In contrast, in more complex injuries, including those with involvement of the coronoid, more extensive exposure is required. In these cases, care must be taken to identify and preserve the insertion of the lateral ligament complex at the supinator crest and the medial collateral ligament at the sublime tubercle.

### Proximal Ulna Fracture Fixation

The proximal ulna fracture that occurs with a transolecranon fracture-dislocation may be a simple oblique or transverse pattern with minimal comminution or a complex injury with significant articular involvement and fragmentation and involvement of the coronoid. Simple transverse or oblique patterns require similar fixation constructs as more complex injuries, specifically a dorsally applied 3.5 mm reconstruction, limited contact dynamic compression or a precontoured olecranon/proximal ulna plate. Tension band or isolated screw fixation are reasonable constructs for simple fracture patterns, either transverse or oblique, in isolation but are at high risk for failure if utilized in the setting of these simpler fracture patterns with a transolecranon fracture-dislocation. Consequently, dorsal plate fixation is a standard treatment for these injuries independent of fracture complexity in these dislocation patterns.

Complex proximal ulna fractures associated with transolecranon fracture-dislocations are associated with higher energy injury, fracture comminution, greater soft tissue injury, and are much more difficult to treat, as well as, more likely to have more guarded outcome expectations. The preoperative assessment should provide the basis for a surgical strategy for fracture exposure, reduction, and fixation. Specifics of the fracture pattern, fragment size, and comminution are critically important to identify and consider. In general, these injuries not only require stable dorsal longitudinal plate fixation, similar to the simpler patterns, but also interfragmentary fixation of comminuted fragments. Complex patterns also often involve the coronoid process and need alternative fixation constructs or added exposure for reduction and fixation.

The goal of surgical treatment of the proximal ulna fracture is to precisely restore anatomic alignment with fixation that allows early range of motion. Early descriptions of plate fixation of the proximal ulna recommended bending a 3.5 mm dynamic compression plate [10]. Subsequently, a variety of precontoured plates with locking screw options are now available. Additional interfragmentary screw fixation can be performed for comminuted injuries using small 1.5, 2.0, or 2.4 mm screws. Small 2.0 or 2.4 mm plates can be applied anteromedially on the coronoid in large comminuted fractures where stable fixation cannot be achieved working "through" the ulna fracture using screws from the plate or outside the plate.

While the fixation of non-comminuted ulna fractures with plates is relatively straightforward, open reduction and internal fixation of comminuted, unstable fractures can be challenging. Restoring appropriate ulnar length can be difficult. Fixation that shortens the greater sigmoid notch will prevent anatomic articulation of the distal humerus and radiocapitellar joint. In some cases, a K-wire drilled through the olecranon, across the ulna fracture, and into the ulna shaft can provide provisional longitudinal stability. Provisional reduction with a distraction device can be very helpful. Reduction and fixation of comminuted fragments helps to restore length and alignment. A small plate placed on the lateral or medial side of the ulnar fracture can be used to support the reduction and maintain length. Once the provisional ulnar reduction is achieved the reduction of the radial head should be confirmed with intraoperative imaging. As stated above, malreduction of the ulna can prevent anatomic reduction of the ulnohumeral and radiocapitellar joints. Likewise, interposed soft tissue or displaced fracture fragments can block reduction of the radial head.

Once the ulnar reduction is confirmed a plate is selected that is long enough to extend beyond the most distal aspect of the fracture by at least three screw holes. A 3.5 mm reconstruction or dynamic compression or precontoured plate should be used. At the proximal end of the olecranon the plate can be placed directly on the triceps, or the triceps tendon insertion can be split to allow the plate to sit directly on bone. It is important when splitting the tendon to sharply elevate only as much of the tendon as needed for the plate to fit. The tendon can then be repaired over the hardware at closure. Initial fixation of the plate can begin proximally or distally and is best determined on an individual case basis. However, beginning the plate fixation by definitively fixing the proximal end at the olecranon increases the risk of distal malposition of the plate. Preliminary positioning of the plate with a proximal k-wire in the olecranon allows for adjustment of the alignment. Next, a screw is placed distal to the ulna fracture in the middle of an oblong screw hole. This allows adjustment of the proximal/distal position of the plate, as well as the angular alignment. Once the final position is determined this screw is tightened.

If the major ulna fracture is non-comminuted the plate can be used to compress the fracture. The plate is fixed with a screw tightened on one side of the fracture, usually proximal, and a non-locking screw is placed in a sliding hole on the other side of the fracture. Non-locking screws can also be used to tighten the plate against the bone. Care should be taken to avoid displacing the fracture when using non-locking screws. Locking screws can be used to further stabilize the fixation, especially in unstable fracture patterns or in cases with osteopenia. Proximal screws directed longitudinally through the plate into the proximal olecranon can further stabilize the fixation. These screws can also be used to support subchondral comminution. Additionally,

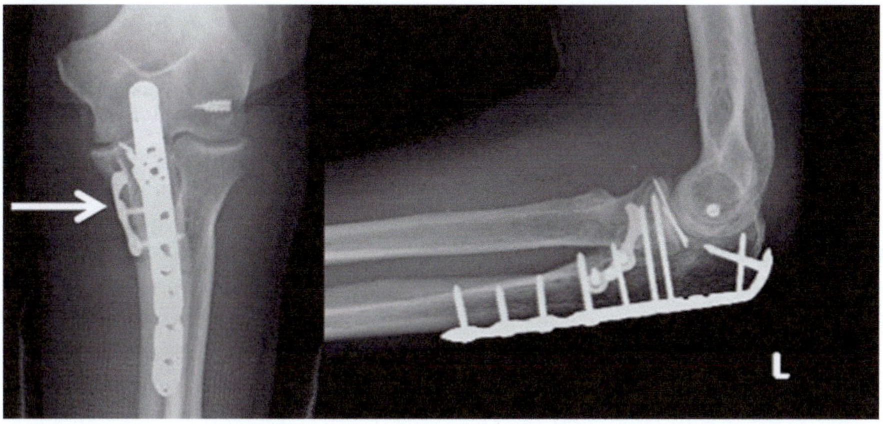


**Fig. 8.1** Buttress plating at the base of the coronoid with small mini-fragment plate can provide additional support for the coronoid fixation (*arrow*). © E. Scott Paxton, MD

longer screws can be placed to further stabilize the entire proximal ulna construct.

After osseous fixation is completed, fluoroscopic imaging is used to assess the accuracy of the fixation and position of the plate and screws. Elbow stability is also evaluated in flexion and extension, and pronation and supination motion, and with application of posterior lateral rotatory stress. Residual ligamentous instability is extremely rare after reconstruction of these injuries but if persistent subluxation or instability is present then the lateral collateral ligament should be explored and repaired if injured. If there is concern about the stability of the internal fixation construct due to comminution or bone loss especially of the coronoid process, external fixation can be used for 4–6 weeks [11].

## Coronoid Fracture Fixation

The coronoid process is critically important for elbow joint stability. Preoperative assessment of the entire proximal ulna fracture will determine how best to approach reduction and fixation of the coronoid. The fracture can be exposed through the ulnohumeral joint for direct visualization of the articular reduction, as well as along the extra-articular aspects. Larger coronoid fragments can be fixed with interfragmentary screws, either outside or through the longitudinal plate used for the ulna fixation. In the later case provisional fixation with a small K-wire can be used to hold the coronoid reduction until the definitive fixation is performed. Interosseous suture or thin wire fixation can be used when there is comminution or smaller fracture fragments. In addition, buttress plating at the base of the coronoid with small mini-fragment or precontoured plates can provide additional support for the coronoid fixation (Fig. 8.1). In most cases, the coronoid is fixed to the more distal aspect of the proximal ulna beyond the primary fracture of the greater sigmoid notch and followed by reduction and internal fixation of the remaining proximal ulna fracture and proximal olecranon fragment with the triceps insertion.

## Articular Impaction and Comminution

The crushing force of the distal humerus impacting the greater sigmoid notch can cause impaction and comminution of the articular surface. This can occur in high energy and low energy injuries. While small areas of comminution and minor incongruities in the transverse groove are well tolerated due to limited load transmission, anatomic reduction of the contour of the greater sigmoid notch and the anterior cortex of the coronoid results in restoration of the ulnohumeral articulation, allowing for a stable elbow joint, and is critical for a successful outcome [5]. While completely displaced and free fragments are obvious, direct exposure and visualization of the greater sigmoid notch is the best means of confirming the presence of articular injury and restoring the anatomy.

Impacted articular fragments should be carefully elevated to avoid creating a free fragment. A small osteotome is placed between the impacted fragment and the underlying stable bone to elevate and reduce the fragment. This creates a cavity that can be filled with bone graft or bone graft substitute to support the reduction. Displaced free osteochondral fragments also need to be reduced and fixed to larger and more stable aspects of the ulna. Fixation can be achieved with small K-wires, absorbable pins, fibrin glue, or cyanoacrylate. Very small chondral and osteochondral fragments can be discarded.

## Postoperative Protocol

A splint is used after surgery for comfort and to protect the elbow during early soft tissue healing. An anteriorly placed extension splint can be utilized to relax posterior soft tissues. Patients should not be splinted longer than 7 days, unless there is a significant soft tissue concern. Stable osseous fixation should allow for early motion of the elbow joint. However, in the case of severely comminuted fractures and poor quality bone, elbow motion may be delayed. Once the initial splint has been removed, assisted passive elbow and forearm motion is initiated. A compressive sleeve that extends from the hand to the upper arm is placed to control edema. A compressive glove can also be worn at night to control hand swelling and frequent wrist, hand, and finger range of motion is encouraged. A hinged elbow brace is utilized for added protection during early stages of healing, as well as also to limit flexion if there is concern about the posterior soft-tissues.

Active motion is progressed after 6 weeks, and carefully controlled passive stretching is initiated to overcome stiffness. Osseous healing is monitored radiographically. Isometric elbow extension and flexion, wrist extension and flexion, and forearm pronation and supination strengthening can be started after 6 weeks. Once motion is recovered, resistive strengthening is begun (typically 10–12 weeks). Patients are generally allowed to return to unrestricted activities at 4–6 months if motion and strength have recovered and there is osseous union.

Osseous healing is monitored with serial plain radiographs. In addition, heterotopic ossification (HO) is a concern for these patients and oral indomethacin can be used for 3–6 weeks to reduce the risk of HO. Radiation therapy should be avoided secondary to risk of fracture nonunion [12].

It is not uncommon for these patients to have limitations of elbow motion at final outcome. If patients are slow at regaining motion, static progressive braces can be used. Late stiffness can be addressed with capsular release and excision of heterotopic bone.

## Outcomes

Good or excellent outcomes can be achieved following management of transolecranon fracture-dislocations [4, 6, 8]. Mortazavi et al. [8] followed patients an average of 37.4 months (range, 10–50 months) after injury. Seven patients were managed with plate fixation and one with tension band. The mean range of flexion was 115° (range, 85–140°), with a mean flexion contracture of 22° (range, 0–45°). There is average arc of rotation measured 157.5° (range, 120–173°), with a mean pronation of 75° (range, 40–90°) and a mean supination of 83° (range, 80–85°). The mean score on the system of Broberg and Morrey was 88 points (range, 71–100 points). There were two excellent, five good, and one fair result. The average score on the American Shoulder and Elbow Surgeons (ASES) system was 89 points.

In a retrospective review of 17 transolecranon fracture-dislocation cases by Ring et al. [4], 15 cases had good or excellent results according to the scale of Broberg and Morrey. The average elbow flexion was 127° (range, 100–140°), with an average elbow flexion contracture of 14° (range, 0–40°). Forearm pronation and supination were normal in all but four patients. Doornberg et al. [5] reported satisfactory results in 9 of 10 patients. In a study by Rommens et al. [13], 65 % of the patients treated with a tension band required removal of hardware after an average of 12 months. Moushine et al. [6] retrospectively evaluated 14 transolecranon fracture-dislocations comparing seven treated with a tension band and seven treated with a plate. In the tension band group, three patients had early complications and had to be revised with a plate and supplemented with bone graft. Two of these patients had comminuted fracture patterns. Consequently, tension band fixation of these injuries should be avoided. Even simple transverse or oblique fractures in the setting of a transolecranon fracture-dislocation should be repaired using a dorsally applied plate.

Poor outcomes are often associated with hardware failure, nonunion, or inadequate postoperative immobilization. Several studies have shown that one-third of tubular plates fail to provide sufficient strength and rigidity for stabilizing more comminuted fractures of the olecranon [3, 4, 10, 14]. Consequently, 3.5 mm reconstruction or dynamic compression plates or precontoured olecranon plates should be used. In cases involving a large type 3 coronoid fracture, a poor outcome is inevitable if the fracture is not recognized and treated [4, 5]. Therefore, anatomic coronoid fixation providing stability to allow early motion is critical for success. Coronoid injuries with severe comminution or poor fixation due to bone quality should be considered for reconstruction utilizing an auto- or allograft with or without the addition of an external fixator. As the olecranon is a subcutaneous bone, hardware may be more prominent and can be painful to patients. In a multicenter study, the need for hardware removal of both plate and screw and tension band constructs was reported as high as 65 % by 18 months after surgery [7].

A long-term outcome study (18 ± 5 years after surgery) by Lindenhovius et al. [14] demonstrated that secure anatomical restoration of the greater sigmoid notch led to durable results. Final flexion arc was 124 ± 30° and final arc of forearm rotation was 133 ± 54°. Outcomes according to the ASES score were 85 ± 19, the Disability of Arm Shoulder and Hand questionnaire (DASH) were 14 ± 17, and Broberg and Morrey were 87 ± 18. The categorical ratings based on the Mayo Elbow Performance Index (MEPI) score were five excellent results, three good results, one fair result, and one poor result. 50 % (5 of 10 patients) developed some degree of ulnar neuropathy and arthrosis. Pain, final flexion arc, and ulnar neuropathy were the most important predictors of poor functional results and outcome. Furthermore, arthrosis did not correlate with final flexion arc and did not affect their evaluation scores. Therefore, despite the complexity of the injury, if stable anatomic reconstruction is achieved, one can be optimistic about the functional result.

## Preferred Treatment Case Presentation

### Simple Transolecranon Fracture-Dislocation

A 53-year-old female presented to the emergency department after a motor vehicle collision, with a chief complaint of left elbow pain. Physical examination of the extremity revealed an obvious deformity of the elbow with an abrasion along the volar forearm. There was no pain with palpation distally in the forearm, wrist, and hand. The skin was intact, except for an abrasion along her forearm. The neurovascular examination demonstrated decreased sensation on the volar aspect of the thumb. Plain AP and lateral radiographs of the elbow demonstrated a simple transolecranon fracture-dislocation (Fig. 8.2). After completion of the examination the extremity was immobilized in a long-arm splint in a position of comfort.

The patient was given a preoperative interscalene nerve block and general laryngeal mask anesthesia. She was positioned supine a padded roll under the ipsilateral thorax so that the operative extremity was draped across her chest on top of folded blankets. A non-sterile tourniquet was placed on the arm well out of the possible operative field. After sterile prep and drape, the operative

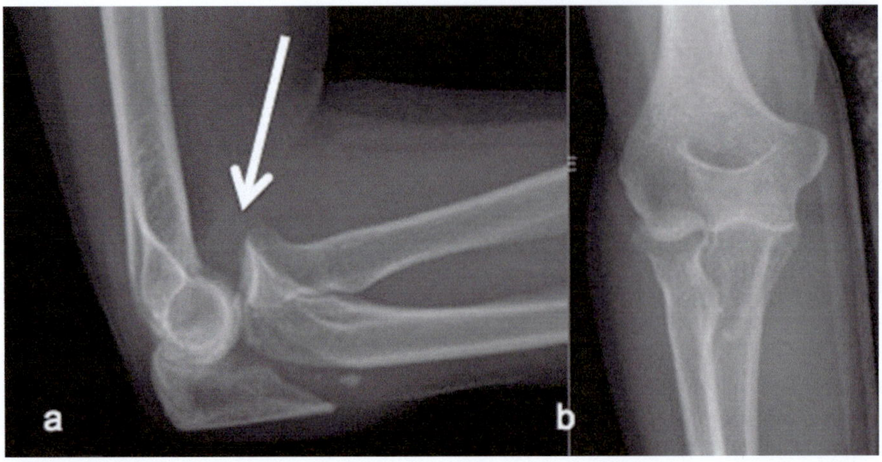


**Fig. 8.2** Plain radiographs of a simple transolecranon fracture-dislocation. (**a**) The lateral view demonstrates the anterior dislocation of the radial head (*arrow*) with minimal comminution of the greater sigmoid notch. (**b**) The anterior-posterior view demonstrates that there is minimal shortening of the ulna fracture. © Andrew Green, MD

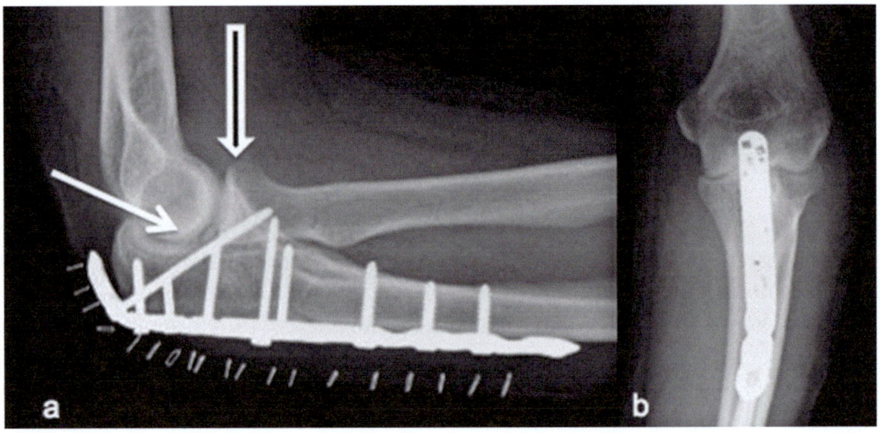


**Fig. 8.3** Plain radiographs after ORIF of the simple transolecranon fracture-dislocation in Fig. 8.2 with a precontoured proximal ulna plate. (**a**) The lateral view demonstrates anatomic reduction of the olecranon fracture (*solid arrow*) and the radiocapitellar joint (*hollow arrow*). (**b**) The anterior-posterior view demonstrates the alignment that the precontoured plated achieves. © Andrew Green, MD

extremity was exsanguinated and the tourniquet inflated to 250 mmHg.

A posterior incision beginning just proximal to the triceps insertion and extending in line with the ulna allowed for exposure of the ulna fracture site. The fracture hematoma was debrided. The periosteum and soft tissue was cleared from the edges of the fracture. The fracture fragments were manipulated and anatomically reduced using a combination of reduction forceps and K-wires. The manipulation and reduction of the ulna fracture resulted in reduction of the radial head dislocation. Fluoroscopy was used to confirm the reduction of the ulna fracture and radial head.

A precontoured proximal ulna locking compression plate was used. The plate was placed on the top of the triceps tendon insertion. A combination of locking and non-locking screws was used to secure the plate and maintain the reduction (Fig. 8.3). Sterile dressings were placed over the incision.

Postoperatively, the extremity was placed into a well-padded, long-arm, posterior splint with the elbow flexed 90° and forearm in neutral rotation.

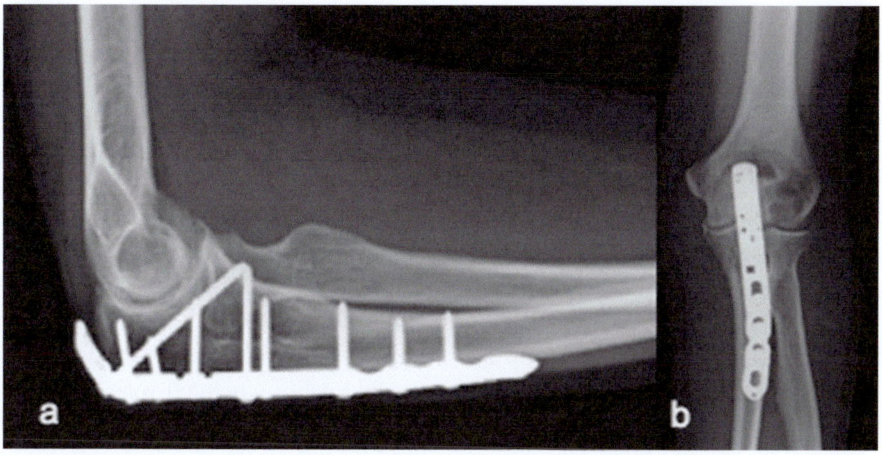

**Fig. 8.4** At 6-month follow-up (**a**) lateral and (**b**) anterior-posterior plain radiographs demonstrated a healed fracture, reduced radiocapitellar joint, intact hardware, and no evidence of HO. © Andrew Green, MD

At her 1-week follow-up appointment, the splint was removed and she was fitted with an elastic compression sleeve, light compression glove, and placed into a hinged elbow brace. The rehabilitation was followed as previously described in the postoperative protocol section of this chapter.

Plain radiographs obtained at 6 months postoperative demonstrated a well-healed fracture, stable hardware, and no evidence of heterotopic ossification (Fig. 8.4). The patient had an elbow flexion arc of 10–155° with full pronation and supination. She had full strength to manual testing. There was some residual posterior elbow pain with resisted flexion and mild tenderness over the plate.

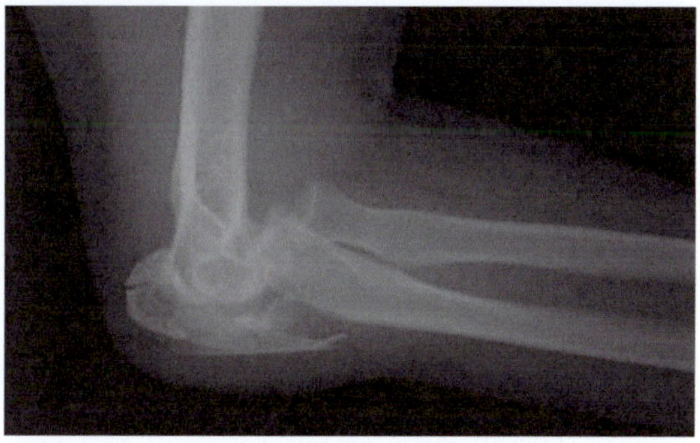

**Fig. 8.5** Lateral radiograph displaying a transolecranon fracture-dislocation with significant comminution of the entire proximal ulna. © E. Scott Paxton, MD

## Complex Transolecranon Fracture-Dislocation

A 27-year-old female presented to the emergency department after a motorcycle collision with a primary complaint of left elbow pain and deformity. Physical examination of the extremity revealed an obvious deformity and swelling of the elbow. There was diffuse ecchymosis about the elbow, but skin was intact. There was tenderness distally in the forearm, wrist, and hand and the neurovascular examination was intact. The lateral plain radiograph (Fig. 8.5) demonstrated a transolecranon fracture-dislocation with marked comminution of the olecranon extending to the coronoid. After stabilizing the patient in a posterior, long-arm splint, a CT scan was obtained to further assess the comminution and potential involvement of the coronoid (Fig. 8.6). The CT confirmed an intact coronoid, but due to the severity of the olecranon comminution, preoperative planning determined that a precontoured proximal ulna locking compression plate, along with interfragmentary fixation and bone grafting, may be required for fracture fixation.

The patient was given a preoperative interscalene nerve block and general laryngeal mask anesthesia. She was placed in the supine position with the operative extremity draped across the body and secured to a sterile articulating arm holder that was fastened to the contralateral side of the operating table. A non-sterile tourniquet was placed on the arm well out of the possible operative field. After sterile prep and drape, the operative extremity was exsanguinated and the tourniquet inflated to 250 mmHg.

The same posterior incision and techniques for exposure of the fracture site were performed as described in the first case. Manipulation and reduction of the ulna resulted in reduction of the radial head. The contour of the greater sigmoid notch was recreated with cancellous bone graft that was placed under the comminuted osteoarticular fragments between the coronoid and olecranon processes to elevate the depressed articular surface. The provisional fracture reduction was held with a combination of reduction forceps and Kirschner wires. Once anatomic alignment was confirmed with fluoroscopy fixation of the ulna was achieved with a precontoured proximal ulna locking compression plate with a combination of locking and non-locking screws. The olecranon fixation was augmented with a single, proximal, 2.7 mm interfragmentary screw. Furthermore, we used #2 FiberWire as offloading sutures through the triceps and into the plate to protect the proximal comminution.

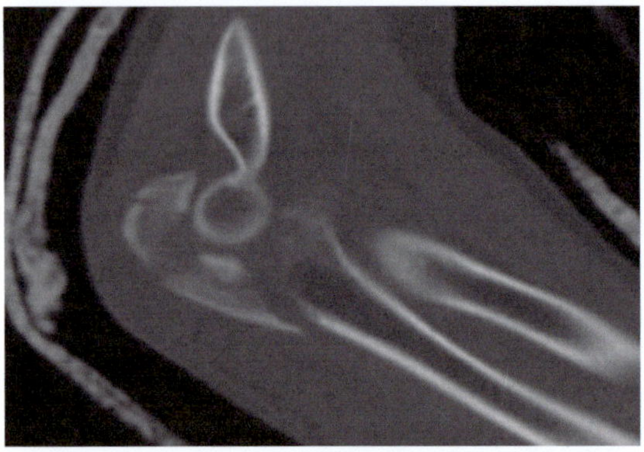

**Fig. 8.6** Sagittal CT image confirming significant comminution of the olecranon, but intact coronoid. © E. Scott Paxton, MD

The skin incision was closed with staples and covered with sterile dressings, the extremity was placed into a well-padded, long-arm, posterior splint with the elbow flexed 90° and forearm in neutral rotation. Postoperative radiographs in the recovery room confirmed the anatomic reduction and fixation (Fig. 8.7).

At 1-week follow-up, the splint was removed and she was fitted with an elastic compression sleeve, light compression glove, and placed into a hinged elbow brace. She began motion at that time and followed the same rehabilitation protocol as previously described.

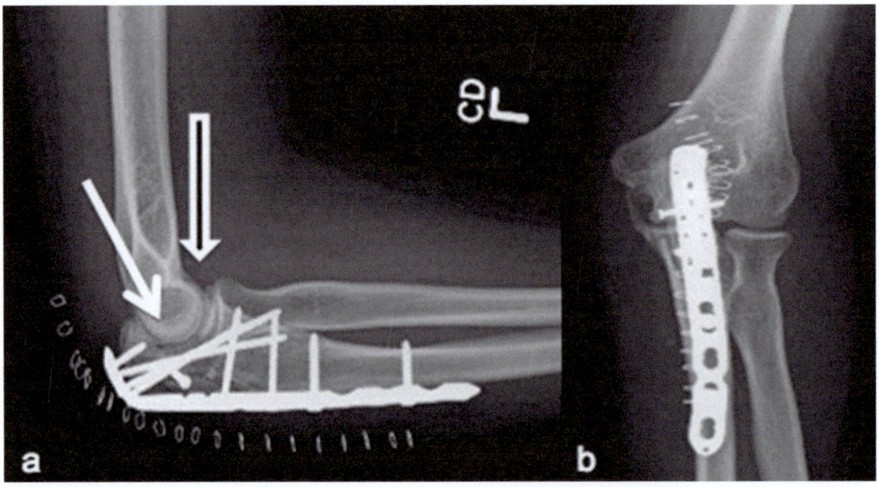


**Fig. 8.7** Postoperative plain radiographs of the case in Fig. 8.6. (**a**) Lateral radiograph demonstrates the anatomic reduction of the proximal ulna (*solid arrow*) as well as the radiocapitellar joint (*hollow arrow*). (**b**) Anterior-posterior radiograph demonstrating the fracture reduction and ulnar plate position. © E. Scott Paxton, MD

## Conclusion

Transolecranon fracture-dislocations are an uncommon injury of the elbow that occurs as the result of an axial load that drives the distal humerus into the greater sigmoid notch. The force of injury creates a proximal ulna fracture while also displacing the forearm anteriorly causing an anterior dislocation of the radiocapitellar joint. Surgical intervention is almost always performed to restore elbow joint anatomy and stability. A dorsally applied plate along the olecranon and proximal ulna allows for the most dependable construct for articular reconstruction combined with stable axial fixation. Satisfactory outcomes after treatment of these injuries are often obtained as long as initial stable fixation allowing early motion is achieved.

## References

1. Biga N, Thomine JM. Trans-olecranal dislocations of the elbow [in French]. Rev Chir Orthop. 1974;60:557–67.
2. Bado JL. The Monteggia lesion. Clin Orthop. 1967;50:71–6.
3. Ring D, Jupiter JB, Sanders RW, Mast J, Simpson NS. Fracture-dislocation of the elbow. J Bone Joint Surg Am. 1998;80:566–80.
4. Ring D, Jupiter JB, Sanders RW, Mast J, Simpson NS. Transolecranon fracture-dislocation of the elbow. J Orthop Trauma. 1997;11(8):545.
5. Doornberg J, Ring D, Jupiter JB. Effective Treatment of fracture-dislocations of the olecranon requires a stable trochlear notch. Clin Orthop Relat Res. 2004;(429):292–300.
6. Mouhsine E, Akiki A, Castagna A, Cikes A, Wettstein M, Borens O, et al. Transolecranon anterior fracture dislocation. J Shoulder Elbow Surg. 2007;16(3):352–7.
7. Edwards SG, Cohen MS, Lattanza LL, Iorio ML, Daniels C, Lodha S, et al. Surgeon perceptions and patient outcomes regarding proximal ulna fixation: a multicenter experience. J Shoulder Elbow Surg. 2012;21(12):1637–43.
8. Mortazavi SMJ, Asadollahi S, Tahririan MA. Functional outcome following treatment of transolecranon fracture-dislocation of the elbow. Injury. 2006;37(3):284–8.
9. Morrey BF. Current concepts in the treatment of fractures of the radial head, the olecranon, and the coronoid. J Bone Joint Surg. 1995;77(2):316–27.
10. Simpson NS, Goodman LA, Jupiter JB. Contoured LCDC plating of the proximal ulna. Injury. 1996;27(6):411–7.
11. Giannicola G, Sacchetti FM, Greco A, Cinotti G, Postacchini F. Management of complex elbow instability. Musculoskelet Surg. 2010;94(S1):25–36.
12. Hamid N, Ashraf N, Bosse MJ, Connor PM, Kellam JF, Sims SH, et al. Radiation therapy for heterotopic ossification prophylaxis acutely after elbow trauma: a prospective randomized study. J Bone Joint Surg Am. 2010;92(11):2032–8.
13. Rommens PM, Küchle R, Schneider RU, Reuter M. Olecranon fractures in adults: factors influencing outcome. Injury. 2004;35(11):1149–57.
14. Lindenhovius AL, Brouwer KM, Doornberg JN, Ring DC, Kloen P. Long-term outcome of operatively treated fracture-dislocations of the olecranon. J Orthop Trauma. 2008;22(5):325–31.

# 9 Treatment of Longitudinal Forearm Instability: Essex-Lopresti Injury

Laura E. Stoll and Ryan P. Calfee

## Background

Longitudinal forearm instability, or Essex-Lopresti injuries, are relatively rare injuries of the forearm axis, but are easily overlooked, with only 25 % of patients being accurately diagnosed at the time of initial presentation [1]. Curr and Coe initially described an injury to the forearm axis resulting in instability in 1946 [2]. Essex-Lopresti went on to describe the pattern of a radial head fracture, disruption of the interosseous membrane, and distal radioulnar joint (DRUJ) injury in 1951 [3]. Failure to recognize these injuries can lead to loss of motion, chronic pain, and ultimately arthrosis of the DRUJ and radiocapitallar joint. While concomitant injuries to the forearm including radial shaft fractures have been described, the injury typically compromises the soft-tissue support structures of the forearm [4].

These injuries can be overlooked as attention is often focused on the radial head fracture [Fig. 9.1]. To reduce the chance of missed diagnosis, all patients with a radial head fracture should undergo radiographic assessment of the wrist to evaluate for disruption of the DRUJ. In the setting of a radial head fracture or radial head resection, lack of interosseous membrane integrity leads to proximal migration of the radial shaft, which in turn leads to ulnar positive variance, distal ulna impaction, abnormal joint reaction forces, pain, and ultimately arthrosis [1] [Fig. 9.2a, b]. Although radial head excision is an acceptable alternative to fixation or arthroplasty in the treatment of isolated radial head fractures, this treatment requires an intact interosseous membrane and TFCC [5].

The radial head primarily prevents proximal migration of the radius, while the interosseous membrane, DRUJ, and TFCC are secondary stabilizers to longitudinal forearm stability [5, 6]. The interosseous membrane is composed of a membranous portion, proximal and distal interosseous bands, and a central band [7]. The central band, otherwise known as the interosseous ligament (IOL), contains thick fibers that lay in a 20–25° oblique proximal radial to distal ulna direction in the mid-aspect of the forearm [8, 9]. The radial origin is an average of 7.7 cm distal to the radial head. The ulnar insertion is 13.7 cm from the olecranon tip. The IOL attaches 3.2 cm proximal to the ulnar styloid. The insertion lengths on the ulna and radius are on average 42–46 and 31–34 mm [8, 9]. The average width is 1.1 cm and it is 0.5–1.85 mm thick [8–11].

The central band of the interosseous membrane contributes to 71 % of the stiffness of the radio-ulnar axis, whereas the triangular fibrocartilage contributes 8 % [6, 12]. There are a variable number of proximal oblique and distal accessory

L.E. Stoll, MD • R.P. Calfee, MD, MSc (✉)
Department of Orthopedic Surgery, Washington University School of Medicine, 660 South Euclid Ave, Campus Box 8233, St. Louis, MO 63110, USA
e-mail: stolll@wudosis.wustl.edu; calfeer@wudosis.wustl.edu

© Springer International Publishing Switzerland 2017

R.Z. Tashjian (ed.), *The Unstable Elbow*, DOI 10.1007/978-3-319-46019-2_9

bands. The distal portion of the interosseous membrane contributes to stability of the DRUJ, especially in 40 % of patients who have a distal oblique cord [13, 14]. It is the central band, or the IOL, which is reconstructed in Essex-Lopresti injuries. With neutral ulnar variance, 80 % of axial load is transmitted to the radiocarpal joint and 20 % to the ulna [15]. The interosseous membrane, primarily the IOL, converts an axial load from the distal radius to the ulna so that the radiocapitellar joint absorbs only 60 % of this original load.

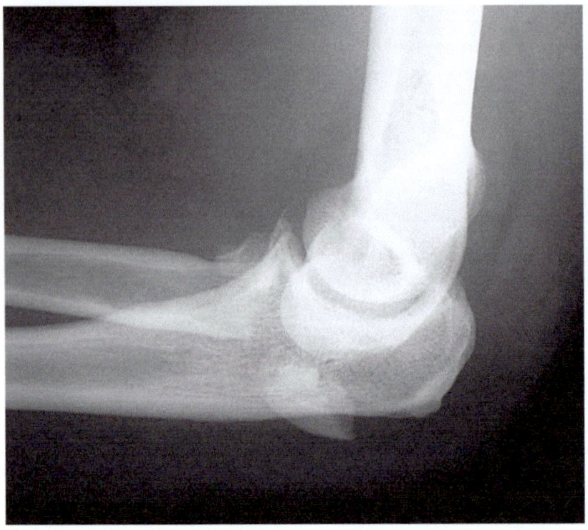

**Fig. 9.1** Lateral radiograph of radial head fracture. Notably, the radial head is comminuted with near contact of the radial neck with the capitellum that should alert to likely Essex-Lopresti injury

The pathoanatomy of the Essex-Lopresti injury lies in the loss of normal conversion of axial forces from the distal radius to the IOL and subsequently to the ulna, creating unequal joint reactive forces at the ulnotrochlear and the radiocapitellar joints. If the radial head support is lost following fracture or excision, and the IOL is disrupted, there is a loss of conversion of the forces and the radius migrates proximally as both the primary and secondary stabilizers are affected [12]. In a cadaveric study, with resection of the radial head, the intraosseous membrane transmits 90 % of the axial load through the forearm, leading to proximal migration of the radius [6]. Proximal radial migration not only leads to impingement proximally, but with every 1 mm of proximal radial migration, there is a 10 % increase in load across the distal ulnar [16]. A recent kinematic analysis suggests that at least a partial lesion of the IOL may precede the radial head fracture in Essex-Lopresti injuries [17]. Even in cases of radial head fracture but incomplete

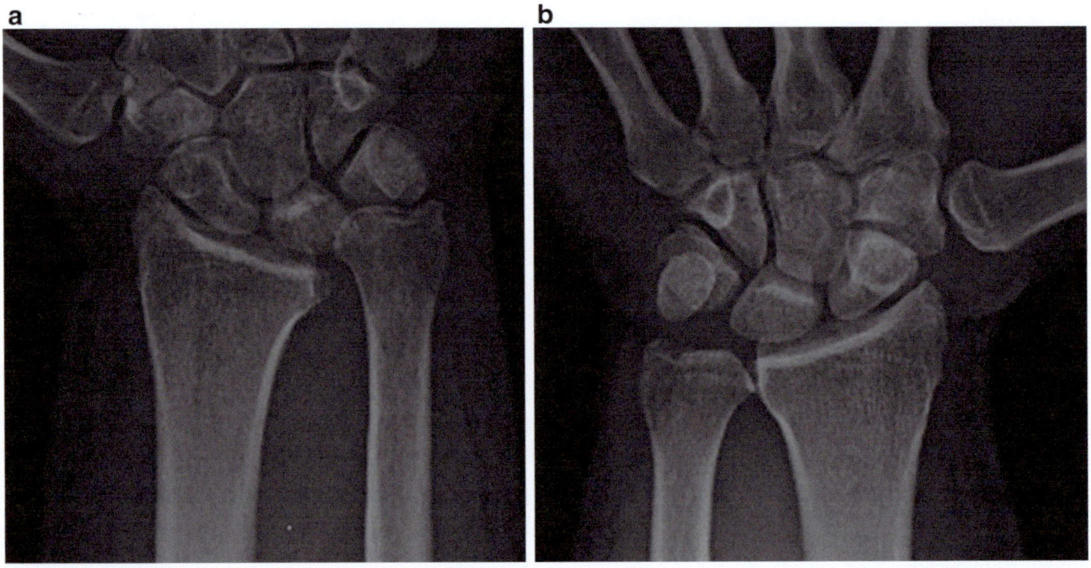

**Fig. 9.2** Posterior-anterior radiographs of the wrist demonstrating pathologic ulnar positive variance in Essex-Lopresti injury on the left (**a**) with comparison uninjured wrist demonstrating minimal ulnar positive variance (**b**)

injury to the interosseous membrane, attenuation of the remaining fibers of the IOM can occur as the IOM becomes responsible for 71 % of the longitudinal stiffness of the forearm [6, 9].

## Evaluation

Patients with Essex-Lopresti injuries usually present after a fall onto an outstretched extremity. Since the disruption of the longitudinal axis of the forearm is primarily a soft tissue injury distal to the radial head, accurate diagnosis is prompted by an astute physical exam. Pain or swelling in the forearm suggests injury to the interosseous membrane. Similarly, pain at the DRUJ in patients with a radial head fracture is indicative of a disruption of the longitudinal axis. The PRUJ and DRUJ should be palpated and manually stressed to evaluate for any instability or pathology. Patients with radial head fractures should have the wrist imaged to evaluate for any associated DRUJ injury, and hence disruption of the soft-tissue supporting structures of the forearm. Radiographic signs of injury at the DRUJ can be subtle so a detailed physical exam and a high suspicion is necessary. A displaced fracture through the base of the ulnar styloid warrants concern for a more extensive forearm axis disruption. In order to accurately determine ulnar variance, a PA of the wrist should be taken with the shoulder abducted and the elbow flexion to 90° (i.e., zero rotation PA view). Contralateral wrist radiographs in the same position are often beneficial as asymmetric alignment is readily appreciated [Fig. 9.2a, b].

If clinical suspicion remains but radiographs are inconclusive, MRI can diagnose injury to the interosseous membrane, with reportedly a greater than 90 % sensitivity and specificity [18, 19]. Alternatively, ultrasound can evaluate interosseous membrane injury [20, 21]. Soubeyrand et al. described the "muscular hernia sign," which is herniation of the forearm musculature through the injured interosseous membrane when a load is placed from anterior to posterior across the forearm [22]. Although less helpful in the acute period, a CT scan can be used to evaluate the integrity of the PRUJ and DRUJ articular surfaces when deciding on reconstructive versus salvage procedures for chronic Essex-Lopresti injuries. In suspected chronic injuries, wrist radiographs should be obtained and examined for asymmetric positive ulnar variance and any signs of ulnar impaction.

When treating radial head fractures, the intraoperative "radius pull test" is described to diagnose Essex-Lopresti injuries [23]. With the shoulder abducted to 90°, the elbow is flexed to 90° with the forearm in neutral. A tenaculum is used to grasp the proximal part of the radius and approximately 20 lb (9.1 kg) is applied in line with the radius while fluoroscopy is used to measure ulnar variance and proximal radial migration at the wrist. Greater than or equal to 3 mm of proximal migration of the radius suggests disruption of the interosseous membrane, whereas greater than or equal to 6 mm of proximal migration indicates disruption of the interosseous membrane and the TFCC. This can be used intraoperatively when contemplating radial head resection, as gross instability of the forearm is a contraindication to radial head resection. Similarly, Soubeyrand et al. reported the "radius joystick test," which involves applying a lateral force to the radial neck with a clamp with the forearm in maximal pronation and the arm firmly held to immobilize the humerus [24]. Lateral displacement of the proximal radius relative to the capitellum under direct visualization indicates disruption of the interosseous membrane.

## Treatment Algorithm (Fig. 9.3)

The choice between repair, reconstruction, and salvage is highly dependent on the timing of presentation as well as the status of the articular surface of the DRUJ, radiocapitellar joint, and radiocarpal joint. In general, those patients who present less than 6 weeks from injury are candidates for repair, while those presenting between 6 and 12 weeks are more likely to undergo reconstruction or salvage procedures. Acute Essex-Lopresti injury is a contraindication to radial head excision as isolated treatment for the radial head fracture.

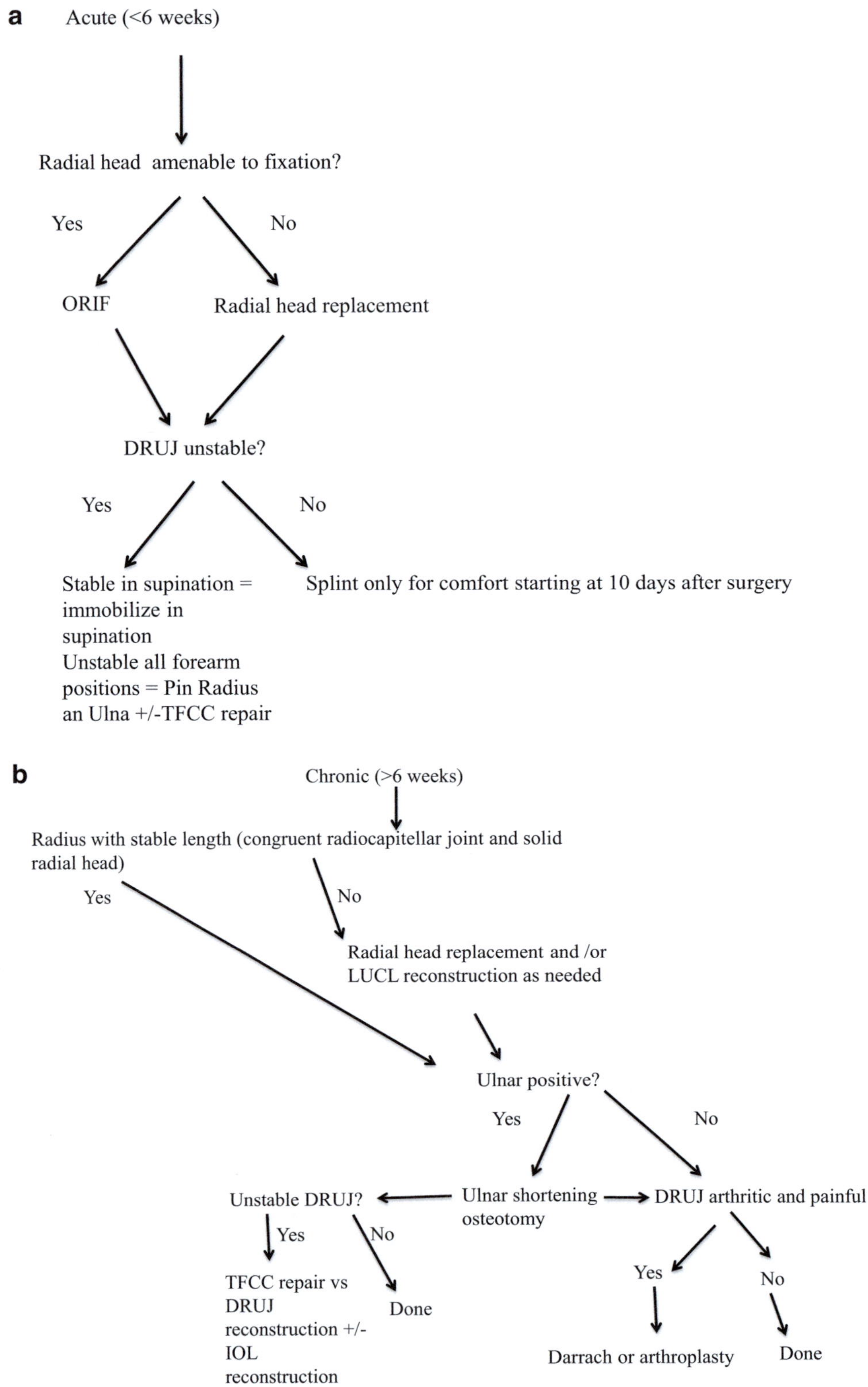


**Fig. 9.3** Algorithm for treatment of Essex-Lopresti injuries—(**a**) Acute injuries (<6 weeks), (**b**) Chronic injuries (>6 weeks)

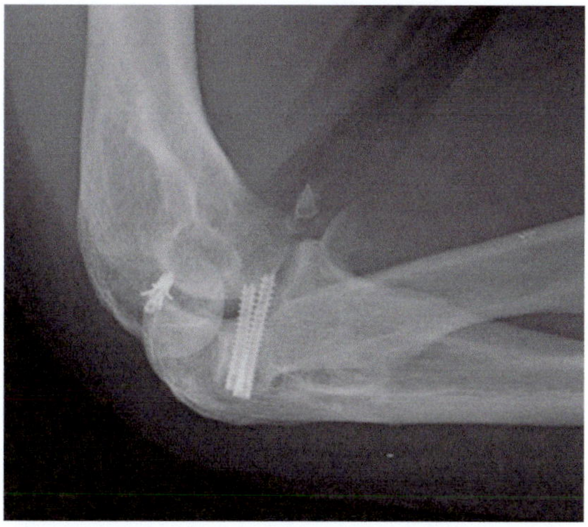

**Fig. 9.4** Patient with challenging case of chronic Essex-Lopresti injury presenting with continued symptoms after failure of radial head fixation resulting in recurrent radius shortening with subluxated radio-capitellar joint

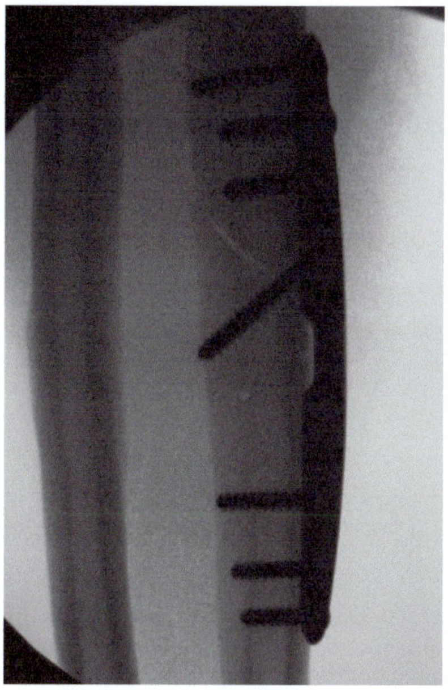

**Fig. 9.5** Ulnar shortening osteotomy with plate and screws across oblique osteotomy used in chronic Essex-Lopresti injury after stabilization of radiocapitellar joint that provided a stable radius length

For those who present late, treatment should initially proceed as if presenting acutely, with radial head replacement [25]. However, in long-standing cases of untreated injuries, or in those who have been treated but are malreduced, there may be radiocapitellar arthritis, which can be worsened symptomatically if a radial head replacement is performed [Fig. 9.4]. If that is the case, one should focus on creating a stable forearm axis and performing a radial head excision.

The DRUJ also needs to be addressed in both acute and chronic cases. Wrist arthroscopy can be used to evaluate the TFCC. In acute cases with an unstable DRUJ, we typically either immobilize in supination (if that affords stability) or simply pin the radius and ulna together (2 0.062″ Kirschner wires just proximal to the DRUJ). As an adjunct in acute cases, the TFCC could be repaired but that would not be our routine. In chronic cases, an ulnar shortening osteotomy addresses ulnar impaction [Fig. 9.5]. An ulnar shortening osteotomy should be considered in chronic injuries to unload the ulnocarpal joint. However, this must be done in conjunction with a stabilization procedure to prevent further proximal migration. An ulnar shortening osteotomy is contraindicated if DRUJ arthritis is present. An excision of the distal ulna or Sauve-Kapandji procedure may be needed when facing a persistently unstable or an arthritic and painful DRUJ to maintain forearm motion.

Reconstruction of the IOL with allograft, autograft, and synthetic materials has been described and should be considered in those cases that fail despite restoration of the radial head through either osteosynthesis or replacement as well as restoration of DRUJ stability. Interestingly, Tejwani and colleagues reported in a cadaveric study that radial head replacement in combination with reconstruction of the IOL with palmaris longus tendon autograft reduces the distal ulnar force better than radial head replacement alone by limiting proximal radial migration [26]. We do not consider reconstruction of the IOL in acute injuries. In chronic injuries that have failed treatment (continued symptomatic longitudinal instability of the forearm) some would consider IOL reconstruction as an alternative to the ultimate salvage of creating a one-bone forearm (radioulnar synostosis creation) [Fig. 9.6].

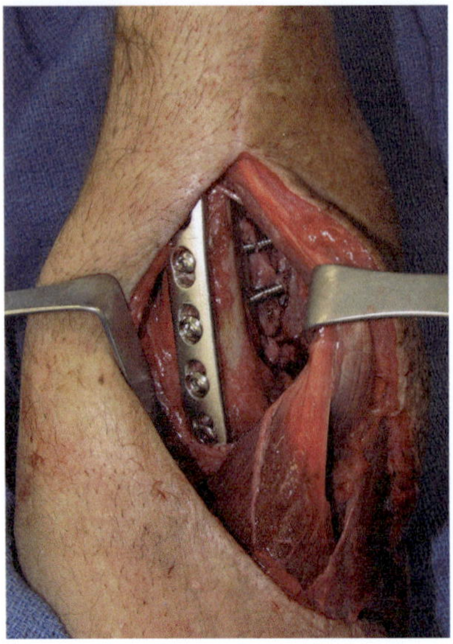

Fig. 9.6 Intraoperative image of creation of one-bone forearm with screws crossing from radius to ulna

## Nonoperative Strategies/Therapy Protocols

There is rarely a role for nonoperative management of Essex-Lopresti injuries. This should only be considered in patients who are medically unfit to undergo an operation.

## Surgical Management/Technique-Based/Surgical Pearls

The key to correct management of Essex-Lopresti injuries is restoration of the relative height of the radial column to the ulna and restoration of the forearm stabilizers. Depending on the extent of radial head injury, management of the acute Essex-Lopresti injury consists of open reduction and internal fixation of the radial head, or radial head arthroplasty if there is comminution. Metallic radial head implants are the most commonly used [Fig. 9.7]. Available literature does not define the role of unipolar versus bipolar metallic radial head arthroplasty. Silicone implants have poor loading characteristics and are prone to failure [27]. Often radial head replacement alone can restore stability [28], although radial head replacement alone theoretically could lead to radiocapitellar pain or prosthesis subluxation if the interosseous membrane and/or TFCC injuries are substantial [25]. Pfaeffle et al. showed decreased radial head prosthesis to capitellum loads if the IOL was also reconstructed [29]. The long-term clinical impact of this finding is unclear. After radial head arthoplasty or repair, there should be an intraoperative assessment of elbow instability, and if present, the posterolateral ligament should be repaired or reconstructed depending on the chronicity of the injury. Lateral collateral ligament injuries greater than 6 weeks from injury should be considered for possible reconstruction as opposed to repair.

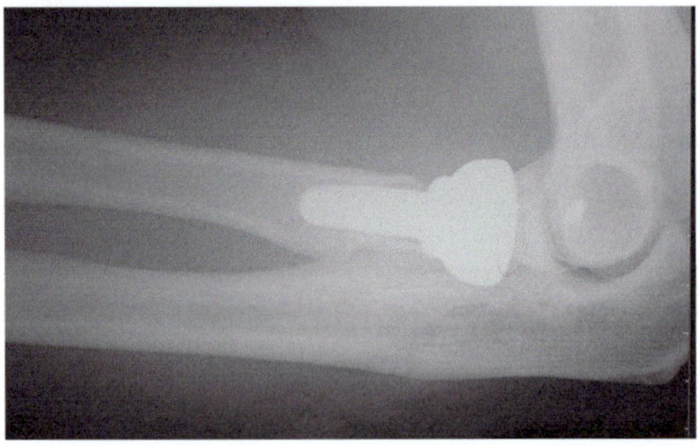

Fig. 9.7 Lateral radiograph of congruent radiocapitellar joint after radial head arthroplasty

The stability of the DRUJ should also be addressed following acute Essex-Lopresti injuries. In acute injuries, the forearm should be immobilized in a position producing maximal stability. This is typically accomplished by splinting in supination postoperatively. If an acute injury is unstable even in supination, the radius and ulnar are reduced and temporarily stabilized by Kirschner wires transfixing the radius and ulna either in isolation or in conjunction with TFCC repair.

Management of chronic Essex-Lopresti injuries is more challenging. Restoration of radial length relative to the forearm axis should be the first treatment goal (if this is not present as indicated by lack of a united radial head and congruent radio-capitellar joint). Regaining pre-injury radius length is readily obtainable in acute situations, but is not possible in chronic injuries secondary to loss of soft tissue compliance. Having established a stable radius length in chronic injuries, if the patient has a symptomatic relatively long ulna, an ulnar shortening osteotomy not only provides a level DRUJ, but also can increase DRUJ stability, if performed proximal to the distal interosseous membrane attachment if a distal oblique band is present [13]. For the ulnar shortening osteotomy, an incision is made over the distal one third ulnar border. The plane of dissection is between the FCU and ECU. There are a number of commercially available shortening systems available. Alternatively, a 6-hole 3.5 mm LCDC plate can be used. The osteotomy can be transverse, oblique, or a step cut [Fig. 9.5]. When planning the amount of bone that needs to be taken to restore negative ulnar variance, one must also take into account the kerf of the saw blade. The plate should be applied in compression mode. If chronic injuries are only complicated by DRUJ instability with congruent radius and ulna lengths, then we would recommend TFCC repair to its foveal insertion or DRUJ ligament reconstruction.

As another approach to Essex-Lopressti injuries, reconstruction of the IOL has been reported for acute and chronic injuries. There is no definitive evidence to suggest the IOL must be repaired to restore longitudinal forearm axis stability acutely or reconstructed in chronic injuries. It is technically challenging and as of yet has not attained widespread use with predictable results.

Multiple different techniques have been reported, including the bone-patellar tendon-bone (BPTB) graft [30], rerouting of the pronator teres [31], FCR [32], semitendinosis [33], palmaris longus [34], and Achilles grafts [35], polyester cords [28, 35], synthetic graft and endobuttons [36, 37], and use of biceps buttons and tenodesis screws [38–40]. BPTB grafts in cadavers had the greatest cross-sectional area, were the most stiff, and allowed the least amount of proximal migration compared to palmaris longus and FCR grafts [11, 26]. However, there was still statistically more proximal migration compared to the native IOL.

If an IOL reconstruction is decided to be performed, independent of the method, an ulnar-shortening osteotomy should be performed first to restore normal ulnar variance if ulnar positive after a chronic injury. For the BPTB technique, an allograft or autograft can be used, with harvest of the BPTB graft being similar to that used for ACL reconstruction. The BPTB graft is first placed on the dorsum of the forearm. The graft is held taut, paralleling the normal fibers of the IOM, and the radial incision is marked out. The ulna is accessed through the ECU/FCU interval. One end of the graft is secured to the ulna with an interfragmentary screw. A small incision is made over the dorsal radial aspect of the forearm, and the interval between the ECRL and ECRB is developed. Alternatively, the interval between the ECRL and brachioradialis can be used, but this puts the superficial radial sensory nerve at risk. The BPTB graft is tunneled beneath the forearm extensors and brought out the radial incision, and finally secured to the posterior radius with an interfragmentary screw. The graft should be tensioned in neutral or supination. Farr et al. determined that the central band was shortest in supination and therefore recommended tensioning the graft in supination [41]. Tejwani reported on IOL reconstruction in conjunction with radial head replacement and found that the forces across the distal ulna were similar to those of an intact forearm [26]. We have not performed any IOL reconstructions but would consider it in cases of chronic injuries having failed other attempts to stabilize the length of the radius (longitudinal forearm stability).

For the persistently unstable forearm having failed primary surgeries including radial head stabilization and possible DRUJ/IOL repairs or reconstructions, creation of a bone-bone forearm is the ultimate salvage technique. Wrist motion and ulnohumeral motion is preserved, though there is loss of pronation/supination. The radius can be transferred to the ulna or a synostosis bridge can be created. One must determine preoperatively the forearm position to provide the most function. If the contralateral forearm is normal, the forearm is placed in a position of neutral to slight pronation. If the contralateral extremity lacks supination, then the forearm should be fused in slight supination. A standard volar Henry approach to the radius is carried out. An osteotomy is made at the mid-shaft level of the radius. The distal radial shaft is pushed to create any distal radius-ulna mismatch. The cortices of the radius and ulna are decorticated at the planned site of fusion. The radius is fixed to the ulna. Cancellous allograft is placed in the interosseous space [Fig. 9.6]. A vascularized free fibula can also be used if additional length or stability is required [42]. Although the radius and ulna can each be osteotomized with the distal radius shaft transferred directly onto the end of the proximal ulna, we have preferred the one-bone-forearm technique of synostosis creation as described.

## Pearls

- Surgery should begin with attempts at recreating the primary stabilizer of the longitudinal axis, the radial head by either internal fixation or arthroplasty.
- Wrist arthroscopy can be used to assess the TFCC for acute injuries and evaluate for potentially reparable TFCC detachments or ulnar impaction syndrome for chronic injuries. Acutely after injury we consider arthroscopy of the wrist for potential TFCC repair infrequently and only in cases of gross DRUJ instability despite restoration of the radius length by the fixation or replacement of the radial head. However, in most cases, we favor pinning the DRUJ in a stable position without attempts to repair the acutely injured TFCC.
- An ulnar shortening osteotomy should be performed prior to the reconstruction of the interosseous ligament if positive ulnar variance is present.
- The incision for the creation of a one-bone forearm includes that used for the ulnar shortening osteotomy of the ulnar side. A second incision is on the radial side of the forearm about 6–8 cm distal the radial head.
- Further clinical studies are needed to support the idea that IOL reconstruction is beneficial in reestablishing forearm stability in Essex-Lopresti injuries.

## Published Outcomes/Complications

*Outcomes*: The outcomes of treatment for Essex-Lopresti injuries are often poor, as a substantial percentage of cases go unrecognized acutely and only 20 % of those treated after a chronic injury having positive outcomes [1]. However, with acute treatment, more encouraging results are seen. Grassman et al. reported an 83 % satisfaction rate at 59 months in those who were treated acutely with DRUJ repair and radial head replacement with no loosening of the radial head prosthesis [43].

Venouziou and colleagues reported a series of seven patients with chronic injuries [44]. All had radial head replacements and ulnar-shortening osteotomies. All had improvement in pain and range of motion of the elbow, forearm, and wrist. Marcotte and Osterman reported improved wrist pain and grip strength in 15 of 16 patients with chronic injuries who were treated with IOL reconstruction using a BPTB graft and ulnar shortening osteotomy without a radial head replacement [30]. Jungbluth et al. reported a series of 13 patients who were diagnosed at least 1 month after initial injury [25]. Ten of the patients underwent radial head replacement and three a Suave-Kapandji procedure. While mean grip strength was 68.5 % that of the unaffected wrist, 11 patients had pain relief. Another option, particularly after a failed Sauve-Kapandji procedure, is a DRUJ implant arthroplasty [45, 46]. The available literature does not define clear indications for DRUJ implant arthroplasty but we would consider this for chronic injuries with a painful DRUJ. Implant arthroplasty may be considered in these cases in the setting of DRUJ arthrosis that would otherwise preclude a joint leveling procedure (ulnar shortening osteotomy).

Allende reported on seven patients treated with the salvage one-bone forearm procedure [47]. All seven patients had a stable and pain-free forearm at 9 years follow-up and all were reportedly satisfied with the position and function of the forearm. However, Peterson et al. reported 19 patients after creation of one-bone forearms with only 69 % of them having good-to-excellent results [48].

*Complications*: Complications include arthritis of the wrist and/or elbow, loss of motion, and pain. Arthritis can not only be the result of the initial injury itself, but also technical failure to correct the longitudinal axis of the forearm correctly, leading to abnormal loading of the proximal and distal joints due to incongruity. Malunion, nonunion, as well as radial head implant loosening can also occur. Compartment syndrome has been reported with creation of a one-bone forearm. A 38 % nonunion rate and 40 % rate of proximal radius impingement has been reported with the one-bone salvage procedure [49].

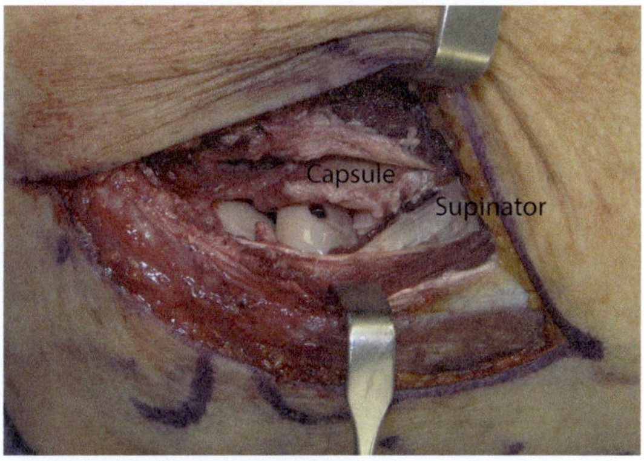


**Fig. 9.8** Intraoperative image of lateral radiocapitellar joint with fixation of the radial head. The confluence of the joint capsule and supinator are well visualized

## Preferred Treatments

We have treated Essex-Lopresti injuries according to their time since injury (acute versus chronic). For acute injuries, key points of history taking include: prior injury to either wrist or elbow, associated musculoskeletal comorbidities, and baseline upper-extremity function. Our examination details tenderness in the forearm and DRUJ as we seek to distinguish isolated radial head fractures from Essex-Lopresti injuries. Initial radiographs examine the injured elbow and forearm and bilateral wrist images taken in identical positions of forearm rotation are used to define the ideal amount of radius length to be restored based on matching ulnar variance.

Our surgical approach starts with restoration of the radius length and stability. When the lateral ulnar collateral ligament is competent we approach the radial head through a lateral ECRB/EDC interval. The surgical window is placed more posteriorly (ECU/anconeus) when repair of the LUCL is needed. We will either primarily fix the radial head or place a metallic arthroplasty. While we will occasionally perform ORIF for comminuted, isolated radial head fractures, we will only pursue ORIF on non-comminuted radial head fractures with solid bone quality when associated with Essex-Lopresti injuries. Our reasoning is that these more substantial injuries are going to place greater amounts of force on the repaired radial head and we believe this increases the chance of failure for tenuous hardware. Second, the impact of lost proximal radius fixation in these injuries has serious implications for forearm and wrist mechanics that once present are often uncorrectable. Internal fixation, when performed, has most commonly been accomplished with headless compression screws that obviate concern over PRUJ impingement, which otherwise may necessitate nonideal hardware placement [Fig. 9.8]. As the radius is grossly mobile in a proximal-distal direction during surgery, implant arthroplasty is sized to produce ulnar variance equal to the opposite contralateral wrist [Fig. 9.9a–e].

After addressing the radius fracture, stability of the radio-capitellar joint is examined to confirm stability. If required, the LUCL is repaired back to the lateral humerus.

Full supination and pronation is confirmed and the DRUJ is tested for stability. In most cases, the DRUJ has been relatively stable after addressing the proximal radius. With a stable DRUJ active motion is initiated at 10 days (wrist flexion/extension, forearm rotation, elbow flexion/extension) using a resting long-arm orthotic for comfort as needed. Passive motion and strengthening are added at 6 weeks [Fig. 9.10a–d]. If the DRUJ is unstable compared to the contralateral wrist, then we determine if one position (usually supination) will stabilize the joint. We prefer to assess DRUJ stability clinically with manual shuck (dorsal and palmar) in pronation, supination, and neutral rotation. We compare the

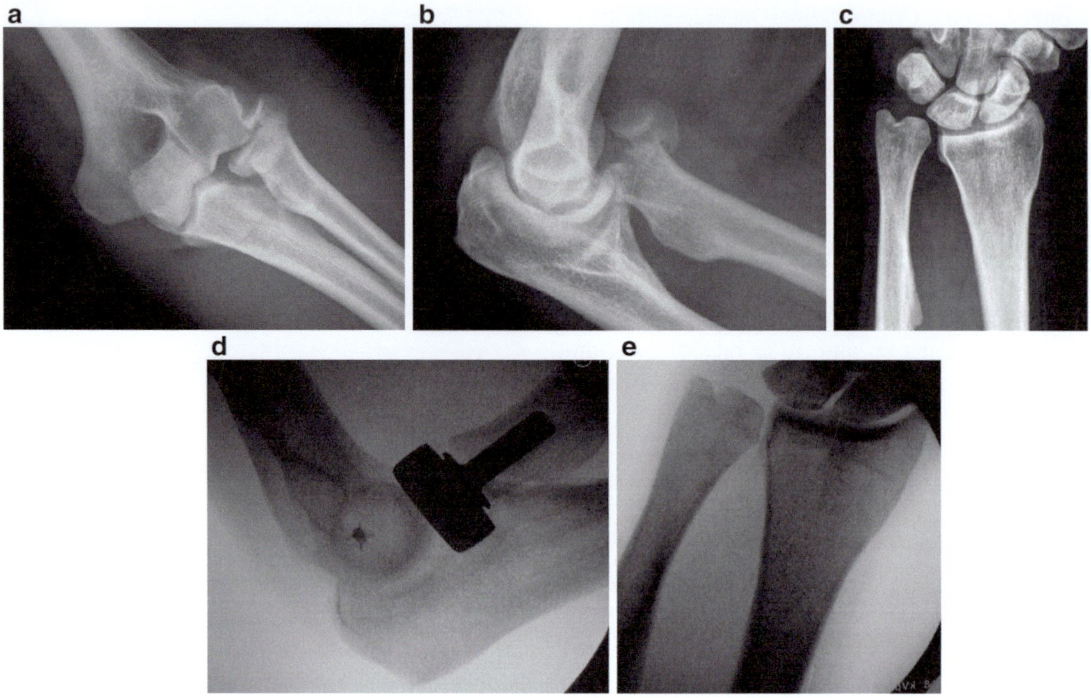


**Fig. 9.9** Anterior posterior (**a**) and lateral (**b**) radiographs of elbow with radial head fracture in Essex-Lopresti injury. Injury wrist radiograph with ulnar positive variance (**c**) secondary to radius shortening. Lateral radiograph (**d**) of elbow after radial head arthroplasty and repair of lateral collateral ligament and final wrist fluoroscopic image (**e**) demonstrating restored ulnar neutral variance

exam to the opposite side to determine if laxity is pathologic. If so, we immobilize in that position and gradually resume forearm rotation 4 weeks after surgery. If unstable in all forearm positions, we proceed with ORIF of any ulnar styloid fracture. Fixing ulnar styloid fractures in these instances has restored stability to the DRUJ reliably when needed. Barring ulnar styloid fracture, we proceed with wrist arthroscopy for examination prior to completing a formal open TFCC repair to the ulnar fovea. We have typically transfixed the radius and ulna with Kirschner wires to protect our TFCC repairs with 2 0.062″ wires placed through four cortices proximal to the DRUJ articular surface. Penetration of four cortices is beneficial to allow for wire removal in the event that wire(s) break prior to planned removal at 4 weeks. We have not repaired or reconstructed the IOM as part of our treatment for these acute injuries.

Chronic Essex-Lopresti injuries have presented for a variety of reasons: elbow or wrist pain, lost forearm rotation, or visible deformity. We discuss the diagnosis at length with the patient as we expect modest improvement when treating these challenging cases. Our radiographic imaging is identical to that of acute injuries but additional attention is paid to arthritic degeneration of the DRUJ and radio-capitellar joint. In cases that have previously been treated surgically, collapse of the radial head or subluxation of the radiocapitellar joint is common. Our first goal is to produce a stable radius length that will not continue to shorten. This usually requires radial head arthroplasty with potential LUCL reconstruction [Fig. 9.11]. In these cases, we do not attempt to re-lengthen the radius back to its native length but instead have a goal of simply setting a stable radius length meaning that the radiocapitellar joint is reduced and stable through motion after placing a metallic radial head arthroplasty (i.e., no further proximal radius migration should occur). Once the radius length is stable we will address the symptomatic wrist. Ulnar impaction

a b c d

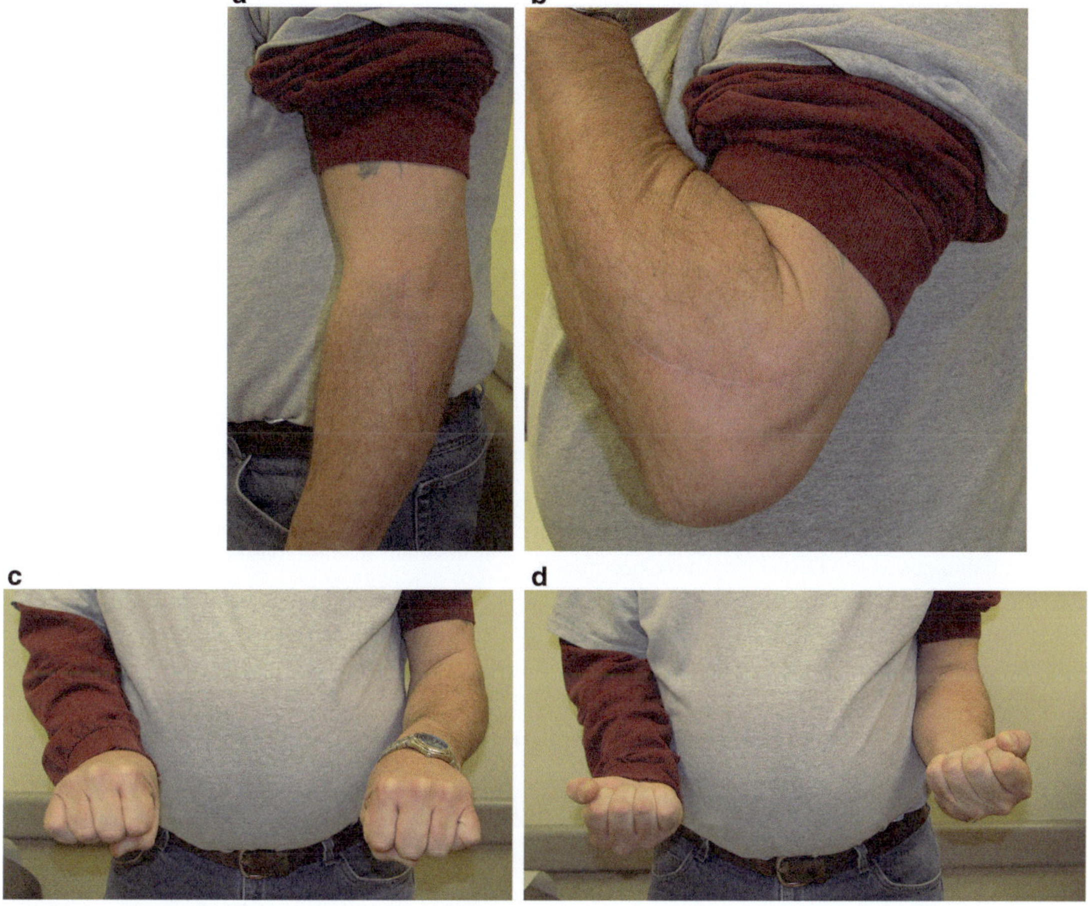

**Fig. 9.10** Excellent outcome at 2 months after surgery for patient from injury images in Fig. 9.9 demonstrating mild restriction in motion of affected left elbow. (**a**) elbow extension, (**b**) elbow flexion, (**c**) pronation, (**d**) supination

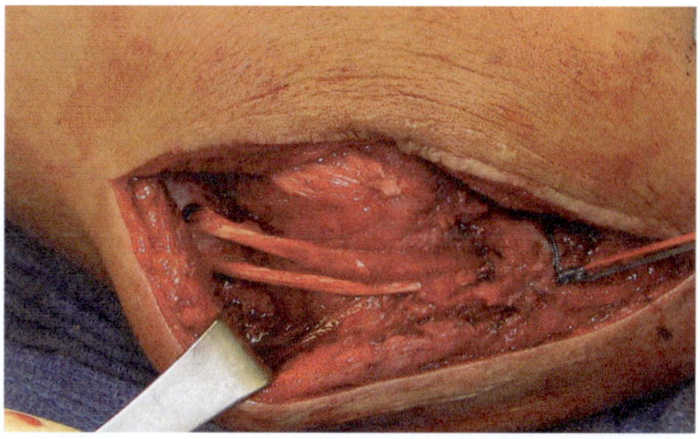

**Fig. 9.11** Intraoperative image of LUCL reconstruction performed with extra-capsular palmaris longus autograft

symptoms are treated with an ulnar shortening osteotomy. Ulnar shortening is also used in isolation for mild DRUJ laxity as it tensions the distal band of the IOM. In our experience 2–3 mm of shortening is enough to improve DRUJ tensioning but in chronic Essex-Lopresti injuries we aim for creating neutral ulnar variance. Shortening is combined with open TFCC repair or reconstruction if the DRUJ is grossly unstable [50]. For the grossly unstable DRUJ and patients with DRUJ arthrosis we consider excision of the distal ulna (Darrach). Although the outcomes are inferior to cases with isolated DRUJ arthrosis, we prefer the Darrach procedure over TFCC repairs/reconstructions in patients reporting impairment from stiffness of forearm rotation. We do not have any experience performing reconstructions of the interosseous membrane or DRUJ implant arthroplasty. For the persistently unstable forearm having failed radial head stabilization and possible DRUJ/IOL repairs or reconstructions, creation of a bone-bone forearm is the ultimate salvage.

## Conclusion

Essex-Lopresti injuries are a complex combination of bony and ligamentous injury. Treatment is first aimed at restoring the longitudinal stability of the forearm by reestablishing a load-bearing radial head and congruent radiocapitellar joint. Second, DRUJ instability is assessed and, if present, is treated with the least invasive sufficient option moving from immobilization, to pinning the radius and ulna or even to include TFCC repair. Chronic Essex-Lopresti injuries present unique challenges as the DRUJ may have become arthritic and the original length of the radius cannot be reestablished if the radius has remained shortened since injury. Treatment of chronic injuries includes the creation of a length stable radius typically with a radial head arthroplasty and distal ulnar reconstructive procedures for ulnar impaction. Indications for IOL reconstruction are still unclear in the acute and chronic settings. Ultimate salvage for a persistently unstable forearm is the creation of a one-bone forearm.

## References


1. Trousdale RT, Amadio PC, Cooney WP, Morrey BF. Radio-ulnar dissociation. A review of twenty cases. J Bone Joint Surg Am. 1992;74(10):1486–97.
2. Curr JF, Coe WA. Dislocation of the inferior radio-ulnar joint. Br J Surg. 1946;34:74–7.
3. Essex-Lopresti P. Fractures of the radial head with distal radio-ulnar dislocation; report of two cases. J Bone Joint Surg Br. 1951;33B(2):244–7.
4. Eglseder WA, Hay M. Combined Essex-Lopresti and radial shaft fractures: case report. J Trauma. 1993;34(2):310–2.
5. Rabinowitz RS, Light TR, Havey RM, Gourineni P, Patwardhan AG, Sartori MJ, et al. The role of the interosseous membrane and triangular fibrocartilage complex in forearm stability. J Hand Surg Am. 1994;19(3):385–93.
6. Hotchkiss RN, An KN, Sowa DT, Basta S, Weiland AJ. An anatomic and mechanical study of the interosseous membrane of the forearm: pathomechanics of proximal migration of the radius. J Hand Surg Am. 1989;14(2 Pt 1):256–61.
7. Noda K, Goto A, Murase T, Sugamoto K, Yoshikawa H, Moritomo H. Interosseous membrane of the forearm: an anatomical study of ligament attachment locations. J Hand Surg Am. 2009;34(3):415–22.
8. Chandler JW, Stabile KJ, Pfaeffle HJ, Li Z-M, Woo SL-Y, Tomaino MM. Anatomic parameters for planning of interosseous ligament reconstruction using computer-assisted techniques. J Hand Surg Am. 2003;28(1):111–6.
9. Skahen JR, Palmer AK, Werner FW, Fortino MD. The interosseous membrane of the forearm: anatomy and function. J Hand Surg Am. 1997;22(6):981–5.
10. McGinley J, Roach N, Gaughan J, Kozin S. Forearm interosseous membrane imaging and anatomy. Skeletal Radiol. 2004;33(10):561.
11. Stabile KJ, Pfaeffle J, Saris I, Li Z-M, Tomaino MM. Structural properties of reconstruction constructs for the interosseous ligament of the forearm. J Hand Surg Am. 2005;30(2):312–8.
12. Birkbeck DP, Failla JM, Hoshaw SJ, Fyhrie DP, Schaffler M. The interosseous membrane affects load distribution in the forearm. J Hand Surg Am. 1997;22(6):975–80.
13. Arimitsu S, Moritomo H, Kitamura T, Berglund LJ, Zhao KD, An K-N, et al. The stabilizing effect of the distal interosseous membrane on the distal radioulnar joint in an ulnar shortening procedure: a biomechanical study. J Bone Joint Surg Am. 2011;93(21):2022–30.
14. Gofton WT, Gordon KD, Dunning CE. Soft-tissue stabilizers of the distal radioulnar joint: an in vitro kinematic study. J Hand Surg Am. 2004;29(3):423–31.
15. Palmer AK, Werner FW. Biomechanics of the distal radioulnar joint. Clin Orthop Relat Res. 1984;(187):26–35.
16. Shepard MF, Markolf KL, Dunbar AM. Effects of radial head excision and distal radial shortening on load-sharing in cadaver forearms. J Bone Joint Surg Am. 2001;83-A(1):92–100.
17. Wegmann K, Engel K, Burkhart KJ, Ebinger M, Holz R, Brüggemann G-P, et al. Sequence of the Essex-Lopresti lesion--a high-speed video documentation and kinematic analysis. Acta Orthop. 2014;85(2):177–80.
18. Fester EW, Murray PM, Sanders TG, Ingari JV. The efficacy of magnetic resonance imaging and ultrasound in detecting disruptions of the forearm interosseous membrane: a cadaver study. J Hand Surg Am. 2002;27(3):418–24.
19. McGinley JC, Roach N, Hopgood BC, Limmer K, Kozin SH. Forearm interosseous membrane trauma: MRI diagnostic criteria and injury patterns. Skeletal Radiol. 2006;35(5):275–81.
20. Failla JM, Jacobson J, van Holsbeeck M. Ultrasound diagnosis and surgical pathology of the torn interosseous membrane in forearm fractures/dislocations. J Hand Surg Am. 1999;24(2):257–66.
21. Jaakkola JI, Riggans DH, Lourie GM, Lang CJ. Ultrasonography for the evaluation of forearm interosseous membrane disruption in a cadaver model. J Hand Surg Am. 2001;26(6):1053–7.
22. Soubeyrand M, Lafont C, Oberlin C, France W, Maulat I, Degeorges R. The "muscular hernia sign":

an original ultrasonographic sign to detect lesions of the forearm's interosseous membrane. Surg Radiol Anat. 2006;28(4):372–8.
23. Smith AM, Urbanosky LR, Castle JA, Rushing JT, Ruch DS. Radius pull test: predictor of longitudinal forearm instability. J Bone Joint Surg Am. 2002; 84-A(11):1970–6.
24. Soubeyrand M, Ciais G, Wassermann V, Kalouche I, Biau D, Dumontier C, et al. The intra-operative radius joystick test to diagnose complete disruption of the interosseous membrane. J Bone Joint Surg Br. 2011; 93(10):1389–94.
25. Jungbluth P, Frangen TM, Arens S, Muhr G, Kälicke T. The undiagnosed Essex-Lopresti injury. J Bone Joint Surg Br. 2006;88(12):1629–33.
26. Tejwani SG, Markolf KL, Benhaim P. Graft reconstruction of the interosseous membrane in conjunction with metallic radial head replacement: a cadaveric study. J Hand Surg Am. 2005;30(2):335–42.
27. Vanderwilde RS, Morrey BF, Melberg MW, Vinh TN. Inflammatory arthritis after failure of silicone rubber replacement of the radial head. J Bone Joint Surg Br. 1994;76(1):78–81.
28. Sellman DC, Seitz WH, Postak PD, Greenwald AS. Reconstructive strategies for radioulnar dissociation: a biomechanical study. J Orthop Trauma. 1995;9(6): 516–22.
29. Pfaeffle HJ, Stabile KJ, Li Z-M, Tomaino MM. Reconstruction of the interosseous ligament unloads metallic radial head arthroplasty and the distal ulna in cadavers. J Hand Surg Am. 2006;31(2):269–78.
30. Marcotte AL, Osterman AL. Longitudinal radioulnar dissociation: identification and treatment of acute and chronic injuries. Hand Clin. 2007;23(2):195–208. vi.
31. Chloros GD, Wiesler ER, Stabile KJ, Papadonikolakis A, Ruch DS, Kuzma GR. Reconstruction of Essex-Lopresti injury of the forearm: technical note. J Hand Surg Am. 2008;33(1):124–30.
32. Skahen JR, Palmer AK, Werner FW, Fortino MD. Reconstruction of the interosseous membrane of the forearm in cadavers. J Hand Surg Am. 1997;22(6):986–94.
33. Soubeyrand M, Oberlin C, Dumontier C, Belkheyar Z, Lafont C, Degeorges R. Ligamentoplasty of the forearm interosseous membrane using the semitendinosus tendon: anatomical study and surgical procedure. Surg Radiol Anat. 2006;28(3):300–7.
34. Tejwani SG, Markolf KL, Benhaim P. Reconstruction of the interosseous membrane of the forearm with a graft substitute: a cadaveric study. J Hand Surg Am. 2005;30(2):326–34.
35. Tomaino MM, Pfaeffle J, Stabile K, Li Z-M. Reconstruction of the interosseous ligament of the forearm reduces load on the radial head in cadavers. J Hand Surg Br. 2003;28(3):267–70.
36. Jones CM, Kam CC, Ouellette EA, Milne EL, Kaimrajh D, Latta LL. Comparison of 2 forearm reconstructions for longitudinal radioulnar dissociation: a cadaver study. J Hand Surg Am. 2012;37(4):741–7.
37. Sabo MT, Watts AC. Reconstructing the interosseous membrane: a technique using synthetic graft and endobuttons. Tech Hand Up Extrem Surg. 2012;16(4): 187–93.
38. Drake ML, Farber GL, White KL, Parks BG, Segalman KA. Restoration of longitudinal forearm stability using a suture button construct. J Hand Surg Am. 2010;35(12):1981–5.
39. Kam CC, Jones CM, Fennema JL, Latta LL, Ouellette EA, Evans PJ. Suture-button construct for interosseous ligament reconstruction in longitudinal radioulnar dissociations: a biomechanical study. J Hand Surg Am. 2010;35(10):1626–32.
40. Miller AJ, Naik TU, Seigerman DA, Ilyas AM. Anatomic interosseus membrane reconstruction utilizing the biceps button and screw tenodesis for Essex-Lopresti injuries. Tech Hand Up Extrem Surg. 2015;20:6.
41. Farr LD, Werner FW, McGrattan ML, Zwerling SR, Harley BJ. Anatomy and biomechanics of the forearm interosseous membrane. J Hand Surg Am. 2015; 40(6):1145–51.e2.
42. Arai K, Toh S, Yasumura M, Okamoto Y, Harata S. One-bone forearm formation using vascularized fibula graft for massive bone defect of the forearm with infection: case report. J Reconstr Microsurg. 2001;17(03):151–6.
43. Grassmann JP, Hakimi M, Gehrmann SV, Betsch M, Kröpil P, Wild M, et al. The treatment of the acute Essex-Lopresti injury. Bone Joint J. 2014;96-B(10):1385–91.
44. Venouziou AI, Papatheodorou LK, Weiser RW, Sotereanos DG. Chronic Essex-Lopresti injuries: an alternative treatment method. J Shoulder Elbow Surg. 2014;23(6):861–6.
45. Kachooei AR, Chase SM, Jupiter JB. Outcome assessment after Aptis distal radioulnar joint (DRUJ) implant arthroplasty. Arch Bone Joint Surg. 2014;2(3):180–4.
46. Martínez Villén G, García Martínez B, Aso VA. Total distal radioulnar joint prosthesis as salvage surgery in multioperated patients. Chir Main. 2014;33(6):390–5.
47. Allende C, Allende BT. Posttraumatic one-bone forearm reconstruction. A report of seven cases. J Bone Joint Surg Am. 2004;86-A(2):364–9.
48. Peterson CA, Maki S, Wood MB. Clinical results of the one-bone forearm. J Hand Surg Am. 1995;20(4): 609–18.
49. Jacoby SM, Bachoura A, Diprinzio EV, Culp RW, Osterman AL. Complications following one-bone forearm surgery for posttraumatic forearm and distal radioulnar joint instability. J Hand Surg Am. 2013; 38(5):976–982.e1.
50. Adams BD, Berger RA. An anatomic reconstruction of the distal radioulnar ligaments for posttraumatic distal radioulnar joint instability. J Hand Surg Am. 2002;27(2):243–51.

# Part III

# Chronic Instabilities of the Elbow

# 10 Evaluation and Management of Posterolateral Rotatory Instability (PLRI)

Pieter Caekebeke, Megan Anne Conti Mica, and Roger van Riet

## Background

The first reports of lateral elbow instability focused on the repair of the lateral elbow ligaments by Osborne and Cotterill [1]. These authors reported on a direct repair of the lateral elbow ligamentous structures in 1966 [1]. They performed a plication of the ligaments in cases with ligament laxity or avulsion of the lateral collateral ligament. They also described an intermittent subluxation of the lateral head into a capsular pocket or capitellar defect (Osbourne-Cotteril lesion), which could easily be reduced by the patient. In retrospect, these signs are consistent with posterolateral instability, now recognized as the most common type of symptomatic chronic instability of the elbow [2]. Laxity of the posterolateral capsule was considered to be the origin of the posterior instability.

Both Hassman et al. and Simeonides et al. reported on recurrent instability of the elbow in 1975 [3, 4]. The former described a patient with a stable ulnohumeral joint despite having required 12 closed reductions of the elbow. Burgess and Sprague reported two cases with posttraumatic radial head subluxation. Post-operative evaluation showed persistent posterior radial head subluxation after annular ligament tightening [5]. Good results were seen in the last three reports using the Osborne and Cotterill technique, which probably involved repair of the insufficient lateral ulnar collateral ligament (LUCL). PLRI, as a formal entity, was not clearly described until 1991 by O'Driscoll et al. who published a case series of five patients, with persistent elbow instability [6]. In general, O'Driscoll's description of PLRI focusing on the LUCL as the primary restraint to PLRI has remained constant with an understanding that the other components of the lateral ligamentous complex (radial collateral ligament, annular ligament) and extensor tendons probably also have secondary stabilizing role.

The lateral collateral ligament complex is comprised of the radial collateral ligament (RCL), the lateral ulnar collateral ligament

---

**Electronic supplementary material** The online version of this chapter (doi:10.1007/978-3-319-46019-2_10) contains supplementary material, which is available to authorized users. Videos can also be accessed at http://link.springer.com/chapter/10.1007/978-3-319-46019-2_10.

P. Caekebeke, MD
Department of Orthopedic, AZ Monica, Deurne, Stevenslei 20, Deurne, Antwerpen 2100, Belgium
e-mail: Caekebeke.pieter@hotmail.com

M.A. Conti Mica, MD
Department of Orthopedics, University of Chicago, 5841 S. Maryland Ave, Chicago, IL 60637, USA
e-mail: mcontimica@bsd.uchicago.edu

R. van Riet, MD, PhD (✉)
Department of Orthopedic Surgery and Traumatology, AZ Monica, Stevenslei 20, Deurne, Antwerpen 2100, Belgium
e-mail: rogervanriet@hotmail.com; drrogervanriet@azmonica.be

© Springer International Publishing Switzerland 2017
R.Z. Tashjian (ed.), *The Unstable Elbow*, DOI 10.1007/978-3-319-46019-2_10

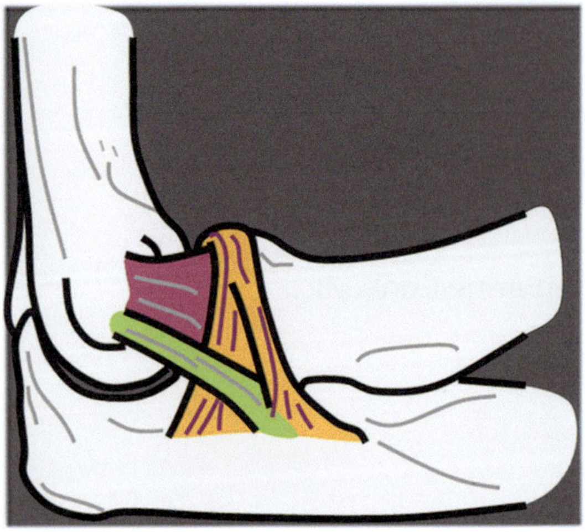

**Fig. 10.1** Schematic overview of the lateral ligamentous anatomy of the elbow. *Purple*: RCL; *Green*: LUCL; *Yellow*: annular ligament (Courtesy of MoRe Foundation)

(LUCL) (Fig. 10.1), the annular ligament, and the accessory lateral collateral ligament. The RCL and LUCL share their origin on the lateral epicondyle and are not individually identifiable at this level [7]. The LUCL arches over the annular ligament and insert on the tubercle of the supinator crest. The insertion has been described as bilobed. The extensor digiti quinti, the extensor carpi ulnaris, and the anconeus muscle cover various portions of the ligament [8].

The LUCL resists external rotation stresses to the elbow [7], but sectioning of the LUCL alone does not induce PLRI. For this to happen, both the RCL and LUCL need to be ruptured [7, 9, 10]. The annular ligament remains intact [11]. Resection of the radial head or coronoid increases the magnitude of PLRI [12]. Muscular constraints play a role maintaining stability of the elbow. Contraction of the extensor muscles has been shown to decrease laxity in LCL deficient elbows [13] and sectioning of the muscles increases laxity [9]. The anconeus muscle has been shown to create a valgus moment and may also play a role in increasing stability of the elbow [14].

The pathoanatomy of an injury leading to lateral elbow instability can be described as a circle with the disruption of soft tissue going from lateral to medial. The soft tissue disruptions are classically described in three stages [6, 15]. Stage 1 encompasses a LUCL disruption. In stage 2, the remainder of the LCL and the anterior and posterior capsules are disrupted. In stage 3A, the posterior bundle of the MCL fails and in stage 3B the anterior bundle of the MCL is also disrupted. The term posterolateral instability characterizes the mechanism of injury in which the ulna externally rotates on the humerus coupled with posterolateral radiohumeral subluxation.

PLRI is the most common cause of residual instability following a simple elbow dislocation. Different mechanisms of injury may lead to chronic PLRI. The LCL complex has a tendency not to heal following injury [16]. Some patients will have a history of one or more simple dislocations. Others may not have had a documented dislocation but a relatively minor trauma, leading to persistent and symptomatic subluxation of the elbow [17]. Some may have a history of repetitive cortisone injections leading to attrition of the lateral ligament complex. PLRI has been described in the setting of cubitus varus deformity of the distal humerus from prior distal humeral malunions with chronic attrition of the LCL. Finally, PLRI can occur following surgery to the lateral side of the elbow, when the LCL is released unintentionally, for example with lateral epicondylitis debridement [18].

## Evaluation

The diagnosis of chronic PLRI is predominantly clinical. Patients will come in complaining of recurrent episodes of elbow dislocations, or more commonly, a sensation of instability, pain, and mechanical symptoms like clicking or catching. Several specific clinical tests have been described to diagnose PLRI.

Varus laxity is present due to rupture of the lateral sided stabilizers but is difficult to quantify clinically. The pivot shift test [19] was originally described by O'Driscoll to detect PLRI and is sensitive but, due to apprehension, the specificity is low in the awake patient. The simplest way to perform this test is with the patient in supine position. The examiner takes the forearm of the patient with both hands, while the shoulder is elevated. The forearm is hypersupinated and a valgus stress and axial load are applied to the elbow. The elbow is then moved from extension to flexion and vice versa. Apprehension or pain is considered to be a positive sign in a patient who is awake. When a patient is placed under general or regional anaesthesia, subluxation or dislocation is considered a positive test [19]. The radial head subluxation usually occurs during extension with the elbow at around 30–45° of flexion (Fig. 10.2). The elbow reduces with further flexion beyond 30° and dislocates with extension beyond 30°.

O'Driscoll has also described the posterolateral rotatory drawer test, similar to the Lachman test of the knee, and has found to be more sensitive and specific than the pivot shift test to detect PLRI [19]. The radiohumeral joint is palpated and the forearm as a whole is externally rotated. In a positive test, the radial head can be felt to rotate posteriorly, relative to the humerus. It is very important not to supinate the forearm during the posterior drawer test as this will result in a false positive test. The cam shape of the radial head will push the finger out of the radiohumeral joint, resembling actual posterior translation of the radial head.

The tabletop test and tabletop relocation tests are carried out with the hand of the patient supported on a table. The forearm is supinated and the patient is asked to support their weight on the arm while flexing the elbow. Pain and apprehension may occur with the elbow at about 40° of flexion. The test is then repeated but the examiner now supports (relocates) the radial head. Pain and apprehension should not occur in a positive test [20] but often the relocation does not completely obliterate the apprehension.

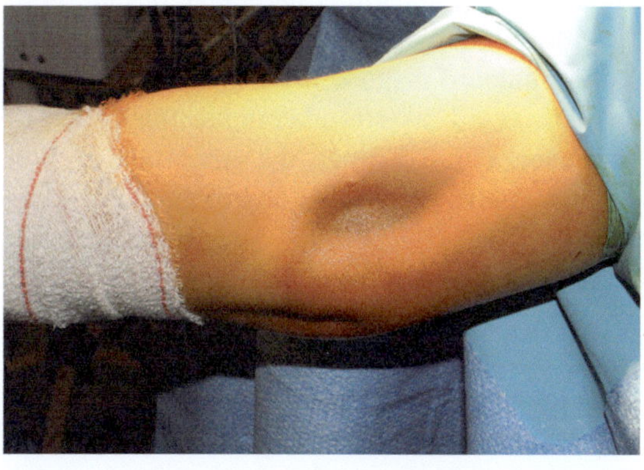

**Fig. 10.2** A positive pivot shift test results in a posterior (sub)luxation of the radial head relative to the humerus. This is apparent by a depression in the skin, proximal to the radial head (Courtesy of MoRe Foundation)

Both the push-up and chair signs have been shown to be sensitive to detect PLRI as well. The patient is asked to perform an active push-up, with the forearm in supination. If the tests are positive, the patient is unable to fully extend the elbow or the patient shows apprehension and guarding while attempting to finish the push-up [21]. It is important to use more than one test. In gross instability, the diagnosis will be clear, but in more subtle cases, some of the tests may be falsely negative. In patients with underlying hyperlaxity, some of the tests may also be falsely positive so one must test for this as well during the physical exam. The diagnosis can only be made if more than one test are considered to be positive. Repeating the tests after an intra-articular injection of local anaesthetic may be considered if the clinical exam is inconclusive.

## Imaging

Radiographs (Fig. 10.3) and CT scans may show indirect signs of ligamentous injury such as calcification of the ligament or subluxation of the joint. In most cases, however, radiographs and CTs will be negative, although in some cases an Osbourne-Cotterill lesion may be visible [1]. MRI scanning is helpful in patients presenting with chronic instability [22]. A ruptured LCL can often be visualized (Fig. 10.4). Scar tissue will be present in most chronic cases. Cartilage lesions are common and these will have a negative effect on the final outcome of treatment.

## Treatment Algorithm

Nonoperative treatment with physical therapy is a reasonable initial treatment for patients with PLRI. It usually includes strengthening of the dynamic stabilizers and activity modification to

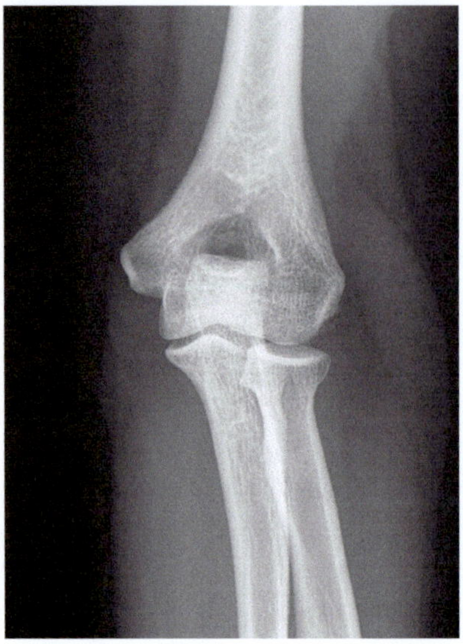

**Fig. 10.3** Anteroposterior radiograph showing a discrete bony avulsion of the lateral collateral ligament complex (Courtesy of MoRe Foundation)

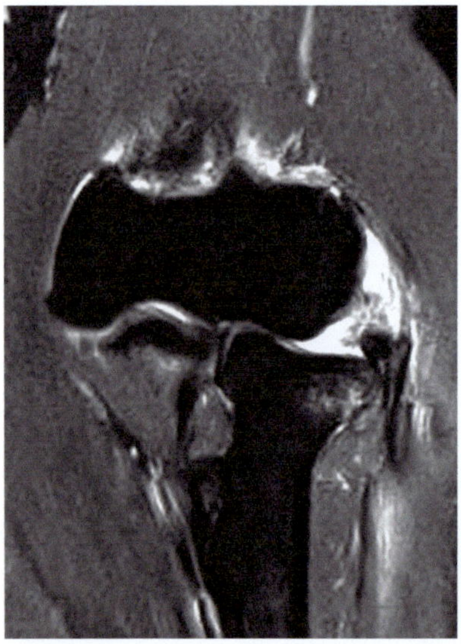

**Fig. 10.4** Magnetic resonance image of the elbow, showing a lateral collateral ligament avulsion (Courtesy of MoRe Foundation)

try to avoid activities with the elbow flexed to prevent subluxation. Bracing is an option and should be discussed with the patient; however, the efficacy of bracing is unknown in cases of chronic instability. Once nonoperative options fail, surgical intervention is indicated.

Surgery is indicated in patients with persistent symptomatic instability of the elbow with pain. Ligament reconstruction has a higher chance of failure if patients have pain only, without symptoms of instability and, in general, should be avoided in these cases. There are several surgical techniques to treat PLRI and, in general, the results are good to excellent in a majority of patients [23]. Primary repair of the chronically ruptured LCL complex depends on the integrity and quality of the remaining tissue. A full arthroscopic repair has been described with good results [24]. Preoperative screening of patients is essential if an arthroscopic technique is contemplated. No comparative data is available on when to imbricate the LCL, when to repair, or when to reconstruct. There is some weak evidence suggesting that reconstruction may be better than repair, in a large group of patients with mixed pathology [17]. Based on the available literature and our personal experiences, we have developed an algorithm (Fig. 10.5).

## Surgical Management

### Arthroscopic Technique

An all-arthroscopic technique has been described for both acute and chronic cases (Video 10.1). We use an adaptation of the original technique that was described by Savoie et al. [24]. It is important to test stability and range of motion of the elbow under anaesthesia. The procedure starts with a standard diagnostic elbow arthroscopy. In order to avoid disastrous complications such as permanent nerve damage, the same standard precautions are followed. We do not recommend an all-arthroscopic technique if the surgeon is not experienced in elbow arthroscopy. The ulnar nerve is palpated and marked and the joint is insufflated.

The arthroscopy starts in the anterior compartment. Some synovitis is almost always present. The elbow is inspected for signs of degenerative changes and cartilage lesions. A distal posterolateral portal is then made at the lateral tip of the olecranon. This portal is slightly more distal than

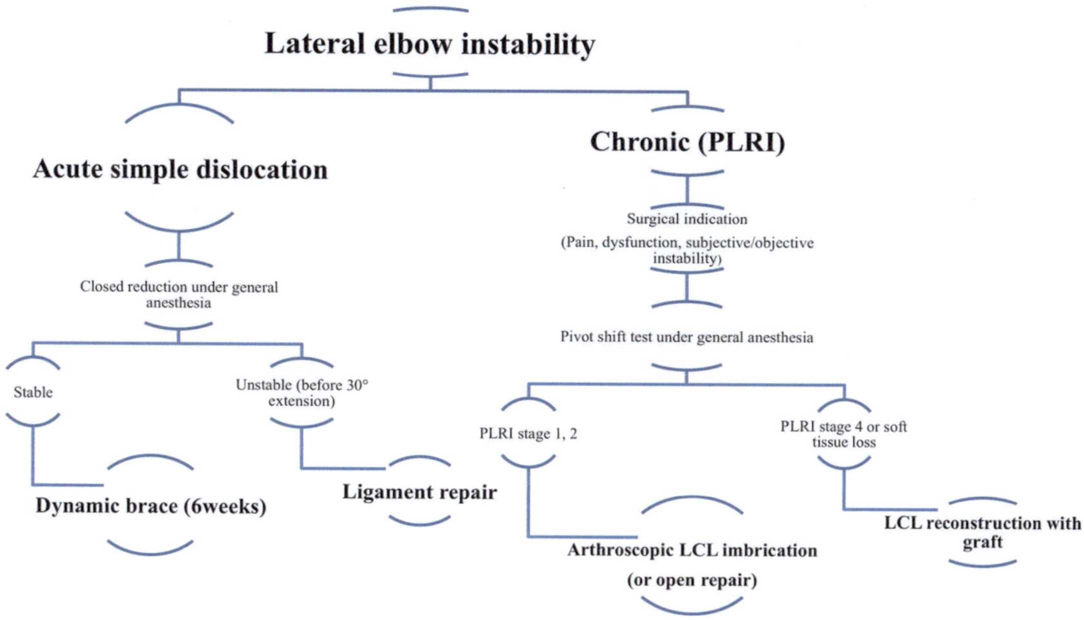


**Fig. 10.5** Treatment algorithm for patients with symptomatic posterolateral rotatory instability (Courtesy of MoRe Foundation)

the classic posterolateral portal, in order to improve the access to the radiohumeral gutter. The scope is first directed to the ulnar gutter, where the posterior band and part of the anterior band of the MCL can be visualized. A valgus stress is applied to the elbow to evaluate the MCL. There should be little or no opening of the medial joint. The olecranon fossa and olecranon tip are inspected. If necessary, a central posterior portal can be made to address posterior pathology. The scope is then brought into the radiohumeral gutter. Typically, there is a synovial fringe that may block a direct view to the radial head. A needle is used to determine the perfect position of the soft spot portal and the portal is made. A shaver is used to remove the synovial fringe and any synovitis. The ulnohumeral joint is inspected and the 'drive through sign' [24] is evaluated. In patients with a clear lateral instability, the scope can be brought from the lateral side to the ulnar gutter. We further evaluate lateral stability by performing a pivot shift test under a direct arthroscopic view. We have found that it is very difficult to perform the actual pivot shift, as the scope prevents a true subluxation/relocation click. We have therefore adapted this test and now perform the pivot shift test with varus stress instead of valgus stress. This frees the radius from the humerus and the posterior translation of the radial head can easily be quantified arthroscopically.

The arthroscopic imbrication of the LCL is then performed. The scope remains in the radiohumeral gutter. A wide lumen spinal needle is loaded with a no. 2 PDS suture. The lateral epicondyle is palpated and the needle punctures the skin at the isometric point of the LCL complex [25]. From there, the needle is directed to the radiohumeral gutter and the suture is shuttled into the joint under a direct arthroscopic view. The PDS suture is brought outside the skin through the soft spot portal and the needle is removed (Fig. 10.6). The suture now runs from the lateral epicondyle to the soft spot. The needle is reloaded with a new strand of PDS suture. The subcutaneous border of the ulna is palpated and the needle punctures the skin on the subcutaneous border, just distal to the radial head. Care is taken to stay on the ulnar bone as the needle is again brought into view in the radiohumeral gutter (Fig. 10.7). The suture is shuttled and again taken out of the soft spot portal,

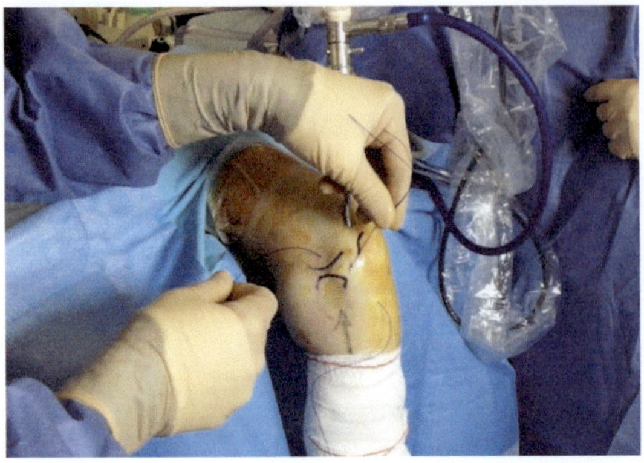

**Fig. 10.6** Image of the lateral side of the elbow. Radial head and capitellum are marked on the skin. A PDS suture enters the joint at the insertion of the LUCL on the lateral epicondyle and exits the skin from the soft spot portal (Courtesy of MoRe Foundation)

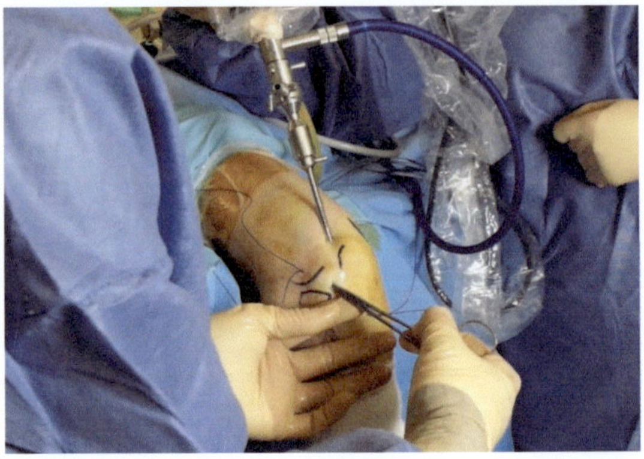

**Fig. 10.8** Both strands of the PDS suture are tunnelled subcutaneously to the soft spot portal. This forms a loop of suture, running from the soft spot portal, subcutaneously to the lateral epicondyle, intra-articularly to the supinator crest and again subcutaneous to the soft spot portal (Courtesy of MoRe Foundation)

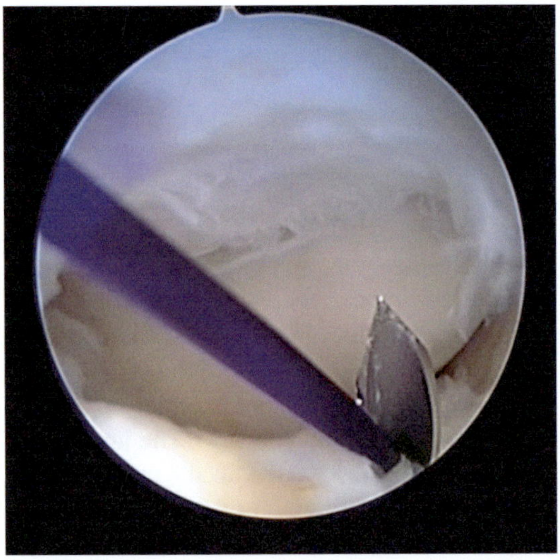

**Fig. 10.7** Arthroscopic view from the radiohumeral gutter. A needle is brought into the gutter from the origin of the LUCL at the supinator crest. A PDS suture is shuttled through the needle, to form the distal half of the imbrication. This suture is then tied to the distal end, to form a single strand of suture (Courtesy of MoRe Foundation)

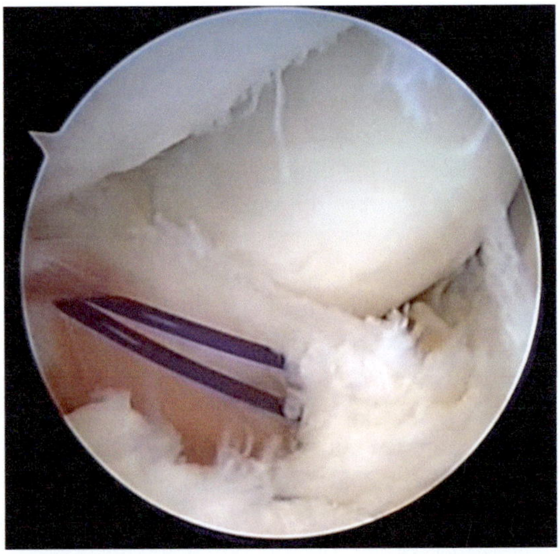

**Fig. 10.9** Arthroscopic view from the radiohumeral gutter, showing the intra-articular portion of the imbrication (Courtesy of MoRe Foundation)

as the needle is removed. We now have two strands of PDS that both represent half of the LUCL. The suture ends, which were taken out of the soft spot portal, are connected and pulled distally. At this moment, there is a single strand of PDS deep to the capsule, exiting the skin at both the origin and the insertion of the LUCL. This suture is used to shuttle a second PDS from distal to proximal, essentially doubling the construction, to a two-strand suture. A mosquito is then brought through the soft spot portal into the subcutaneous tissue and both the proximal and distal ends of the sutures are pulled subcutaneously (Fig. 10.8). This creates a loop with two sutures from the soft spot, superficial to the LCL complex to the lateral epicondyle, then deep to the LCL (Fig. 10.9) towards the origin on the ulna and again out of the soft spot portal superficially to the LCL. Both sutures are then tightened and the arthroscopic adaptation of the pivot shift is repeated with the sutures relaxed and tightened. The scope is removed if adequate stability is obtained and both sutures are tied individually. The knots are buried away from the portal. Besides irritation of the knot and stiffness requiring a manipulation under anaesthesia, we have not had any complications related to this technique.

The first 20 patients who were treated with this technique were followed for an average of 21 months (12–30 months). A traumatic incident was the cause of instability in 16 patients. Tennis elbow surgery was the cause of instability in three patients. One patient had multiple prior surgeries due to an OCD lesion. The delay between the onset and the arthroscopic imbrication was 48 months on average (range 3–386 months). The pivot shift, posterior drawer, and table-top tests were used to clinically evaluate the stability of the elbow. Two out three tests were positive in all patients, with the posterior drawer test being the most sensitive test. This was positive in 18 patients. Range of motion was preserved in most with an average extension deficit of 5° (range 0–40°). Average flexion was 140° (range 120–145). Preoperative Mayo Elbow Performance score (MEPS) was 48 (range 20–75). The Quick DASH score was 54 (range 25–82). At the final follow-up there was a significant improvement in Quick DASH and MEPS scores. The average post-operative MEPS was 91 with average improvement of 43 points. Average post-operative QuickDQSH was 10, with an average improvement of 43 points. Average extension improved to 2° (range −5° to 20°) and flexion remained 140° (120–145°). A revision to an open reconstruction was performed 7 months following the arthroscopic procedure in one patient, due to persistent pain. No subjective or objective signs of instability were found in any of the other patients.

## Open Technique

### Primary Repair

Acute ligament repairs are indicated in patients in whom a closed reduction is not possible or if the elbow remains unstable after a successful closed reduction. The elbow is moved from flexion to extension following the reduction. If the elbow dislocates before 30° of extension can be reached, we feel that an acute repair is indicated. Finally, surgical repair may also be indicated for active patients in certain professions or sports.

An open ligament repair can be performed under general or regional anaesthesia. An ultrasound-guided supraclavicular block is the preferred technique in our institution. The patient is placed in a supine position with the arm on a hand table since a lateral approach is preferred. A pivot shift test is performed under anaesthesia. PLRI is often difficult to determine in an awake patient, due to pain and apprehension but may become apparent once the arm is anaesthetized (Fig. 10.10). Alternatively, the patient can be placed in lateral decubitus or prone position if the surgeon prefers to approach the elbow through a posterior incision [26]. We prefer to use a 2 cm lateral incision and an extensor tendon split anterior to the remnant of the

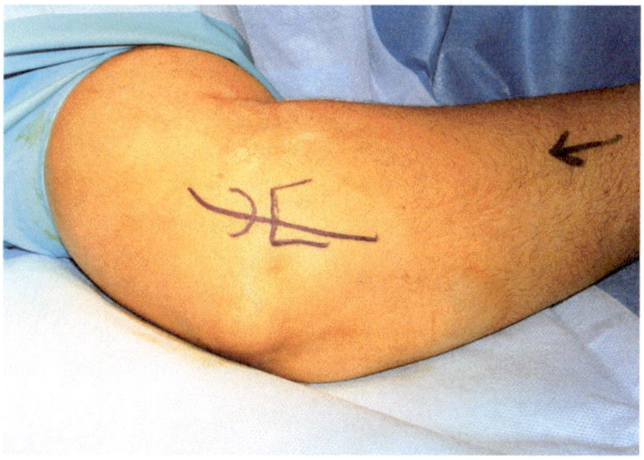

Fig. 10.10 A lateral incision is used. The incision is centred on the lateral condyle and directed, over the posterior one-third of the radial head, to the supinator crest of the ulna (Courtesy of MoRe Foundation)

LCL (Fig. 10.11). Most commonly, it is avulsed from the humerus [27]. In the acute situation, it is not uncommon to have an avulsion of the common extensor tendon mass [27], allowing for direct access to the joint once the fascia is incised.

The isometric point on the capitellum is determined. It is situated just anterior to the circle made by the articular surface of the capitellum [25]. The exact location of the avulsion can often be identified in acute cases. The LCL can be reattached using bone tunnels or a bone anchor, depending on the preference of the surgeon. As subcutaneous knots often cause irritation due to their subcutaneous location, the extensor tendon split is closed with running sutures, so that there is only one single knot distally. The knot is buried in the extensor tendon mass.

## Post-operative Protocol

The arm is placed in a removable splint for 24 h, with the elbow in 90°. On the first post-operative day, the arm is protected with a dynamic elbow brace and both passive and active motion is started. Unlimited flexion of the elbow is allowed immediately. Extension is blocked at 60° for the first 2 weeks, to 30° for the following 2 weeks and full extension in the brace is allowed from weeks 4 to 6. The dynamic brace is worn for a total of 6 weeks after which strengthening exercises of the arm are started. Unrestricted activity is permitted at 3 months.

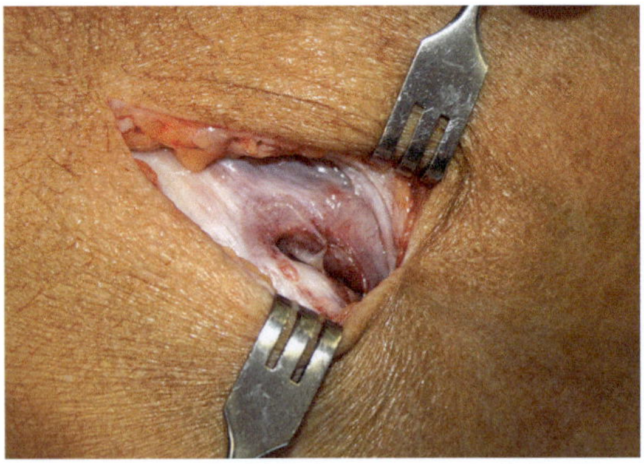

**Fig. 10.11** Intraoperative view of the lateral elbow. After incision of the skin only, both an avulsion of the LCL complex, together with an avulsion of the extensor tendons became apparent (Courtesy of MoRe Foundation)

## LCL Reconstruction

A formal reconstruction is indicated in patients with severe chronic instability. This can occur after a single or multiple elbow dislocations or when the instability occurs following surgery to the lateral elbow.

In 1992, Nestor, O'Driscoll and Morrey first described reconstructing the LUCL with a series of 11 patients using a modified Kocher and elevating the common extensor origin, along with the anconeus and extensor carpi ulnaris [28]. If the LUCL was identified to be insufficient, reconstruction with autologous tendon graft consisting of the palmaris longus was performed. The supinator crest is palpated and the origin of the LUCL is identified. Two converging bone tunnels based off the supinator crest of the ulna are created and the graft is passed through the tunnel. The isometric point of the lateral epicondyle is identified and two tunnels are made diverging from the insertion on the lateral epicondyle. The graft is passed through the tunnels, reflected back across the joint and sutured back onto itself [28].

Various techniques have since been published. Jones et al. described an adaptation of the original technique, using a similar ulnar tunnel with a proximal docking technique through the humerus [29]. Using a autologous palmaris longus looped through the ulna at the level of the supinator crest, it is then tunnelled through the isometric point. Two small drill holes exit the humerus for two sutures attached to both graft limbs. These are used to dock the graft in the tunnel [29].

Beyond the configuration of tunnels, the number of strands of the LUCL reconstructed has been explored, with single strand reconstruction versus double stranded showing equal outcomes [6, 11, 15, 28]. Different grafts, both auto and allografts, including Achilles, triceps fascia, gracilis and Palmaris longus have been used. All grafts have been shown to be of sufficient strength [30] and no clear differences have been found in clinical studies.

Our preferred method of reconstruction of the ligament begins using a 4 cm lateral incision—identical to the incision used during an acute repair but continuing slightly more distal towards the supinator crest of the ulna. The Kocher interval (Fig. 10.12) is identified between the anconeus and the extensor carpi ulnaris (ECU). There is a strip of fatty tissue between these two muscles that allows easy identification of the interval. This can usually be identified through the fascia. The fascia is incised over the interval and the plane between the anconeus and ECU is developed. Kocher's interval is followed onto the proximal ulna. There are always three small blood vessels on the ulna at the distal part of the approach. These are best coagulated, to avoid post-operative bleeding. The supinator crest on the ulna is palpated and followed proximally. A small tubercle can often be palpated on the most proximal part of the crest, just distal to the radial head, at the base of the annular ligament. This is the insertion of the LUCL. The annular ligament is typically intact, as is the lateral capsule, which may be lax. It is hard to identify the LCL, in chronic cases, as the whole of the lateral capsule and ligament complex will often be very fibrotic. The lateral epicondyle is then approached and the common extensor tendon is released from posterior to anterior. The entire LCL will no longer be attached to the lateral epicondyle most of these patients and any remnants are released sharply for later fixation to the graft. The lateral capsule is then opened. The capsule should be opened slightly anterior to allow interposition between the final graft and radial head to prevent abrasion on the graft.

The choice of graft depends on the preference of the surgeon. A variety of allograft, autograft or synthetic grafts have all been described [17]. All are of sufficient strength to reconstruct the LCL complex [30]. We use an allograft extensor hallucis longus (EHL) tendon of approximately 20 cm. There are multiple ways to fix the graft to the humerus and the ulna. Bone tunnels can be used, as well as anchors, interference screws, or cortical buttons. The graft can be placed in a yoke or docking configuration and single- or multiple strands of graft can be used. No differences between these techniques have been shown in the literature. We use a cortical bone button with a retractable loop to fix the graft (ToggleLoc, Zimmer Biomet, Warsaw, Indiana).

A unicortical drill hole with a diameter of 4.5 mm is made at the insertion of the LUCL at the supinator crest on the ulna (Fig. 10.13). The button is placed intramedullary. The button is inserted longitudinally through the tunnel. The button is then flipped in the canal and secured by pulling the button onto the intramedullary side of the lateral cortex of the ulna. The EHL graft is then placed in the retractable loop. The graft has a length of about 20 cm and is pulled halfway through the loop. This means that approximately 10 cm of graft will be at either side, once the graft

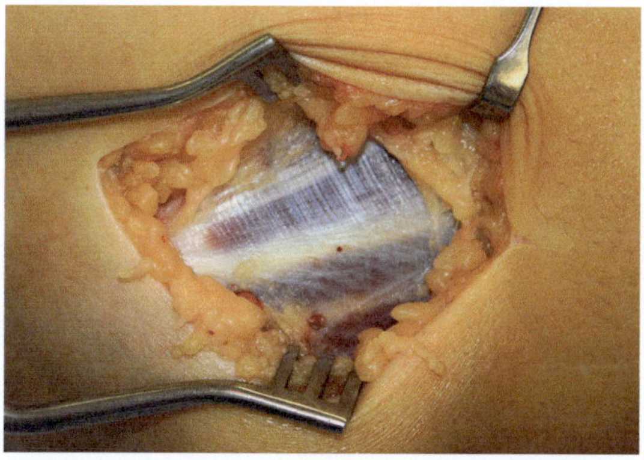

**Fig. 10.12** Kocher's interval is identified between the anconeus and the extensor carpi ulnaris (Courtesy of MoRe Foundation)

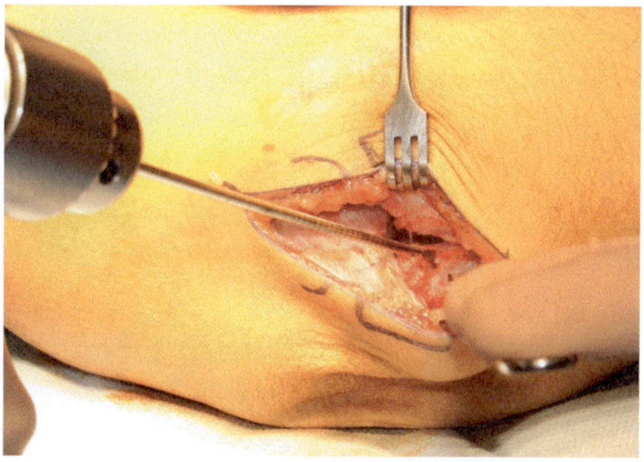

**Fig. 10.13** The supinator crest can easily be palpated on the ulna. A guidewire is drilled unicortically through the lateral cortex of the ulna (Courtesy of MoRe Foundation)

is inserted in the loop. The loop is then closed and by doing this, the middle portion of the graft is pulled into the drill hole at the insertion of the LUCL. This essentially leaves two limbs of graft on either side of the tunnel.

The isometric point on the capitellum is then determined. It is situated just anterior to the circle made by the articular surface of the capitellum [25]. A small suture can be used to determine this isometric point, while the elbow is moved through flexion and extension [23]. A guidewire is drilled from the isometric point, bicortically, through the posterior cortex of the humerus (Fig. 10.14). Care should be taken not to exit in the olecranon fossa as this could later lead to impingement of the button between the ulna and the humerus. The first cortex is overdrilled up to, but not through the second cortex, with a 6 mm canulated drill. This creates a tunnel for the graft. The posterior cortex is overdrilled with a 4.5 mm drill, so that the button can exit the tunnel past the second cortex. The humeral button is then pushed through the tunnel from distal to proximal and secured on the posterior cortex. Part of the loop will remain distally, outside the tunnel. The position of the buttons can be checked with fluoroscopy or, the humeral button, can be visualized directly if necessary.

The capsule is closed in order to avoid friction between the radial head and lateral side of the capitellum, once the graft is placed and tensioned. Both limbs of the graft are then fixed to the button. The first limb is pulled through the loop from medial to lateral. The second limb is pulled through the loop from medial to lateral. Kocher type clamps are attached to the ends of both limbs. Both limbs are then tightened manually. The elbow is fully reduced and held with the forearm in pronation as the graft is tightened. The sliding loop is then closed, tightening the graft further and pulling a part of both limbs into the humeral tunnel (Fig. 10.15). Usually the graft is long enough, so that the ends of both limbs will remain outside the tunnel. The ends of both limbs are folded proximally and used to suture the limbs back onto the tightened part of the graft (Fig. 10.16). All lateral structures are then closed over the graft. Although the LCL is isometric, the LUCL has been shown to be lax in extension and tighten in flexion [25]. We therefore tighten the graft in approximately 30° of flexion, allowing the reconstruction to tighten even more when the elbow is flexed.

## Post-operative Protocol

The post-operative regimen is identical to the primary repairs. Radiographs may be used to confirm the correct position of the buttons (Fig. 10.17). Post-operatively, patients are instructed to mobilize the elbow in a dynamic

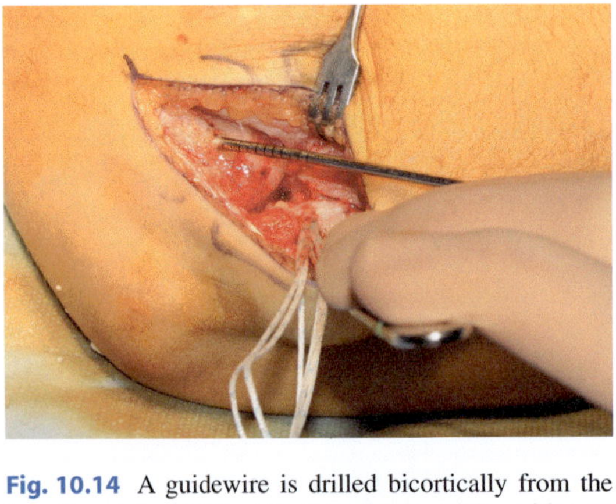

**Fig. 10.14** A guidewire is drilled bicortically from the insertion of the LUCL at the lateral epicondyle, exiting on the posterior cortex of the humerus (Courtesy of MoRe Foundation)

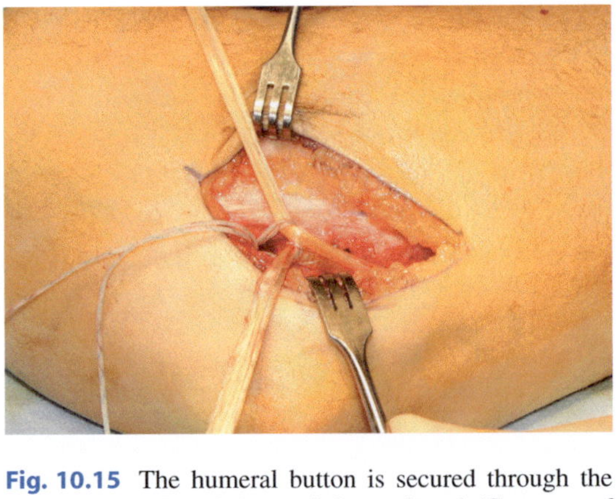

**Fig. 10.15** The humeral button is secured through the humeral tunnel and the graft is tensioned (Courtesy of MoRe Foundation)

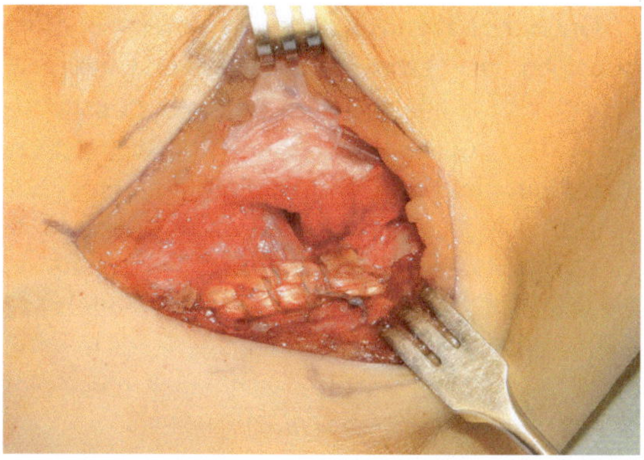

**Fig. 10.16** The remaining graft is doubled back and sutured onto itself for additional fixation (Courtesy of MoRe Foundation)

elbow brace for 6 weeks. Extension is progressively allowed with increments of 30° every 2 weeks, starting with a 60° extension block.

## Outcomes After Surgical Treatment of PLRI

Results after reconstruction for PLRI are overall good to excellent in about 85 % of patients. Instability is the most common complication despite accurate repair or reconstruction [17, 31]. Several authors have reported results after reconstruction with a majority of patients remaining stable with worse outcomes in patients with degenerative arthritis, pain only without symptoms of instability and prior surgery [16, 29, 30].

Jones et al. reported on eight patients at a mean of 7 years post-operative from LUCL reconstruction using a palmaris autograft with two distal ulnar tunnels and a proximal docking technique [29]. The authors reported complete resolution of instability in six patients and recurrence in two of eight (25 %). Despite recurrence, all the patients were reported to be satisfied at final follow-up. Nestor et al. evaluated 11 patients (three repairs and eight reconstructions) who underwent surgery for PLRI [28]. The reconstructions were performed using a 5-tunnel technique (three in the humerus and two in the ulna) and a palmaris autograft. They noted three patients with fair outcomes and one with a poor outcome according to their classification. The patients who underwent repair had good results; however, they had less severe disease than the patients who underwent reconstruction. Prior surgery and the presence of radiocapitellar arthrosis were noted to be risk factors for poor outcomes. They suggest that all patients are counselled regarding these risks and that the quality of the joint is assessed preoperatively and during surgery.

a b

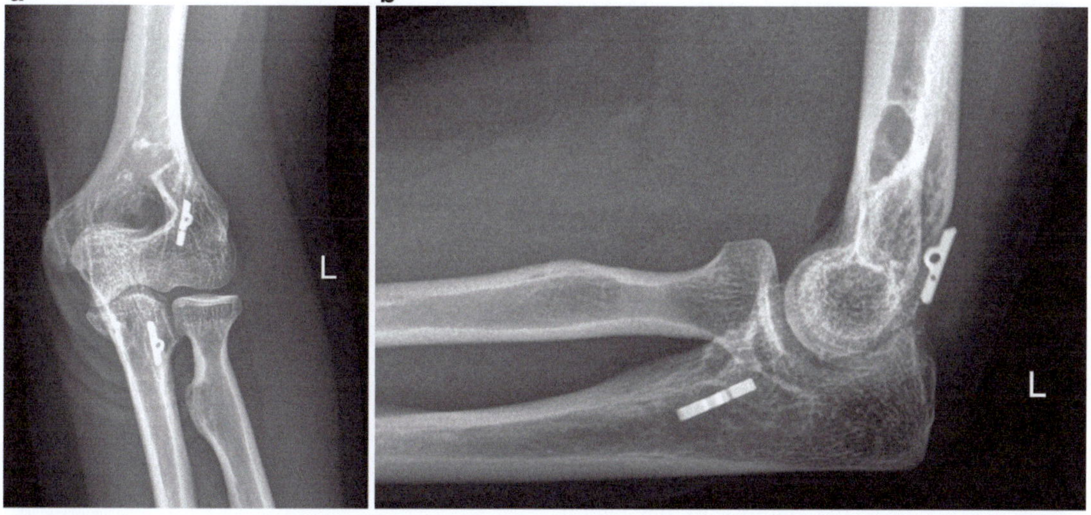


**Fig. 10.17** (**a**, **b**) Post-operative anteroposterior and lateral radiographic view of the elbow, showing correct placement of the buttons (Courtesy of MoRe Foundation)

Sanchez-Sotelo et al. reported their outcomes in 44 (12 repairs and 33 reconstructions) patients who underwent surgery for PLRI. Five patients (11%) noted further instability, and 27% of patients described fair or poor results [17]. Better results were noted in patients with a post-traumatic etiology, subjective instability and in those patients in whom a graft was utilized. Most recently, Baghdadi et al. reported on 11 patients who had a revision LUCL reconstruction for a failed prior reconstruction utilizing an allograft tendon [30]. The revision reconstructions were performed at a mean of 3 years after the initial LUCL reconstruction. Osseous deficiency was identified at some level in 8 of 11 patients. At an average of 5 years status post-revision reconstruction, 8 of 11 elbows remained stable. All patients who remained stable had a good or excellent result whereas all patients who had persistent instability were noted to have some degree of bone loss. The authors concluded that revision LUCL reconstruction is an option for persistent instability although it must be recognized that almost half of the patients either had persistent instability after revision or a fair or poor outcome.

## Conclusions

Posterolateral rotatory instability is caused by an insufficiency of both the lateral collateral ligament and the lateral ulnar collateral ligament of the elbow. The proximal ulna and radial head externally rotate about the distal humerus when the forearm is positioned in supination and slight flexion and when axial compression is applied to the forearm. It typically occurs from a fall on the outstretched hand causing a subluxation or dislocation, rupturing the stabilizers of the elbow. Failure to heal may lead to symptomatic PLRI. Surgery to the lateral elbow may also injure the lateral structures and is a relatively common cause of PLRI.

Four stages of PLRI exist and treatment may be tailored to severity of instability. The diagnosis of PLRI is mainly clinical. Several specific tests are used to evaluate the stability of the lateral elbow. Further evaluation usually includes MRI scanning.

Once the diagnosis is made, surgery is often indicated in chronic cases. Several surgical options exist, depending on the stage of instability. Arthroscopic imbrication of the lateral ligaments can yield excellent results in milder cases. A formal reconstruction is usually indicated in more severe stages of instability. Depending on the severity of instability and the preoperative status of the elbow, surgery usually leads to good or excellent results with a very small chance of recurrence.

## References


1. Osborne G, Cotterill P. Recurrent dislocation of the elbow. J Bone Joint Surg. 1966;48(2):340–6.
2. Charalambous CP, Stanley JK. Posterolateral rotatory instability of the elbow. J Bone Joint Surg. 2008;90(3):272–9.
3. Hassmann GC, Brunn F, Neer 2nd CS. Recurrent dislocation of the elbow. J Bone Joint Surg Am. 1975;57(8):1080–4.
4. Symeonides PP, Paschaloglou C, Stavrou Z, Pangalides T. Recurrent dislocation of the elbow. Report of three cases. J Bone Joint Surg Am. 1975;57(8):1084–6.
5. Burgess RC, Sprague HH. Post-traumatic posterior radial head subluxation. Two case reports. Clin Orthop Relat Res. 1984;(186):192–4.
6. O'Driscoll SW, Bell DF, Morrey BF. Posterolateral rotatory instability of the elbow. J Bone Joint Surg Am. 1991;73(3):440–6.
7. Dunning CE, Zarzour ZD, Patterson SD, Johnson JA, King GJ. Ligamentous stabilizers against posterolateral rotatory instability of the elbow. J Bone Joint Surg Am. 2001;83-A(12):1823–8.
8. Cohen MS, Hastings 2nd H. Rotatory instability of the elbow. The anatomy and role of the lateral stabilizers. J Bone Joint Surg Am. 1997;79(2):225–33.
9. McAdams TR, Masters GW, Srivastava S. The effect of arthroscopic sectioning of the lateral ligament complex of the elbow on posterolateral rotatory stability. J Shoulder Elbow Surg. 2005;14(3):298–301.
10. Olsen BS, Sojbjerg JO, Nielsen KK, Vaesel MT, Dalstra M, Sneppen O. Posterolateral elbow joint instability: the basic kinematics. J Shoulder Elbow Surg. 1998;7(1):19–29.
11. King GJ, Dunning CE, Zarzour ZD, Patterson SD, Johnson JA. Single-strand reconstruction of the lateral ulnar collateral ligament restores varus and posterolateral rotatory stability of the elbow. J Shoulder Elbow Surg. 2002;11(1):60–4.
12. Schneeberger AG, Sadowski MM, Jacob HA. Coronoid process and radial head as posterolateral rotatory stabilizers of the elbow. J Bone Joint Surg Am. 2004;86-A(5):975–82.

13. Dunning CE, Zarzour ZD, Patterson SD, Johnson JA, King GJ. Muscle forces and pronation stabilize the lateral ligament deficient elbow. Clin Orthop Relat Res. 2001;(388):118–24.
14. Buchanan TS, Delp SL, Solbeck JA. Muscular resistance to varus and valgus loads at the elbow. J Biomech Eng. 1998;120(5):634–9.
15. O'Driscoll SW, Morrey BF, Korinek S, An KN. Elbow subluxation and dislocation. A spectrum of instability. Clin Orthop Relat Res. 1992; (280):186–97.
16. Steinmann SP. Elbow trauma. Preface. Orthop Clin North Am. 2008;39(2):1. ix.
17. Sanchez-Sotelo J, Morrey BF, O'Driscoll SW. Ligamentous repair and reconstruction for posterolateral rotatory instability of the elbow. J Bone Joint Surg. 2005;87(1):54–61.
18. Kalainov DM, Cohen MS. Posterolateral rotatory instability of the elbow in association with lateral epicondylitis. A report of three cases. J Bone Joint Surg Am. 2005;87(5):1120–5.
19. O'Driscoll SW. Classification and evaluation of recurrent instability of the elbow. Clin Orthop Relat Res. 2000; (370):34–43.
20. Arvind CH, Hargreaves DG. Table top relocation test--new clinical test for posterolateral rotatory instability of the elbow. J Shoulder Elbow Surg. 2006;15(4):500–1.
21. Regan W, Lapner PC. Prospective evaluation of two diagnostic apprehension signs for posterolateral instability of the elbow. J Shoulder Elbow Surg. 2006;15(3):344–6.
22. Potter HG, Weiland AJ, Schatz JA, Paletta GA, Hotchkiss RN. Posterolateral rotatory instability of the elbow: usefulness of MR imaging in diagnosis. Radiology. 1997;204(1):185–9.
23. Mehta JA, Bain GI. Posterolateral rotatory instability of the elbow. J Am Acad Orthop Surg. 2004;12(6):405–15.
24. Savoie 3rd FH, O'Brien MJ, Field LD, Gurley DJ. Arthroscopic and open radial ulnohumeral ligament reconstruction for posterolateral rotatory instability of the elbow. Clin Sports Med. 2010;29(4):611–8.
25. Moritomo H, Murase T, Arimitsu S, Oka K, Yoshikawa H, Sugamoto K. The in vivo isometric point of the lateral ligament of the elbow. J Bone Joint Surg Am. 2007;89(9):2011–7.
26. Mehta JA, Bain GI. Surgical approaches to the elbow. Hand Clin. 2004;20(4):375–87.
27. McKee MD, Schemitsch EH, Sala MJ, O'Driscoll SW. The pathoanatomy of lateral ligamentous disruption in complex elbow instability. J Shoulder Elbow Surg. 2003;12(4):391–6.
28. Nestor BJ, O'Driscoll SW, Morrey BF. Ligamentous reconstruction for posterolateral rotatory instability of the elbow. J Bone Joint Surg Am. 1992;74(8):1235–41.
29. Jones KJ, Dodson CC, Osbahr DC, Parisien RL, Weiland AJ, Altchek DW, et al. The docking technique for lateral ulnar collateral ligament reconstruction: surgical technique and clinical outcomes. J Shoulder Elbow Surg. 2012;21(3):389–95.
30. Baumfeld JA, van Riet RP, Zobitz ME, Eygendaal D, An K-N, Steinmann SP. Triceps tendon properties and its potential as an autograft. J Shoulder Elbow Surg. 2010;19(5):697–9.
31. Olsen BS, Sojbjerg JO. The treatment of recurrent posterolateral instability of the elbow. J Bone Joint Surg. 2003;85(3):342–6.

# 11 Evaluation and Nonoperative Treatment of the Unstable Throwing Elbow

Paul Sethi and Craig J. Macken

## Abbreviations

UCL Ulnar collateral ligament
VEO Valgus extension overload
ROM Range of motion

## Introduction

Instability of the throwing elbow represents a continuum of a microinstability of the ulnar collateral ligament (UCL). While UCL insufficiency has been reported in lacrosse, tennis, wrestling, European handball, and javelin throwers, the majority of these injuries are seen in American baseball players, particularly pitchers. In fact, medial elbow symptoms account for up to 97 % of injuries in major league pitchers [1]. This chapter reviews the diagnosis and nonoperative treatment of the unstable elbow in throwing athletes.

P. Sethi, MD (✉)
Department of Orthopedic Surgery, ONS Foundation for Clinical Research and Education, Greenwich, CT, USA
e-mail: sethi@onsmd.com

C.J. Macken, BS
ONS Foundation for Clinical Research and Education, Greenwich, CT, USA
e-mail: Cjmacken15@yahoo.com

## Background

### Elbow Stability

The elbow joint is a synovial hinge joint consisting of three articulations: the ulnotrochlear, radiocapitellar, and proximal radioulnar joint [2]. The primary stabilizers include the ulnotrochlear articulation, the UCL, and the radial collateral ligament. The secondary stabilizers consist of the radial head, the anterior and posterior joint capsule, and the common flexor and extensor muscle origins. The dynamic stabilizers are the anconeus, biceps, brachialis, and the triceps [3].

The UCL consists of three bands: anterior, posterior, and transverse. The anterior band is the primary valgus stabilizer of the elbow [4–7]. The biceps, brachialis, and triceps contribute to valgus stability by a joint compression effect [8]. The flexor–pronator mass—flexor carpi ulnaris, flexor digitorum superficialis, pronator teres—provide dynamic stability by direct muscle action to resist valgus torque of the elbow [9]. The ulnar nerve lies in close proximity to the UCL and flexor–pronator mass, so the unstable throwing elbow can often manifest with ulnar nerve symptoms.

### Injury Mechanism

Injury to the throwing elbow is thought to be the result of cumulative stress from repetitive throwing [10]. Approximately 22–26 % of all

© Springer International Publishing Switzerland 2017
R.Z. Tashjian (ed.), *The Unstable Elbow*, DOI 10.1007/978-3-319-46019-2_11

injuries to major league baseball pitchers involve the elbow joint [11, 12]. The forces behind the throwing motion elucidate the injury mechanism behind repetitive throwing. Valgus forces have been estimated to reach 64 Nm during the acceleration and late cocking phase of throwing [13–16]. Additionally, the elbow extends at over 2300° per second during the pitching motion, producing a medial shear force of 300 N and compressive force of 900 N [13, 14]. These forces put extreme pressure on the UCL, ultimately exceeding its native tensile strength of 34 Nm [7, 15–27]. As such, repetitive throwing in athletes can lead to partial or complete tears in the ligament [1, 16, 23–26, 28].

In conjunction with the UCL, the flexor–pronator mass is susceptible to injury during activities of repeated valgus stress such as throwing. Flexor–pronator mass injuries typically occur during the acceleration and follow-through stages of the throwing motion, when forceful extension of the elbow and pronation of the forearm occur [1]. The close proximity of the UCL and flexor–pronator mass puts the ulnar nerve at risk of injury when these structures are damaged. A significant number of athletes presenting with UCL insufficiency develop ulnar neuritis [23, 29, 30]. Injuries occur by compressing or stretching the nerve between two fixed points and most commonly occurs during the late cocking and early acceleration stages of throwing [31].

## Evaluation

### History

A specific, detailed history should be taken of the athlete to aid in the diagnosis and treatment of the injured elbow. A detailed throwing history that includes arm dominance, duration, intensity, location, phase of the throwing motion, and activities that elicit symptoms should be noted as well as any associated symptoms [23, 32, 33]. Occasionally, athletes can recall a specific throwing event, accompanied by a "pop" in the elbow, which led to the injury [10]. Most athletes experience a gradual onset of symptoms during the acceleration stage of throwing with some loss of velocity and or accuracy [10, 23]. Studies have shown that different pitches cause varying degrees of symptoms in the elbow [16, 21, 34]. The curveball generates the greatest valgus stress, while the fastball and slider generate the greatest force; the changeup generates the least stress [35].

Ulnar nerve function is a critical part of the throwing elbow; therefore a detailed history of any neurologic conditions is necessary. Early warning signs of neural pathology include cold intolerance, numbness or tingling in the hand or fingertips, shooting sensations, and a tendency to drop objects [36]. Intrinsic muscle hand weakness, clumsiness with fine motor movements, parasthesias or dysesthesias in the distribution of the ulnar nerve, commonly felt in the ring and little finger are symptoms pertaining to the ulnar nerve [37, 38].

### Physical Exam

A thorough examination of the entire upper extremity and cervical spine of the throwing athlete should be performed [38]. In throwing athletes, particular attention should be paid to the medial elbow. The inspection begins by assessing the resting position of the elbow and its carrying angle. The normal carrying angle is 11° and 13° of valgus in men and women, respectively [15, 39], although, carrying angles greater than 15° of valgus have been reported in overhead athletes [40]. It is important to note any swelling, ecchymosis, effusion, scars, developmental abnormalities, and any previous signs of trauma to the elbow [37, 38].

The normal ROM in the joint is from full extension of 0–140° flexion and from 75° pronation to 85° supination [41]. Throwers will often have a loss of 10–15° of extension that is often directly related to the duration of throwing career. Cain et al. described the "end-feel" at the extremes of motion in the throwing athlete [15]. Normal extension ends with a firm sensation of the posterior bony articulation coming in contact with the olecranon fossa. Normal flexion ends when the soft tissues of the distal humerus and proximal forearm come into contact [15]. Loss of motion may be due to effusion, soft tissue swelling, bony hypertrophy, or osteophyte formation [37].

Palpation of specific structures of the elbow should be carried out in a sequential manner to determine the site of discomfort. Palpation of the UCL is carried out with the elbow flexed 70–90° and palpated along its entire course [37] [Fig. 11.1]. Then palpation of the medial epicondyle and flexor–pronator mass should be performed, by moving distal and slightly anterior to the medial epicondyle [37]. Next, palpation of the lateral structures including the radial head, capitellum, lateral epicondyle, and extensor mass, should be performed [37]. Palpation of the anterior soft tissues, including the biceps tendon, brachialis tendon, and anterior capsule, and posterior tissues, including the olecranon tip and triceps tendon, should be performed [37].

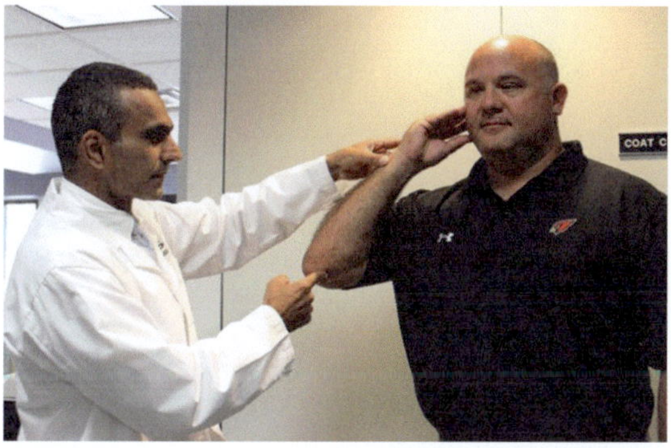

Fig. 11.1 Palpation of the medial elbow during the physical exam. The UCL and flexor–pronator mass are palpated along their course to determine the site of pain. The subject is asked to apply pressure towards his face, activating the flexor mass. Tenderness or pain at the site suggests tendon or muscular pathology (Image courtesy of ONSF—ONS Foundation for Clinical Research and Education)

Tenderness posteromedially, over the olecranon and olecranon fossa, upon palpation with the elbow in full extension, is common in valgus extension overload (VEO). Posterior pain with forced gentle hyperextension suggests posterior impingement. Posteromedial elbow pain during a milking maneuver test, during which the patient's forearm is flexed and supinated while the patient's thumb is pulled downward towards the shoulder, may be suggestive of VEO or UCL insufficiency [38]. A valgus stress test should also be performed between 20° and 30° of flexion to assess the quality of the UCL. A moving valgus stress test should also be performed, by maintaining valgus stress while moving from 30° of flexion to full extension [38]. According to O'Driscoll et al. [42], the moving valgus stress test was highly sensitive (100 %, 17 of 17 patients) and specific (75 %, 3 of 4 patients) when compared to assessment of the UCL by either surgical exploration or arthroscopic valgus stress testing. We find this test to be particularly helpful [Fig. 11.2].

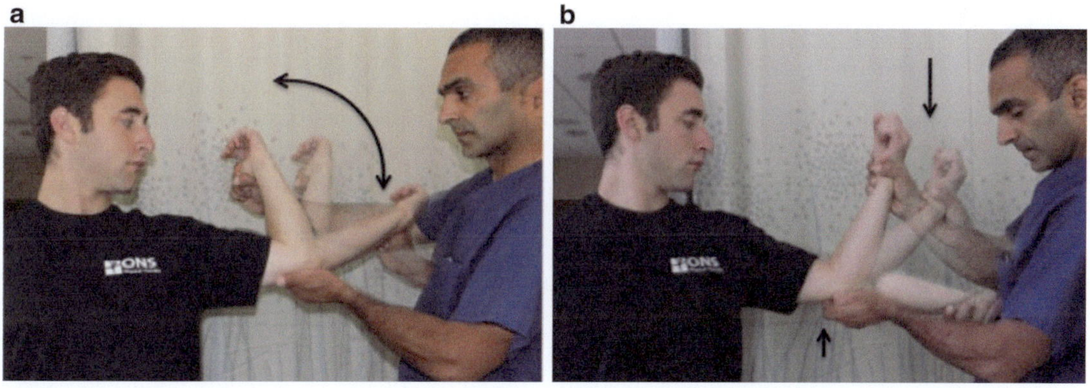

Fig. 11.2 Physical exam tests (a) The moving valgus stress test is performed to access the UCL. The supinated forearm starts with 30° of flexion, then fully extends while valgus stress is placed on the elbow. A positive finding results in pain during the arc of motion or reproducing symptoms on the medial elbow. (b) The hyperextension test is performed to access the stability of the capsule as well as posterior impingement. The supinated forearm starts with 0° of flexion, then fully extended until no further motion is available. This should include comparison to the contralateral side. Pain, end feel, firm or soft, are assessed and are suggestive of posterior impingement and VEO (Images courtesy of ONSF—ONS Foundation for Clinical Research and Education)

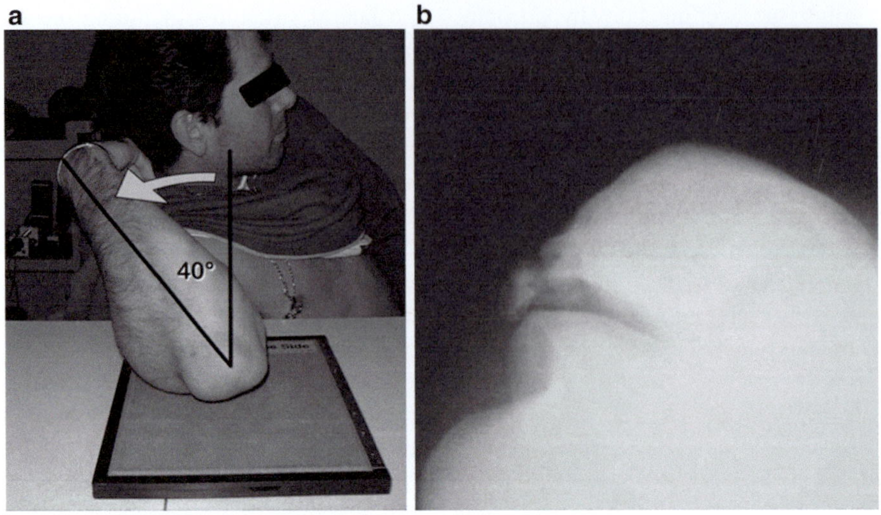


**Fig. 11.3** Special radiographs to assess posterior impingement. (**a**) The Conway X-ray is performed to visualize the posteromedial olecranon and associated osteophytes. An AP X-ray is taken with the elbow in full flexion with 40° of external rotation. (**b**) The result of a Conway test demonstrating posteromedial osteophyte, not always visualized on straight axial radiograph (Image courtesy of John Conway, MD)

The ulnar nerve should also be carefully assessed during physical exam. Palpation of the ulnar nerve should start at the medial epicondyle and travel distally into the flexor carpi ulnaris muscle [37]. Any neurologic symptoms in the two ulnar digits, as well as instability or subluxation of the ulnar nerve, or a Tinel sign should be identified [32].

## Imaging

Proper imaging should supplement the history and physical examination when diagnosing injuries to the elbow. Radiographs, including AP, lateral, and oblique views with the elbow in flexion can be used to identify osteophytes. Imaging of the contralateral arm is useful in skeletally immature athletes and may help to identify stress and avulsion fractures. Wilson et al. found that posterior osteophytes were easily found in a standard lateral radiograph in all their presurgical patients, but noted that identification of the problematic posteromedial osteophyte using radiographic imaging was difficult [43]. They found that with the elbow in 110° of flexion and the beam angled at 45° to the ulna, the symptomatic osteophyte was most easily seen [43]. Conway recommended an AP view with the elbow in full flexion with 40° of external rotation for complete visualization of the posteromedial olecranon and osteophytes [44] [Fig. 11.3]. CT scans and/or MRI can be utilized to identify stress fractures or avulsion fractures in the elbow [37, 45]. MRI remains the best option when evaluating soft tissue damage to muscles, tendons, ligaments, and articular cartilage [Figs. 11.4 and 11.5] [37, 38]. Intra-articular contrast medium improves the yield of detecting tears in the UCL, especially undersurface tears [45–47]. Ultrasonography and dynamic ultrasonography can be used to evaluate the UCL and can detect increased laxity with valgus instability [32, 48].

## Nonoperative Treatment

Instability of the UCL represents a wide spectrum of injuries. The treatment of these injuries is guided by a complex interplay of the patient age, level of participation, concomitant injuries, degree of instability and dysfunction, patient and family expectations, and response to rest and therapeutic exercise.

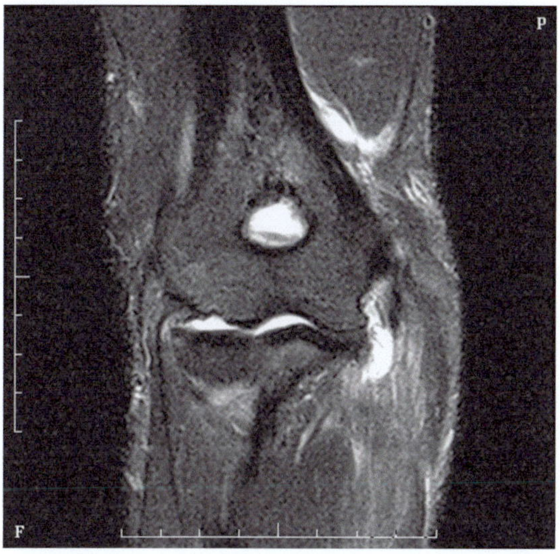

**Fig. 11.4** T2 weighted Coronal MRI demonstrating acute avulsion of the distal UCL. This is a 19-year-old dominant arm of a college football wide receiver treated nonoperatively following the guidelines in Table 11.1. Player returned to full sports with no symptoms

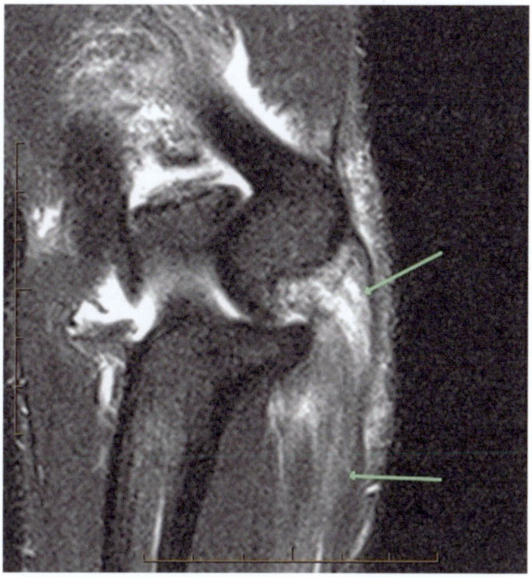

**Fig. 11.5** T2 weighted coronal MRI demonstrating insertional and intrasubstance partial tearing of the flexor mass in a collegiate pitcher. Player was able to return to pitching after nonoperative management

Age is useful parameter to help guide treatment. Youth baseball players, 16 years old and younger, frequently present with overuse symptoms in the medial elbow. The overwhelming majority of youth injuries, especially those seen in younger side of this cohort, are treated with rest, player and family education, and rehabilitation concluding with a graduated return to sport. Stress fractures are seen in both youth and elite players. These can be uniformly treated with rest and nonoperative management. In contrast, rest and therapy may not be the ideal for the acute displaced sublime or medial epicondyle fracture [Fig. 11.6]. Open reduction and internal fixation of medial epicondyle fractures with displacement of 5–10 mm of the fragment has been suggested in the competitive youth athlete [49]. There is a lack of defined parameters for sublime tubercle fractures, but 2 mm displacement may be an indication for surgery. Prior to surgical intervention some youth athletes may be encouraged to change positions, away from pitching, or even consider switching sports if the youth athlete is not committed to the requisite rehabilitation and the desire for participation at the university level.

VEO is an important part of medial elbow instability. VEO is characterized by posteromedial elbow pain with osteophytes that form in the posteromedial joint as a result of ligament attenuation and abutment of the ulna against the olecranon fossa [Fig. 11.7]. It is sometimes useful to think of VEO as a prodromal syndrome to frank UCL insufficiency. Importantly, this prodrome may last for many years or may never manifest into overt UCL incompetence, even in the setting of a complete tear of the UCL. The pathological osteophytes may actually be protective against UCL incompetence. While seen in young athletes, VEO is seen more often in an older athlete. Acute pain and loss of extension may lead to alteration in throwing mechanics and a subsequent earlier release of the ball, perpetuating the stress seen on the elbow. Treatment for this entity involves cessation of throwing until the inflammatory phase is resolved, regaining pain-free pre-injury motion along with guided therapy followed by a gradual resumption of sports. As a rough guideline, the period of shutdown is doubled to estimate the ease back into sports. So if a player needs 2 weeks of shutdown to regain pain-free range motion, that player will need 4

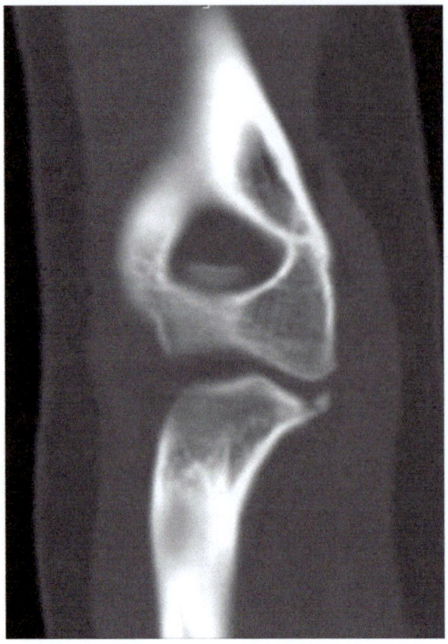

**Fig. 11.6** CT scan image of the elbow demonstrating a nondisplaced sublime tubercle fracture in a high school pitcher. This was treated nonoperatively with full return to throwing

additional weeks of a graduated throwing program. The MRI appearance of the ligament should not guide the treatment in the absence of clinically overt symptoms, especially in the older elite player who may recover and return to play with an overtly abnormal ligament. Judicious use of intra articular corticosteroid injection may also be helpful in the early phase of treatment of VEO.

Isolated partial and complete soft tissue tears of the UCL in the youth population should be considered for nonoperative management, particularly in the 11–15 year old age group. The diagnosis of a partial tear may be facilitated by MRI arthrogram; CT arthrogram is also an option. Once again, player age, chronicity and degrees of dysfunction help to guide treatment and period of shutdown, ranging from a few weeks to 3 months. The majority of acute tears are from the ulnar insertion of the UCL; recent biomechanical data suggests that tears just proximal to the sublime tubercle, as opposed to just

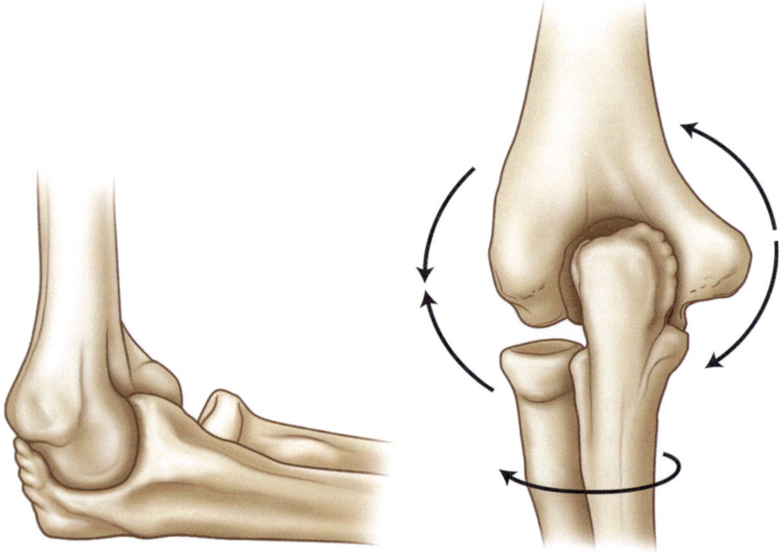

**Fig. 11.7** Image demonstrating posteromedial osteophyte formation on the olecranon tip. This osteophyte is formed when increased UCL laxity increases compressive forces. These osteophytes cause impingement of the olecranon fossa and may result in pain and discomfort during throwing. Identification of the tidemark between normal articular cartilage and the osteophyte is the hallmark of surgical resection, and overly aggressive resection may result in further instability of the UCL. The osteophyte may even be protective in the older asymptomatic throwing athlete (Image courtesy of Christian Caliboso)

distal, may be associated with greater degrees of instability [50]. Hassan et al. conducted a study where 13 specimens had their UCL detached at 50 % and then 100 % from the ulna in a proximal-to-distal fashion and 12 specimens followed the converse tear pattern, distal-to-proximal [50]. There was a significant change in contact area and movement of the center of pressure in partial proximal versus partial distal simulated rupture, suggesting that the proximal half of the distal UCL has a primary role in maintaining posteromedial stability of the elbow [50]. Earlier data had suggested that partial tears in elite athletes should be considered for early surgical reconstruction [51–53]. In contrast, Podesta et al. conducted a study involving 34 athletes with partial UCL tears, who failed at least 2 months of nonoperative treatment as well as an interval throwing program [54]. Each patient was injected with platelet-rich plasma and asked not to take any NSAIDs after the procedure [54]. After injection, each patient underwent a progressive course of physical therapy designed for eventual return to play [54]. The results of this study showed an 88 % return to play without complaints, with an average return to play at 12 weeks [54]. There is promise to this technique in soft tissue injuries. The rehabilitation program is not to be understated in this study.

While some may advocate for operative treatment of acute traumatic tears of the UCL, the extremes of age of the throwing athlete, the very young, ages 11–15, and the older elite athletes, ages 35–40, may undergo a trial of nonsurgical treatment. The patient may be placed in hinged elbow brace, locking out the terminal 30° of extension for 4–6 weeks, followed by a therapy and guided throwing program with a goal for return to sports at 3–4 months.

Acute traumatic avulsions in contact athletes such as football and lacrosse may also be braced with an extension block. Return to sport may be faster than the 3–4 month program for throwing. Return to contact sports is more guided by symptoms and function, with players returning to play in just a few weeks.

## Specific Guidelines Have Been Developed for Supervised Physical Therapy and Gradual Return to Throwing [Tables 11.1 and 11.2]

### Phase 1: Immediate Motion

This phase is to be completed after a period of rest, use of NSAIDS and ice. The goals of this phase are to minimize effects of immobilization, reestablish nonpainful ROM, decrease pain and inflammation, and retard muscle atrophy of the elbow [55]. It is important to manage pain and inflammation during this phase. Cryotherapy, laser, and high-voltage stimulation may be used in the acute response [55]. Following the acute response, moist heat, warm whirlpool, and ultrasound may be used to prepare the tissue for stretching [55]. Early ROM exercises are performed in all planes of elbow and wrist motions to minimize the formation of scar tissue and adhesions, while nourishing articular cartilage and assisting in the synthesis, alignment, and organization of collagen tissue [56–63]. Additionally, joint mobilizations may be performed to minimize joint contractures at this time [55]. If the patient is having difficulty reaching full ROM, low-load, long-duration stretching may be incorporated to produce a deformation of the collagen tissue, resulting in tissue elongation [64–67] [Fig. 11.8]. Slowing muscle atrophy plays an important role during this phase. It is important to perform subpainful and submaximal isometrics for the elbow flexor and extensor, as well as the wrist flexor, extensor, pronator, and supinator muscle groups [55].

### Phase 2: Intermediate

In order to proceed to phase 2, full throwing ROM, minimal pain and tenderness, and a good manual muscle test of the elbow flexor and extensor muscle groups must be achieved [55]. The goals of this phase are maintaining and enhancing elbow and upper extremity mobility, improving

**Table 11.1** Rehabilitation protocol for medial elbow pain

| | |
|---|---|
| Phase I | Acute Phase (week 1) |
| Goals | • Improve motion |
| | • Diminish pain and inflammation |
| | • Retard muscle atrophy |
| Exercises | • Stretching for wrist, elbow, and shoulder joints |
| | • Strengthening exercises: isometrics for wrist, elbow and shoulder musculature |
| | • Pain and inflammation control: cryotherapy, HVGS, ultrasound, and whirlpool |
| Phase II | Subacute Phase (weeks 2–4) |
| Goals | • Normalize motion |
| | • Improve muscular strength, power, and endurance |
| Exercises | Week 2 |
| | • Initiate isotonic strengthening for wrist and elbow muscles |
| | • Initiate tubing exercises for shoulder |
| | • Continue use of cryotherapy, HVGS, ultrasound, and whirlpool |
| | Week 3 |
| | • Initiate rhythmic stabilization drills for elbow and shoulder joints |
| | • Progress isotonic strengthening for entire upper extremity |
| | • Initiate isokinetic strengthening exercises for elbow flexion/extension |
| | Week 4 |
| | • Initiate Thrower's Ten Program |
| | • Emphasize eccentric biceps work, concentric triceps and wrist flexor work |
| | • Program endurance training |
| | • Initiate light plyometric drills |
| | • Initiate swinging drills |
| Phase III | Advanced Phase (weeks 5–6) |
| Goals | • Preparation of athlete for return to functional activities |
| Exercises | Week 5–6 |
| | • Continue strengthening exercises, endurance drills, and flexibility exercises daily |
| | • Thrower's Ten Program (Advanced) |
| | • Progress plyometric drills emphasize maintenance program based on pathology |
| | • Progress swinging drills (i.e., hitting) |
| Phase IV | Return to Activity Phase (weeks 7–10) |
| Goals | • Return to play, depends on condition and progress of injury and physician determination of safety |
| Exercises | Week 7 |
| | • Initiate interval sports program once determined by physician (phase I) |
| | Weeks 8–10 |
| | • Continue strengthening program, Thrower's Ten Program (Advanced) and flexibility program |
| | • Progress functional drills (phase II) to unrestricted play |

*Source*: Wilk KE, Macrina LC, Cain EL, Dugas JR, Andrews JR. Rehabilitation of the overhead athlete's elbow. *Sports Health*. 2012;4(5):404–414. Doi: 10.1177/1941738112455006

muscular strength and endurance, and reestablishing neuromuscular control of the elbow complex [55]. More aggressive mobilization techniques are applied to the joint as well as stretching exercises that focus on wrist, elbow, and shoulder flexibility [55]. Strengthening exercises during this phase include isotonic contractions, starting with concentric eventually reaching eccentric [55]. Exercises focus on elbow flexion and extension, wrist flexion and extension, and forearm pronation and supination [55]. If elbow pain is absent, the glenohumeral and scapulothoracic muscles may be placed on a progressive resistance program [55]. While working the shoulder, strengthening should focus on the external rotators and periscapular muscles [55]. The Thrower's Ten Program

**Table 11.2** Modified rehabilitation protocol for acutely traumatic avulsion

| | |
|---|---|
| Phase I | Immediate Motion Phase (weeks 0–2) |
| Goals | • Increase ROM |
| | • Promote healing of UCL |
| | • Retard muscle atrophy |
| | • Decrease pain and inflammation |
| Exercises | ROM |
| | • Brace (optional) nonpainful ROM [20–90°] |
| | • AAROM, PROM elbow and wrist (nonpainful range) |
| | Exercises |
| | • Isometrics—wrist and elbow musculature |
| | • Shoulder strengthening (no external rotation strengthening) |
| | Ice and compression |
| Phase II | Intermediate Phase (weeks 3–6) |
| Goals | • Increase ROM |
| | • Improve strength/endurance |
| | • Decrease pain and inflammation |
| | • Promote stability |
| Exercises | ROM |
| | • Gradually increase motion 0–135° (increase 10° per week) |
| | Exercises |
| | • Initiate isotonic exercises: wrist curls, wrist extensions, pronation/supination, biceps/triceps dumbbells, external rotation, deltoid, supraspinatus, rhomboids, internal rotation (Thrower's Ten Program) |
| | Ice and compression |
| Phase III | Advanced Phase (weeks 6–12) |
| Goals | • Increase strength, power, and endurance |
| | • Improve neuromuscular control |
| | • Initiate high speed exercise drills |
| Exercises | Exercises |
| | • Initiate exercise tubing, shoulder program, biceps/triceps program, supination/pronation, wrist extension/flexion (Advanced Thrower's Ten Program) |
| | • Plyometrics |
| | • Throwing drills |
| Phase IV | Return to Activity Phase (weeks 13–14) |
| Goals | • Return to functional activity |
| Exercises | Exercises |
| | • Initiate interval throwing, continue Advanced Thrower's Ten Program, continue plyometrics |

*Source*: Wilk KE, Macrina LC, Cain EL, Dugas JR, Andrews JR. Rehabilitation of the overhead athlete's elbow. *Sports Health*. 2012;4(5):404–414. Doi: 10.1177/1941738112455006

[Table 11.3] may be utilized during this phase, which has shown to illicit activity of muscles most needed for dynamic stability of the elbow [68–70] [Fig. 11.9]. Neuromuscular control exercises are initiated to enhance the muscles' ability to control the elbow joint during athletics, using proprioceptive neuromuscular facilitation with rhythmic stabilizations and manual resistance elbow/wrist flexion drills [55].

## Phase 3: Advanced Strengthening

Before progressing to stage 3, the patient must have full nonpainful external and internal rotation total ROM, no pain or tenderness, and 70 % strength compared to the contralateral extremity [55]. The goals of this phase are to increase strength, power, endurance, and neuromuscular control in preparation for return to activity [55].

Exercises during this phase are meant to progress to higher resistance, functional movements, eccentric contraction, and plyometric activities [55]. Eccentric contraction is the focus of elbow flexion during this phase [55]. The use of weight machines may be incorporated during this phase, if appropriate weight is used [55]. The Advanced Thrower's Ten Program [Table 11.4] may be incorporated to emphasize exercises specific to throwing [71]. During this phase, side-lying external rotation neuromuscular control exercises may be performed, with manual resistance [55]. Plyometric drills have shown to be beneficial to the recovery of the throwing elbow [72, 73]. During later stages of plyometric training, incorporating a weighted ball is important to train the shoulder and elbow to withstand high levels of stress [55] [Fig. 11.10].

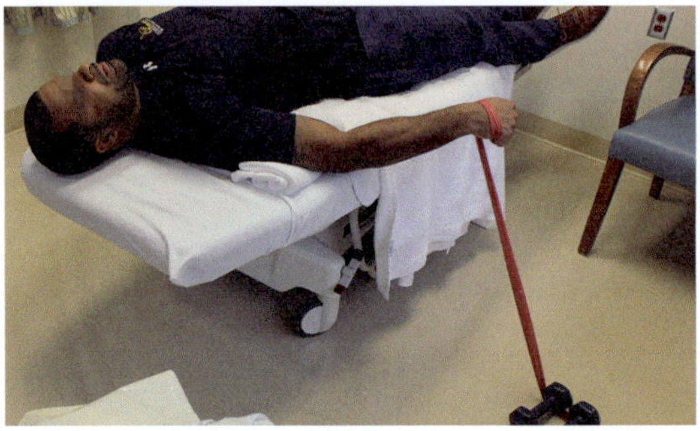

**Fig. 11.8** Low-load, long-duration stretch into elbow extension using light resistance is performed by having the shoulder internally rotated while the forearm is pronated to best isolate and maximize the stretch on the elbow joint. Patients having difficulty reaching full ROM use this progressive stretch into extension (Image courtesy of ONSF—ONS Foundation for Clinical Research and Education)

**Table 11.3** Thrower's Ten Program

| Thrower's Ten Program | |
|---|---|
| 1 | (A) Diagonal pattern D2 extension |
| | (B) Diagonal pattern D2 flexion |
| 2 | (A) External rotation at 0° abduction |
| | (B) Internal rotation at 0° abduction |
| 3 | Shoulder abduction to 90° |
| 4 | Scaption, external rotation |
| 5 | Sidelying external rotation |
| 6 | (A) Prone horizontal abduction (Neutral) |
| | (B) Prone horizontal abduction (Full ER, 100° ABD) |
| | (C) Prone row |
| | (D) Prone row into external rotation |
| 7 | Press-ups |
| 8 | Push-ups |
| 9 | (A) Elbow flexion |
| | (B) Elbow extension |
| 10 | (A) Wrist extension |
| | (B) Wrist flexion |
| | (C) Wrist supination |
| | (D) Wrist pronation |

*Source*: Wilk KE, Macrina LC, Cain EL, Dugas JR, Andrews JR. Rehabilitation of the overhead athlete's elbow. *Sports Health*. 2012;4(5):404–414. Doi: 10.1177/1941738112455006

a b

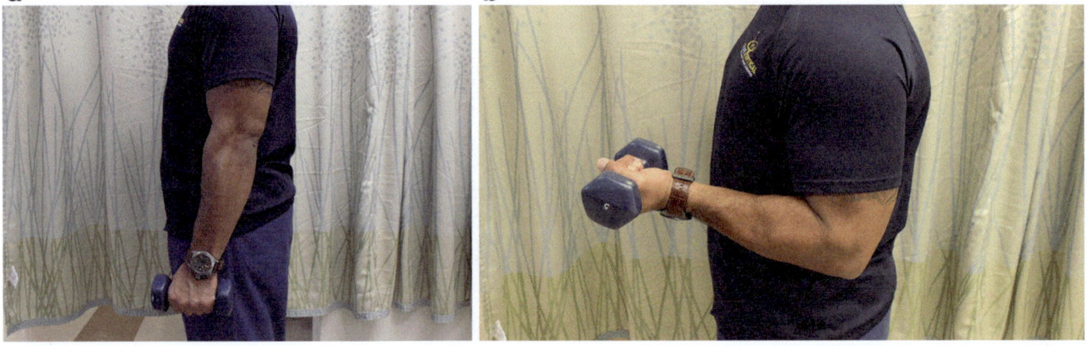

**Fig. 11.9** An important exercise in the Thrower's Ten Program as part of rehabilitation is elbow flexion. To perform this exercise, (**a**) stand with an arm against the side and palm facing inward, then (**b**) bend the elbow upward turning the palm as the exercise progresses. The exercise is used to strengthen the biceps muscle, one of the dynamic stabilizers of the elbow (Image courtesy of ONSF—ONS Foundation for Clinical Research and Education)

## Phase 4: Return to Activity

The goal of this phase is for the athlete to progressively return to competition using an interval throwing program [55]. In order to proceed to this phase, the athlete must have full pain-free throwing ROM, no tenderness, a satisfactory isokinetic test, and medical clearance from a physician [55]. If no symptoms are present, the athlete can participate in a long-toss interval throwing program beginning at 45 ft and progressing through 180 ft [74] [Tables 11.5 and 11.6]. When distance and intensity increase, stress of the medial elbow and anterior shoulder increase as well [74]. An important note to mention is with increased distance comes increased forces on the joints; therefore, it is important to stretch beforehand [75]. If the player is a pitcher, he or she should proceed to phase II of the program throwing off a mound [74] [Table 11.7]. During this phase, the number of throws, intensity, and type of pitch gradually progress to increase stress on the elbow and shoulder joints [55].

**Table 11.4** Advanced Thrower's Ten Program

| Advanced Thrower's Ten Program (Performed on stability ball) | |
|---|---|
| 1 | (A) External rotation at 0° Abduction |
| | (B) Internal rotation at 0° Abduction |
| 2 | (A) External rotation at 0° abduction with sustained hold |
| | (B) Internal rotation at 0° abduction with sustained hold |
| 3 | Shoulder abduction to 90° with sustained hold |
| 4 | Scaption, external rotation |
| 5 | Sidelying external rotation (No stability ball) |
| 6 | (A) Prone horizontal abduction (Neutral) |
| | (B) Prone horizontal abduction (Full ER, 100° ABD) |
| | (C) Prone row |
| | (D) Prone row into external Rrotation |
| 7 | (A) Seated scapular retraction into ER |
| | (B) Seated low trap |
| | (C) Seated neuromuscular control |
| 8 | Tilt-board push-ups |
| 9 | (A) Elbow flexion |
| | (B) Elbow extension (Abduction) |
| 10 | (A) Wrist extension |
| | (B) Wrist flexion |
| | (C) Wrist supination |
| | (D) Wrist pronation |

*Source*: Wilk KE, Macrina LC, Cain EL, Dugas JR, Andrews JR. Rehabilitation of the overhead athlete's elbow. *Sports Health*. 2012;4(5):404–414. Doi: 10.1177/1941738112455006

## Conclusion

Overhead throwing athletes are at risk of injury to the elbow due to cumulative stress of repetitive throwing particularly given that forces generated during the throwing motion ultimately exceed the native tensile strength of the UCL. The flexor–pronator mass and ulnar nerve are closely linked to the UCL; therefore injuries to these structures can be seen as well.

A detailed history and physical examination are necessary for a proper diagnosis, along with supplemented imaging studies. It is important to take a detailed throwing history that includes arm

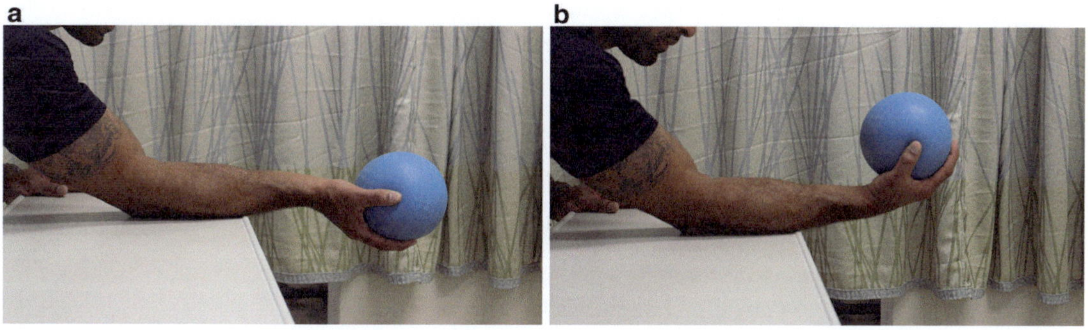

**Fig. 11.10** Plyometric wrist flexion flips using a weighted medicine ball to strengthen wrist flexors; (**a**) relaxed, (**b**) flexed. The exercise is particularly important for elbow rehabilitation because of the emphasis on forearm and hand musculature (Image courtesy of ONSF—ONS Foundation for Clinical Research and Education)

**Table 11.5** Interval Throwing Program for positional players

| | |
|---|---|
| 45′ Phase | |
| • Step 1 | • Step 2 |
| 1. Warm-up throwing | 1. Warm-up throwing |
| 2. 45′ (25 throws) | 2. 45′ (25 throws) |
| 3. Rest 5–10 min. | 3. Rest 5–10 min. |
| 4. Repeat 1–3 one more time | 4. Repeat 1–3 two more times |
| 60′ Phase | |
| • Step 3 | • Step 4 |
| 1. Warm-up throwing | 1. Warm-up throwing |
| 2. 60′ (25 throws) | 2. 60′ (25 throws) |
| 3. Rest 5–10 min. | 3. Rest 5–10 min. |
| 4. Repeat 1–3 one more time | 4. Repeat 1–3 two more times |
| 90′ Phase | |
| • Step 5 | • Step 6 |
| 1. Warm-up throwing | 1. Warm-up throwing |
| 2. 90′ (25 throws) | 2. 90′ (25 throws) |
| 3. Rest 5–10 min. | 3. Rest 5–10 min. |
| 4. Repeat 1–3 one more time | 4. Repeat 1–3 two more times |
| 120′ Phase | |
| • Step 7 | • Step 8 |
| 1. Warm-up throwing | 1. Warm-up throwing |
| 2. 120′ (25 throws) | 2. 120′ (25 throws) |
| 3. Rest 5–10 min. | 3. Rest 5–10 min. |
| 4. Repeat 1–3 one more time | 4. Repeat 1–3 two more times |
| 150′ Phase | |
| • Step 9 | • Step 10 |
| 1. Warm-up throwing | 1. Warm-up throwing |
| 2. 150′ (25 throws) | 2. 150′ (25 throws) |
| 3. Rest 3–5 min. | 3. Rest 3–5 min. |
| 4. Repeat 1–3 one more time | 4. Repeat 1–3 two more times |
| 180′ Phase | |
| • Step 11 | • Step 12 |
| 1. Warm-up throwing | 1. Warm-up throwing |
| 2. 180′ (25 throws) | 2. 180′ (25 throws) |
| 3. Rest 3–5 min. | 3. Rest 3–5 min. |
| 4. Repeat 1–3 one more time | 4. Repeat 1–3 two more times |
| • Step 13 | • Step 14 |
| 1. Warm-up throwing | 1. Return to respective position |
| 2. 180′ (25 throws) | |
| 3. Rest 3–5 min | |
| 4. Repeat 1–3 one more time | |
| 5. Repeat 1–3 with 20 throws | |
| 6. Warm-up throwing | |
| 7. 15 throws progressing from 120′ to 90′ | |

*Notes*

- All throws should be on an arc with a crow-hop
- Warm-up throws consist of 10–20 throws at approximately 30 ft
- Throwing program should be performed every other day, three times per week unless otherwise specified by your physician or rehabilitation specialist
- Perform each step two times before progressing to next step

*Source*: Wilk KE, Macrina LC, Cain EL, Dugas JR, Andrews JR. Rehabilitation of the overhead athlete's elbow. *Sports Health*. 2012;4(5):404–414. Doi: 10.1177/1941738112455006

**Table 11.6** Interval Throwing Program for Pitchers Phase I

| 45′ Phase | |
|---|---|
| • Step 1 | • Step 2 |
| 1. Warm-up throwing | 1. Warm-up throwing |
| 2. 45′ (25 throws) | 2. 45′ (25 throws) |
| 3. Rest 3–5 min. | 3. Rest 3–5 min. |
| 4. Repeat 1–3 one more time | 4. Repeat 1–3 two more times |
| 60′ Phase | |
| • Step 3 | • Step 4 |
| 1. Warm-up throwing | 1. Warm-up throwing |
| 2. 60′ (25 throws) | 2. 60′ (25 throws) |
| 3. Rest 3–5 min. | 3. Rest 3–5 min. |
| 4. Repeat 1–3 one more time | 4. Repeat 1–3 two more times |
| 90′ Phase | |
| • Step 5 | • Step 6 |
| 1. 60′ (10 throws) | 1. 60′ (7 throws) |
| 2. 90′ (20 throws) | 2. 90′ (18 throws) |
| 3. Rest 3–5 min. | 3. Rest 3–5 min. |
| 4. Repeat 1–3 one more time | 4. Repeat 1–3 two more times |
| 120′ Phase | |
| • Step 7 | • Step 8 |
| 1. 60′ (5–7 throws) | 1. 60′ (5 throws) |
| 2. 90′ (5–7 throws) | 2. 90′ (10 throws) |
| 3. 120′ (15 throws) | 3. 120′ (15 throws) |
| 4. Rest 3–5 min. | 4. Rest 3–5 min. |
| 5. Repeat 1–4 one more time | 5. Repeat 1–4 two more times |
| • Step 9 | • Step 10 |
| 1. 60′ (10–15 throws) | 1. 60′ (10–15 throws) |
| 2. 90′ (10 throws) | 2. 90′ (10 throws) |
| 3. 120′ (10 throws) | 3. 120′ (10 throws) |
| 4. 60′ (flat ground) using pitching mechanics (20–30 throws) | 4. 60′ (flat ground) using pitching mechanics (20–30 throws) |
| | 5. Rest 3–5 min. |
| | 6. 60′–90′ (10–15 throws) |
| | 7. 60′ (flat ground) using pitching mechanics (20 throws) |

*Notes*
• All throws should be on an arc with a crow-hop
• Warm-up throws consist of 10–20 throws at approximately 30 ft
• Throwing program should be performed every other day, with 1 day of rest between steps, unless otherwise specified by your physician
• Perform each step two times before progressing to next step
*Source*: Wilk KE, Macrina LC, Cain EL, Dugas JR, Andrews JR. Rehabilitation of the overhead athlete's elbow. *Sports Health*. 2012;4(5):404–414. Doi: 10.1177/1941738112455006

dominance and duration, intensity and location of symptoms as well as the phase of the throwing motion and activities that elicit symptoms. Clinical tests to evaluate valgus instability of the elbow should be performed in the throwing athlete. X-ray and MRI are often the preferred diagnostic imaging techniques.

Rehabilitation of the thrower's elbow follows a strict multiphasic approach. The first phase is meant to improve motion, diminish pain and inflammation, and slow muscle atrophy of the elbow. The goals of the next phase are to normalize motion and improve muscular strength, power, and endurance. The following phase

**Table 11.7** Interval Throwing Program for Pitchers Phase II

| | |
|---|---|
| Stage One: Fastballs Only | • Step 1 |
| | 1. Interval throwing |
| | 2. 15 throws off mound (50 %) |
| | • Step 2 |
| | 1. Interval throwing |
| | 2. 30 throws off mound (50 %) |
| | • Step 3 |
| | 1. Interval throwing |
| | 2. 45 throws off mound (50 %) |
| | • Step 4 |
| | 1. Interval throwing |
| | 2. 60 throws off mound (50 %) |
| | • Step 5 |
| | 1. Interval throwing |
| | 2. 70 throws off mound (50 %) |
| | • Step 6 |
| | 1. 45 throws off mound (50 %) |
| | 2. 30 throws off mound (75 %) |
| | • Step 7 |
| | 1. 30 throws off mound (50 %) |
| | 2. 45 throws off mound (75 %) |
| | • Step 8 |
| | 1. 10 throws off mound (50 %) |
| | 2. 65 throws off mound (75 %) |
| Stage Two: Fastballs Only | • Step 9 |
| | 1. 60 throws off mound (75 %) |
| | 2. 15 throws in batting practice |
| | • Step 10 |
| | 1. 50–60 throws off mound (75 %) |
| | 2. 30 throws in batting practice |
| | • Step 11 |
| | 1. 45–50 throws off mound (75 %) |
| | 2. 45 throws in batting practice |
| Stage Three | • Step 12 |
| | 1. 30 throws off mound (75 %) |
| | 2. 15 throws off mound (50 %, begin breaking balls) |
| | 3. 45–60 throws in batting practice (fastball only) |
| | • Step 13 |
| | 1. 30 throws off mound (75 %) |
| | 2. 30 breaking balls (75 %) |
| | 3. 30 throws in batting practice |
| | • Step 14 |
| | 1. 30 throws off mound (75 %) |
| | 2. 60–90 throws in batting practice (gradually increase breaking balls) |
| | • Step 15 |
| | 1. Simulated game: progressing by 15 throws per workout (pitch count) |

*Notes*

- All throwing off the mound should be done in the presence of your coach or sport biomechanist
- Stress proper throwing mechanics
- Use interval program 120′ phase as warm-up

*Source*: Wilk KE, Macrina LC, Cain EL, Dugas JR, Andrews JR. Rehabilitation of the overhead athlete's elbow. *Sports Health*. 2012;4(5):404–414. Doi: 10.1177/1941738112455006 begins the process to a functional recovery by preparing the athlete for throwing. The final phase is meant to prepare the athlete for a return to play by including an interval throwing program.

## References

1. Chen FS, Rokito AS, Jobe FW. Medial Elbow problems in the overhead-throwing athlete. J Am Acad Orthop Surg. 2001;9(2):99–113.
2. Bain GI, Mehta JA. Anatomy of the elbow joint and surgical approaches. In: Baker Jr CL, Plancher KD, editors. Operative treatment of elbow injuries. New York, NY: Springer; 2001. p. 1–27.
3. O'Driscoll SW, Jupiter JB, King GJW, et al. The unstable elbow. J Bone Joint Surg Am. 2000;82:724–38.
4. Callaway GH, Field LD, Deng XH, Torzilli PA, O'Brien SJ, Altchek DW, Warren RF. Biomechanical evaluation of the medial collateral ligament of the elbow. J Bone Joint Surg Am. 1997;79:1223–31.
5. Hotchkiss RN, Weiland AJ. Valgus stability of the elbow. J Orthop Res. 1987;5:372–7.
6. Regan WD, Korinek SL, Morrey BF, An KN. Biomechanical study of ligaments around the elbow joint. Clin Orthop Relat Res. 1991;(271):170–9.
7. Morrey BF, An KN. Articular and ligamentous contributions to the stability of the elbow joint. Am J Sports Med. 1983;11:313–9.
8. Morrey BF, Tanaka S, An KN. Valgus stability of the elbow. A definition of primary and secondary constraints. Clin Orthop Relat Res. 1991;(265):187–95.
9. Park MC, Ahmad CS. Dynamic contributions of the flexor-pronator mass to elbow valgus stability. J Bone Joint Surg Am. 2004;86-A(10):2268–74.
10. Murthi AM, Keener JD, Armstrong AD, Getz CL. The recurrent unstable elbow: diagnosis and treatment. J Bone Joint Surg Am. 2010;92(8):1794–804.
11. Conte S, Requa RK, Garrick JG. Disability days in major league baseball. Am J Sports Med. 2001;29(4):431–6.
12. Posner M, Cameron KL, Wolf JM, Belmont PJ, Owens BD. Epidemiology of major league baseball injuries. Am J Sports Med. 2011;39(8):1676–80.
13. Fleisig GS, Escamilla RF. Biomechanics of the elbow in the throwing athlete. Oper Tech Sports Med. 1994;4(2):62–8.
14. Werner SL, Fleisig GS, Dillman CJ, Andrews JR. Biomechanics of the elbow during baseball pitching. J Orthop Sports Phys Ther. 1993;17(6):274–8.
15. Cain E, Dugas J, Wolf R, Andrews J. Elbow injuries in throwing athletes: a current concepts review. Am J Sports Med. 2003;31:621–35.
16. Fleisig GS, Andrews JR, Dillman CJ, et al. Kinetics of baseball pitching with implications about injury mechanisms. Am J Sports Med. 1995;23:233–9.
17. Dillman CJ, Smutz P, Werner S. Valgus extension overload in baseball pitching. Med Sci Sports Exerc. 1991;23:S135.
18. Schickendantz M. Diagnosis and treatment of elbow disorders in the overhead athlete. Hand Clin. 2002;18:65–75. doi:10.1016/S0749-0712(02)00007-0.
19. Morrey BF. Applied anatomy and biomechanics of the elbow joint. Instr Course Lect. 1986;35:59–68.
20. Morrey BF, An KN. Functional anatomy of the ligaments of the elbow. Clin Orthop Relat Res. 1985;(201):84–90.
21. Dillman CJ, Fleisig GS, Andrews JR. Biomechanics of pitching with emphasis upon shoulder kinematics. J Orthop Sports Phys Ther. 1993;18:402–8.
22. Pappas A, Zawacki R, Sullivan T. Biomechanics of baseball pitching: a preliminary report. Am J Sports Med. 1985;13:216–22.
23. Conway JE, Jobe FW, Glousman RE, et al. Medial instability of the elbow in throwing athletes. J Bone Joint Surg. 1992;74A:67–83.
24. Jobe FW, Kvitne RS. Elbow instability in the athlete. Instr Course Lect. 1991;40:17–23.
25. Jobe FW, Stark H, Lombardo SJ. Reconstruction of the ulnar collateral ligament in athletes. J Bone Joint Surg. 1986;68A:1158–63.
26. Timmerman LA, Schwarts ML, Andrews JR. History and arthroscopic anatomy of the ulnar collateral ligament of the elbow. Am J Sports Med. 1994;22:667–73.
27. Ahmed CS, Lee TQ, ElAttrache NS. Biomechanical evaluation of a new ulnar collateral ligament reconstruction technique with interference screw fixation. Am J Sports Med. 2003;31(3):332–7.
28. Hariri S, Safran MR. Ulnar collateral ligament injury in the overhead athlete. Clin Sports Med. 2010;29(4):619–44.
29. Boatright JR, D'Alessandro DF. Nerve entrapment syndromes at the elbow. In: Jobe FW, Pink MM, Glousman RE, Kvitne RE, Zemel NP, editors. Operative techniques in upper extremity sports injuries. St. Louis, MO: Mosby-Year Book; 1996. p. 518–37.
30. Gabel GT, Morrey BF. Operative treatment of medial epicondylitis: influence of concomitant ulnar neuropathy at the elbow. J Bone Joint Surg Am. 1995;77:1065–9.
31. Harris JD, Lintner DM. Nerve injuries about the elbow in the athlete. Sports Med Arthrosc. 2014;22(3):e7–15. doi:10.1097/JSA.0000000000000038.
32. Hammond J, Cole BJ. Elbow injuries and the throwing athlete. In: Nicholson GP, editor. Orthopedic knowledge update: shoulder and elbow 4. Rosemont, IL: American Academy of Orthopedic Surgeons; 2013. p. 495–503.
33. Andrews JR, Wilk KE, Satterwhite YE, et al. Physical examination of the thrower's elbow. J Orthop Sports Phys Ther. 1993;17:296–304.
34. Azar FM, Andrews JR, Wilk KE, et al. Operative treatment of ulnar collateral ligament injuries of the elbow in athletes. Am J Sports Med. 2000;28:16–23.

35. Fleisig GS, Kingsley DS, Loftice JW, et al. Kinetic comparison among the fastball, curveball, change-up, and slider in collegiate baseball pitchers. Am J Sports Med. 2006;34(3):423–30.
36. Dugas JR, Weiland AJ. Vascular pathology in the throwing athlete. Hand Clin. 2000;16:477–85.
37. McCall BR, Cain Jr EL. Diagnosis, treatment, and rehabilitation of the thrower's elbow. Curr Sports Med Rep. 2005;4(5):249–54.
38. O'Holleran JD, Altchek DW. The thrower's elbow: arthroscopic treatment of valgus extension overload syndrome. HSS J. 2006;2(1):83–93.
39. Beals RK. The normal carrying angle of the elbow. Clin Orthop Relat Res. 1976;(119):194–6.
40. King JW, Brelsford HJ, Tullos HS. Analysis of the pitching arm of the professional baseball pitcher. Clin Orthop Relat Res. 1969;(67):116–23.
41. American Academy of Orthopedic Surgeons. Joint motion: method of measuring and recording. Chicago, IL: American Academy of Orthopedic Surgeons; 1965.
42. O'Driscoll SW, Lawton RL, Smith AM. The "moving valgus stress test" for medial collateral ligament tears of the elbow. Am J Sports Med. 2005;33(2):231–9.
43. Wilson FD, Andrews JR, Blackburn TA, McClusky G. Valgus extension overload in the pitching elbow. Am J Sports Med. 1983;11:83–8.
44. Ahmed CS, Conway JE. Elbow arthroscopy: valgus extension overload. Instr Course Lect. 2011;60:191–7.
45. Timmerman LA, Schwartz ML, Andrews JR. Preoperative evaluation of the ulnar collateral ligament by magnetic resonance imaging and computed tomography. Evaluation in 25 baseball players with surgical confirmation. Am J Sports Med. 1994;22:26–32.
46. Cotton A, Jacobson J, Brossman J, Pedowitz R, Haghighi P, Trudell D, Resnick D. Collateral ligaments of the elbow: conventional MR imaging and MR arthrography with coronal oblique plane and elbow flexion. Radiology. 1997;204:806–12.
47. Munshi M, Pretterblieber ML, Chung CB, Haghighi P, Cho JH, Trudell DJ, Resnick D. Anterior bundle of ulnar collateral ligament: evaluation of anatomic relationships by using MR imaging, MR arthrography, and gross anatomic and histologic analysis. Radiology. 2004;231:797–803.
48. Sasaki J, Takahara M, Ogino T, Kashiwa H, Ishigaki D, Kanauchi Y. Ultrasonographic assessment of the ulnar collateral ligament and medial elbow laxity in college baseball players. J Bone Joint Surg Am. 2002;84:525–31.
49. Osbahr DC, Chalmers PN, Frank JS, Williams III RJ, Widmann RF, Green DW. Acute, avulsion fractures of the medial epicondyle while throwing in youth baseball players: a variant of Little League elbow. J Shoulder Elbow Surg. 2010;19:951–7.
50. Hassan SE, Parks BG, Douoguih WA, Osbahr DC. Effect of distal ulnar collateral ligament tear pattern on contact forces and valgus stability in the posteromedial compartment of the elbow. Am J Sports Med. 2014;43(2):447–52.
51. Cain Jr EL, Andrews JR, Dugas JR, et al. Outcome of ulnar collateral ligament reconstruction of the elbow in 1281 athletes: results in 743 athletes with minimum 2-year follow-up. Am J Sports Med. 2010;38:2426–34.
52. Savoie III FH, Trenhaile SW, Roberts J, Field LD, Ramsey JR. Primary repair of ulnar collateral ligament injuries of the elbow in young athletes: a case series of injuries to the proximal and distal ends of the ligament. Am J Sports Med. 2008;36:1066–72.
53. Vitale MA, Ahmad CS. The outcome of elbow ulnar collateral ligament reconstruction in overhead athletes: a systematic review. Am J Sports Med. 2008;36:1193–205.
54. Podesta L, Crow SA, Volkmer D, Bert T, Yocum LA. Treatment of partial ulnar collateral ligament tears in the elbow with platelet-rich plasma. Am J Sports Med. 2013;41(7):1689–95. doi:10.1177/0363546513487979.
55. Wilk KE, Macrina LC, Cain EL, Dugas JR, Andrews JR. Rehabilitation of the overhead athlete's elbow. Sports Health. 2012;4(5):404–14. doi:10.1177/1941738112455006.
56. Coutts RD, Toth C, Kaita JH. The role of continuous passive motion in the rehabilitation of the total knee patient. In: Hungerford DS, Krackow KA, Kenna RV, editors. Total knee arthroplasty: a comprehensive approach. Baltimore, MD: Williams & Wilkins; 1984. p. 126–32.
57. Dehne E, Torp RP. Treatment of joint injuries by immediate mobilization: based upon the spinal adaption concept. Clin Orthop Relat Res. 1971;(77):218–32.
58. Haggmark T, Eriksson E. Cylinder or mobile cast brace after knee ligament surgery. A clinical analysis and morphologic and enzymatic studies of changes in the quadriceps muscle. Am J Sports Med. 1979;7(1):48–56.
59. Noyes FR, Mangine RE, Barber S. Early knee motion after open and arthroscopic anterior cruciate ligament reconstruction. Am J Sports Med. 1987;15(2):149–60.
60. Perkins G. Rest and movement. J Bone Joint Surg Br. 1953;35(4):521–39.
61. Salter RB, Hamilton HW, Wedge JH, et al. Clinical application of basic research on continuous passive motion for disorders and injuries of synovial joints: a preliminary report of a feasibility study. J Orthop Res. 1984;1(3):325–42.
62. Salter RB, Simmonds DF, Malcolm BW, Rumble EJ, MacMichael D, Clements ND. The biological effect of continuous passive motion on the healing of full-thickness defects in articular cartilage: an experimental investigation in the rabbit. J Bone Joint Surg Am. 1980;62(8):1232–51.
63. Wilk KE, Arrigo C, Andrews JR. Rehabilitation of the elbow in the throwing athlete. J Orthop Sports Phys Ther. 1993;17(6):305–17.
64. Kottke FJ, Pauley DL, Ptak RA. The rationale for prolonged stretching for correction of shortening of connective tissue. Arch Phys Med Rehabil. 1966; 47(6):345–52.

65. Sapega AA, Quedenfeld TC, Moyer RA, Butler RA. Biophysical factors in range-of-motion exercise. Phys Sports Med. 1981;9(12):57–65.
66. Warren CG, Lehmann JF, Koblanski JN. Heat and stretch procedures: an evaluation using rat tail tendon. Arch Phys Med Rehabil. 1976;57(3):122–6.
67. Warren CG, Lehmann JF, Koblanski JN. Elongation of rat tail tendon: effect of load and temperature. Arch Phys Med Rehabil. 1971;52(10):465–74.
68. Reinold MM, Macrina LC, Wilk KE, et al. Electromyographic analysis of the supraspinatus and deltoid muscles during 3 common rehabilitation exercises. J Athl Train. 2007;42(4):464–9.
69. Reinold MM, Wilk KE, Fleisig GS, et al. Electromyographic analysis of the rotator cuff and deltoid musculature during common shoulder external rotation exercises. J Orthop Sports Phys Ther. 2004;34(7):385–94.
70. Wilk KE, Obma P, Simpson CD, Cain EL, Dugas JR, Andrews JR. Shoulder injuries in the overhead athlete. J Orthop Sports Phys Ther. 2009;39(2):38–54.
71. Wilk KE, Yenchak AJ, Arrigo CA, Andrews JR. The advanced throwers ten exercise program: a new exercise series for enhanced dynamic shoulder control in the overhead throwing athlete. Phys Sports Med. 2011;39(4):90–7.
72. Schulte-Edelmann JA, Davies GJ, Kernozek TW, Gerberding ED. The effects of plyometric training of the posterior shoulder and elbow. J Strength Cond Res. 2005;19(1):129–34.
73. Wilk KE, Voight ML, Keirns MA, Gambetta V, Andrews JR, Dillman CJ. Stretch-shortening drills for the upper extremities: theory and clinical application. J Orthop Sports Phys Ther. 1993;17(5):225–39.
74. Reinold MM, Wilk KE, Reed J, Crenshaw K, Andrews JR. Interval sport programs: guidelines for baseball, tennis, and golf. J Orthop Sports Phys Ther. 2002;32(6):293–8.
75. Fleisig GS, Bolt B, Fortenbaugh D, Wilk KE, Andrews JR. Biomechanical comparison of baseball pitching and long-toss: implications for training and rehabilitation. J Orthop Sports Phys Ther. 2011;41(5):296–303.

# Operative Strategies for Ulnar Collateral Ligament Insufficiency

12

Kyle R. Duchman, Robert W. Westermann, and Brian R. Wolf

## Background

### History of Ulnar Collateral Ligament Injury and Reconstruction

The first report in the literature of a medial ulnar collateral ligament (UCL) injury was provided in 1946 by Waris, describing medial elbow pain and instability in a cohort of javelin throwers [1]. Since that time, reports of UCL injury have been described in a variety of athletes, most notably overhead throwing athletes. Within this population, UCL injury was frequently noted in baseball pitchers, where repetitive valgus forces can lead to chronic attenuation or acute injury to the medial ligamentous structures of the elbow. Prior to modern diagnostic and therapeutic techniques, UCL injury was almost certainly a career-ending injury for professional baseball pitchers. While attempts at UCL repair were described, the results in the baseball pitcher were less than satisfying [2]. The first described UCL reconstruction was performed in 1974 by Dr. Frank Jobe on Los Angeles Dodgers pitcher Tommy John. The first operation was generally accepted as a success, as Tommy John returned to pitching and made several All-Star game appearances after the procedure. The results of Dr. Jobe's initial UCL reconstruction technique were published in 1986 [3], setting the stage for multiple technique and rehabilitation modifications to be made to his original description of UCL reconstruction, now popularly referred to as Tommy John surgery in reference to Jobe's first patient.

## Epidemiology

As most UCL injuries in non-throwing athletes are managed conservatively without surgical intervention, the true prevalence of UCL injury is unknown. Within the general population, UCL injury requiring surgical intervention is rare, with as few as 4 in 100,000 individuals undergoing surgical intervention. The incidence of UCL reconstruction procedures appears to be highest in young patients, aged 15–19 years, where the incidence of reconstruction approaches 22 in 100,000 patients [4]. The majority of today's UCL reconstruction procedures are performed in baseball players, where as many as 10 % of minor league and professional players have undergone UCL reconstruction [5]. The prevalence is even

---

**Electronic supplementary material** The online version of this chapter (doi:10.1007/978-3-319-46019-2_12) contains supplementary material, which is available to authorized users. Videos can also be accessed at http://link.springer.com/chapter/10.1007/978-3-319-46019-2_12.

K.R. Duchman, MD • R.W. Westermann, MD
B.R. Wolf, MD, MS (✉)
Department of Orthopedics and Rehabilitation, University of Iowa Hospitals and Clinics, 200 Hawkins Drive, 01008 JPP, Iowa City, IA 52242, USA
e-mail: kyle-duchman@uiowa.edu; robert-westermann@uiowa.edu; brian-wolf@uiowa.edu

© Springer International Publishing Switzerland 2017

R.Z. Tashjian (ed.), *The Unstable Elbow*, DOI 10.1007/978-3-319-46019-2_12

higher in professional baseball pitchers, where nearly 25 % of current professional pitchers describe a history of UCL reconstruction. Over the last decade, there has been an estimated annual increase in UCL reconstruction procedures of 4 %, with annual growth rates approaching 10 % for patients aged 15–19 years [4]. Given the high prevalence of UCL reconstruction procedures in elite baseball players as well as the increasing incidence in young patients over the last decade, it is safe to assume that team physicians, athletic trainers, and rehabilitation specialists will be managing a record number of post-UCL reconstruction athletes in the coming years. Fortunately, while primary UCL reconstruction procedures continue to increase, the incidence of revision UCL reconstructions is decreasing, presumably secondary to improved techniques and rehabilitation protocols [6]. If recent trends continue to hold true, preventative strategies, including throwing programs and pitch limits for youth baseball players [7], will be important to implement in order to protect our young athletes in future years.

## Relevant Anatomy

The UCL is comprised of three components, including the anterior, posterior and transverse bundles [8]. The anterior bundle of the ligament originates at the anteroinferior portion of the medial epicondyle of the humerus. Moving distally from its relatively broad-based origin, the anterior bundle narrows in the sagittal plane prior to inserting on the sublime tubercle of the ulna and fanning out along the medial ulnar collateral ridge [9]. The anterior bundle of the UCL can be identified as a distinct structure from the underlying elbow joint capsule [10], which distinguishes it from the other bundles of the UCL. The anterior bundle of the UCL provides the primary restraint to valgus force between 20° and 120° [11–14]. Outside of this range, the osseous anatomy of the elbow serves as the primary restraint to valgus laxity. The posterior bundle is essentially a fan-shaped thickening of the elbow joint capsule, coursing between the medial epicondyle of the humerus and the semilunar notch of the ulna. The fan-shaped posterior bundle has been found to have a relatively insignificant role, described as a secondary or tertiary restraint in mid-flexion, with respect to elbow stability [12, 13]. The transverse bundle both originates and inserts on the ulna. It connects the medial olecranon to the inferomedial coronoid process. As it does not cross the ulnohumeral joint, it does not act as a valgus restraint. As the anterior bundle of the UCL has been shown to be the primary static stabilizer to resist valgus stress, the majority of UCL reconstruction procedures have aimed to reproduce this anatomy.

## Evaluation

### History

Obtaining a detailed history is the first step toward diagnosis of UCL. The presentation almost invariably includes medial sided elbow pain that is aggravated by activity. A patient's age, activity, sport, and level of competition are all important to ascertain during the initial history and may help narrow the diagnosis. UCL injuries are frequently described in baseball players, particularly pitchers, javelin throwers, tennis players, and volleyball players but may occur during a variety of other sporting and non-sporting activities. A prior history of elbow injury or surgery should be elucidated, as should any previous upper extremity injury, surgery, or cervical spine pathology. Determining whether or not a patient's symptoms resolved with appropriate treatment in the setting of prior injury or surgery is important, as surgical failure, reinjury, underlying concomitant injury, or missed diagnosis should all be considered.

The duration and context of the pain is also important to note. With UCL injury, presentations often fit two classic scenarios. The first and most common presentation is an acute onset of pain [15], which is frequently described as a popping sensation. In the competitive overhead athlete, this presentation may coincide with a specific throw or pitch followed by the inability to continue with competition. This scenario likely represents an acute rupture or acute on chronic presentation in the setting of a previously attenuated ligament. The second scenario is also described as medial elbow pain, but in a more chronic setting with more ambiguous symptoms which may be accompanied by a gradual decline in performance, such as decreased throwing velocity, control, or endurance in a pitcher, as well as a noticeable or perceived change in mechanics to accommodate for underlying symptoms. In this type of presentation, it is important to note the timing of the symptoms relative to training regimens and pitch counts.

In the case of baseball pitchers, pain is often noted most during the late cocking and early acceleration phases of throwing when the most stress is placed on the UCL [16]. Despite the complexity of the overhead throwing motion, overhead athletes can fairly reliably describe the location of their symptoms as well as the phase of throwing that those symptoms occur during. Both the location of the pain as well as phase of the throwing motion are important components of the history, with medial-sided symptoms occurring during the late cocking or early acceleration phase frequently described by patients who ultimately are determined to have a UCL injury at the conclusion of their diagnostic workup [2].

While the history is the first step toward diagnosis of a UCL injury, UCL pathology can occur independently or concomitantly with several other diagnoses not limited to valgus extension overload [17], osteochondral defects with or without loose bodies, ulnar neuritis or subluxation [18], olecranon stress fracture [19], and flexor–pronator mass strains or tendonitis which need to be identified for appropriate treatment. These diagnoses as well as other diagnoses, including medial epicondylitis, little leaguer's elbow, or a variety of nerve entrapment syndromes, may also occur independent of UCL injury, further confounding the diagnosis. In this setting, additional questions including the presence or absence of radiating symptoms or paresthesias, loss of hand intrinsic strength, or vascular complaints [20] are all important to note. Additional clinical testing and diagnostic imaging can help clarify the diagnosis when in question or when concomitant pathology is a significant concern.

## Physical Examination

A thorough understanding of the bony anatomy as well as the active and passive soft tissue stabilizers of the elbow is a prerequisite to completing a systematic exam of the elbow when there is suspicion of UCL injury. Physical examination begins with visual inspection of the elbow. Comparison of muscle mass and distribution as well as gross alignment should be made to the contralateral limb and should not be limited to the region of the elbow alone but should include the shoulder and hand, where intrinsic muscle wasting may be indicative of underlying ulnar nerve or systemic pathology. Depending on the nature and timing of the injury, visible swelling or ecchymosis may be seen along the medial aspect of the elbow. Additionally, the posture of the elbow should be noted, as an effusion will often lead to the patient holding the elbow in flexion to accommodate increased intracapsular volume [21]. The natural carrying angle of the elbow is in slight valgus, approximately 10° in males [22], which may be increased in the dominant arm of the throwing athlete and should not be confused with pathology in this population [23]. Also noted should be any prior surgical scars along the elbow, which may provide clues to previous injuries if the patient is unable to provide sufficient detail. In cases where UCL reconstruction is likely, inspection of the wrist and determination of the presence or absence of a palmaris longus tendon may influence graft choice.

Following inspection of the elbow, palpation of the elbow can be performed. The most prominent structure on the medial aspect of the elbow is the medial epicondyle, serving as the origin of the flexor–pronator mass. The UCL sits deep to the proximal flexor–pronator mass and it may be tender along its entire course. The ligament should be palpated from its origin at the medial epicondyle, along the mid-substance of the ligament, all the way to the insertion on the sublime tubercle of the ulna. Flexing the elbow to 50–70° of flexion moves the bulk of the flexor–pronator mass anteriorly, making the underlying UCL more accessible [24]. As the medial epicondyle is the common origin for many structures about the elbow, tenderness to palpation is a relatively nonspecific finding [25]. Palpation of other bony landmarks, including the posteromedial aspect of the ulna, lateral epicondyle, posterolateral soft triangle, and radiocapitellar joint may help identify concomitant pathology, such as valgus extension overload [17] or olecranon stress fracture. Additionally, the ulnar nerve assumes a relatively subcutaneous position at the elbow and should be palpated throughout an entire range of motion in order to assess the stability of the ulnar nerve. Anterior subluxation, or less commonly anterior dislocation, of the nerve may be identified, contributing to symptoms and potentially altering management at the time of surgical intervention if indicated. The ulnar nerve can also be lightly percussed or gently compressed within the cubital tunnel in order to provoke paresthesias or abnormal sensation in the ring and small finger of the affected extremity, which may indicate underlying ulnar neuritis.

Following inspection and palpation of the elbow, assessment of both active and passive range of motion is important. As a ginglymoid joint, the ulnohumeral articulation acts as a simple hinge with varus and valgus motion limited by a combination of bony and soft tissue restraints. In the sagittal plane, the elbow typically has 0–140° of motion [21]. The radiocapitellar joint accommodates pronation and supination at the level of the elbow, and should also be assessed. The contralateral elbow can serve as a readily available comparison when any concerns arise. Additionally, pain, crepitus, or mechanical symptoms should be noted during range of motion testing. In the throwing athlete, it is not uncommon to have a loss of motion [23], particularly terminal extension, which may not represent injury in this population. Assessment of elbow stability has been described previously through the use of several special tests. Assessing valgus stability of the elbow is best done in the supine position, allowing stabilization of the scapula and humerus. Valgus stress can be applied to the elbow at a variety of elbow flexion and shoulder abduction angles, with flexion of the arm to approximately 70° while maintaining neutral forearm rotation has been found to result in the greatest valgus laxity [26]. Valgus stress testing that is asymmetric compared to the contralateral elbow, painful, or lacks a firm endpoint is concerning for a UCL injury. Pain is often the most important indicator, as clinically unperceivable valgus opening can be associated with a partial or complete tear of the UCL [27, 28]. Alternatively, where available and technically an option, stress ultrasonography can provide a dynamic evaluation of the UCL [29]. Other tests, including the milking maneuver [24] and modified milking maneuver [30], can be performed with the patient in the seated position and 90° of shoulder abduction while a valgus load is applied by the patient themselves or the examiner (Fig. 12.1). O'Driscoll and colleagues have

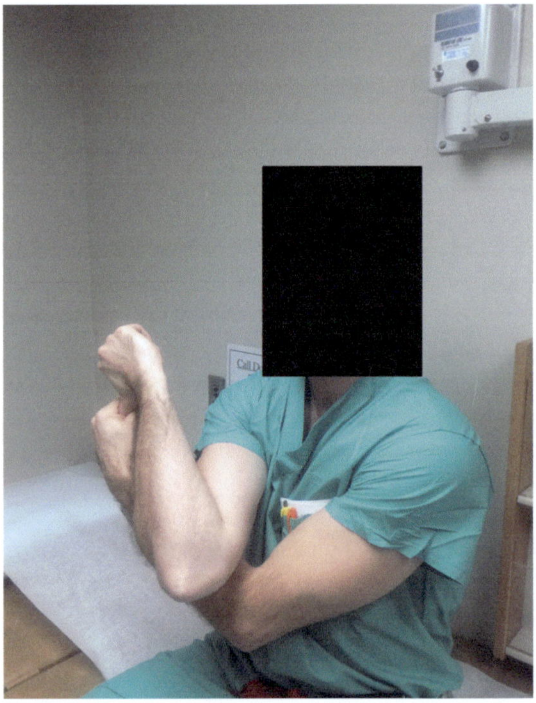

**Fig. 12.1** The milking maneuver can be performed by the patient or examiner. Valgus stress is applied while maintaining the forearm in supination. A positive test elicits pain at the medial elbow

described the moving valgus stress test, which places the elbow in full flexion and the shoulder in 90° of abduction followed by rapid extension of the elbow while a valgus load is applied [31]. This was originally described in the seated position, but can also reliably be performed in the supine position (Fig. 12.2), which is preferred by the authors. Supine positioning allows the examining table to stabilize the shoulder and arm while stressing the elbow. Using this test, pain or apprehension as the elbow is extended from 120° to 70° of flexion while a valgus load is applied is concerning for UCL injury with good sensitivity and specificity reported.

In addition to examination of the elbow, examination of the adjacent shoulder and wrist should also be performed. For example, pain at the medial elbow with resisted flexion of the wrist may represent flexor–pronator strain or tendonitis. Additionally, UCL injuries have been associated with decreased shoulder motion including deficits in total shoulder range of motion as well as glenohumeral internal rotation deficit. These deficits in motion may be secondary to adaptive changes in the throwing shoulder and are common among throwing athletes [32, 33]. As such, these findings may be less of a diagnostic clue when attempting to diagnosis UCL injury, but rather serve as a potential therapeutic intervention either prophylactically or as part of nonoperative or post-surgical management in the throwing athlete to prevent subsequent injury or reinjury, respectively.

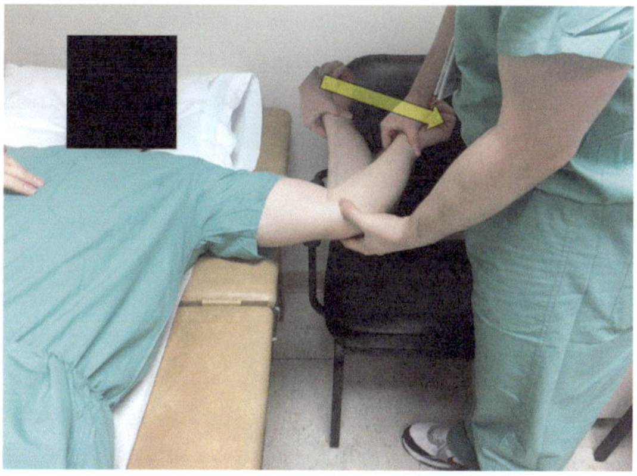

**Fig. 12.2** The moving valgus stress test performed in the supine position. The arm is extended from 120° to 70° of flexion while a valgus force is applied. Pain in this range of motion is consistent with a positive test

## Diagnostic Imaging

Imaging of the painful elbow is indicated with persistent pain or concern for acute injury. Standard anteroposterior and lateral radiographs of the elbow are useful as they may identify avulsion at the sublime tubercle in acute cases [34] or heterotopic ossification adjacent to the ligamentous insertion in more chronic cases of UCL insufficiency [35]. Additionally, radiographs can help identify concomitant pathology including loose bodies, osteochondral defects, or posteromedial olecranon osteophytes associated with valgus extension overload [17]. Additional radiographs, include internal and external oblique views as well as oblique axial views can be obtained depending on the concern for concomitant pathology. Historically, valgus stress radiographs have also been described. However, increased valgus laxity may be a normal finding in some overhead athletes [36], and the absolute amount of medial opening that indicates pathology is unclear. Because of this, the reported benefit of stress radiographs are inconsistent throughout the literature [15, 37], and their role in practice is limited, particularly given the improvement and widespread availability of advanced imaging techniques.

With widespread availability and improved quality, magnetic resonance imaging (MRI) of the elbow has become the study of choice for evaluation of UCL injury. MRI without contrast has been shown to have both sensitivity and specificity approaching 100 % in detecting full-thickness UCL injuries with good interrater reliability [38], but may be limited in detecting partial-thickness tears. Sensitivity and specificity are both improved with the addition of intraarticular gadolinium contrast in the form of a magnetic resonance arthrogram (MRA). MRA is particularly useful given the spectrum of pathology that can exist within the UCL, ranging from degenerative changes, partial-thickness tears, and full-thickness tears that may be difficult to distinguish with standard MRI sequences [25, 39–41]. With MRA, the undersurface of the UCL can be better visualized, improving sensitivity for partial thickness tears [38, 40], and any contrast extravasation from the joint is indicative of a UCL injury. With the widespread availability of MRI, the role for computed tomography (CT) either alone or with intraarticular contrast has become limited. However, in patients who cannot undergo MRI due to implanted medical devices or severe claustrophobia, or those with significant osteophytes or loose bodies, CT arthrography remains an option.

The use of ultrasound in imaging the UCL continues to evolve. Ultrasound provides the benefit of a dynamic, real-time evaluation, but may be limited by operator experience and availability. In the competitive throwing athlete, the UCL is often thickened [42], and areas of heterogeneity within the ligament must be distinguished from pathology. Dynamic ultrasound in the form of valgus stress ultrasound is limited by many of the same factors that limit interpretation of stress radiographs, namely increased laxity in the throwing elbow of the asymptomatic thrower [36, 43] and the lack of a definitive amount of medial opening to indicate a tear. Ultrasound remains an evolving technology, and its diagnostic and therapeutic uses in the setting of UCL injury will require further evaluation in years to come.

## Treatment Algorithm

### Injury Prevention

With the increased rate of UCL reconstruction over the last decade [4], efforts to reduce injuries have been made, particularly at the level of youth baseball. Efforts to reduce injury in young pitchers have primarily focused on reducing pitch quantity, as the amount of pitching has been shown to correlate with the risk of subsequent elbow injury [44, 45]. Additionally, injuries are more likely to occur in baseball pitchers who express symptoms of fatigue or overuse. Fatigue has been shown to alter pitching kinematics, potentially setting the stage for future injury [46]. Based on these findings, pitch count recommendations for youth baseball players have been made at the national level as well as local and regional levels. Despite these efforts, a lack of knowledge and compliance with pitch count recommendations has been noted, with both youth baseball players and coaches deficient in this area, suggesting that further education on this topic is necessary [47, 48]. Further hindering compliance is the fact that players frequently play in multiple leagues with multiple coaches, which has also been shown to be a risk factor for injury, likely serving as a surrogate for overall pitch volume [45]. While pitch choice has often been implicated as a risk factor for elbow injury in youth pitchers, there is little solid evidence to support that throwing curveballs or sliders increases the risk of injury, although it may increase the incidence of arm pain [45, 49]. However, increased pitch velocity has been associated with an increased risk of elbow injury [44]. In light of these findings, several recommendations have been made to reduce the risk of elbow injury in youth pitchers and include responding to fatigue and pain with rest, avoid pitching more than 100 innings in a calendar year, encourage non-pitching activities for at least 4 months of the year, teach and reinforce proper mechanics, and encourage compliance with pitch count regulations [7, 49]. In order to address the increased rates of shoulder and elbow injuries in youth baseball pitchers, several organizations guided by expert panels, including Little League® and USA Baseball, have provided age-specific pitch count and rest recommendations for young pitchers [50, 51] (Table 12.1). Additionally, optimizing shoulder and elbow health in the throwing athlete with a dedicated program focused on range of motion, core and lower extremity strengthening, and scapular stabilization can help correct kinematic abnormalities and prevent deficits, such as glenohumeral internal rotation deficits [52], which may reduce the risk of UCL injury.

**Table 12.1** Age-based daily pitch count recommendations and rest recommendations [50, 51]

| *Pitch count recommendations* | |
|---|---|
| Age | Pitches per day |
| 7–8 | 50 |
| 9–10 | 75 |
| 11–12 | 85 |
| 13–16 | 95 |
| 17–18 | 105 |
| 19–22 | 120 |
| *Rest recommendations* | |
| Pitches per day | |
| <14 years of age | Rest days required |
| 1–20 | 0 |
| 21–35 | 1 |
| 36–50 | 2 |
| 51–65 | 3 |
| ≥66 | 4 |
| 15–18 years of age | |
| 1–30 | 0 |
| 31–45 | 1 |
| 46–60 | 2 |
| 61–75 | 3 |
| ≥76 | 4 |
| 19–22 years of age | |
| 1–30 | 0 |
| 31–45 | 1 |
| 46–60 | 2 |
| 61–75 | 3 |
| 76–105 | 4 |
| ≥106 | 5 |

## Nonoperative Management

Nonoperative management of UCL injuries remains the treatment of choice for non-throwing athletes. Nonoperative management in the non-throwing athlete includes rest for 4–6 weeks, activity modification, physical therapy, pain control with nonsteroidal anti-inflammatory medications, and possible hinged bracing as athletes return to play depending on their level of competition, sport, and position. Using this protocol, nonoperative management has even been shown to be effective in some throwing populations, including professional quarterbacks, where 90 % were able to return to sport without surgical intervention [53]. While the vast majority of the current literature has focused on failures of nonoperative management in baseball players, specifically pitchers, nonoperative management remains the treatment of choice for non-throwing and even some throwing athletes.

Nonoperative management of UCL injuries in baseball players have historically produced less than satisfying results. However, the literature frequently fails to distinguish between partial-thickness and full-thickness tears, limiting the applicability of findings. In one of the largest case series detailing the results of nonoperative treatment in the throwing athlete, Rettig et al. found that only 42 % of athletes were able to return to sport at a preinjury level [54]. The non-operative protocol utilized in their study included two stages. The first stage consisted of complete rest from throwing for 2–3 months, pain control with anti-inflammatory medications, ice, and active and passive elbow range of motion with bracing at night. The second stage of the protocol was initiated after the athlete was pain free and included upper extremity strengthening, a progressive throwing program, and an elbow hyperextension brace. While their overall results would be considered poor, the inability to distinguish athletes with partial-thickness and full-thickness tears limits conclusions.

While nonoperative management of full-thickness tears is unlikely to produce satisfying results, nonoperative management of partial-thickness tears remains a viable option. Nonoperative protocols for partial-thickness UCL strains typically include a minimum of 3 months of no throwing activity, with immediate initiation of non-painful active and passive range of motion, progressing toward exercises to increase strength, power, and endurance while incorporating a thrower's ten program [55]. A brace can be used during range of motion exercises to prevent valgus loading and restrict motion to a non-painful arc. Progression to throwing activities at 3 months only occurs if the athlete has non-painful and full range of motion and no increased valgus laxity on exam. With these requirements satisfied, the throwing athlete can initiate an interval throwing program while still focusing on the thrower's ten program, core strengthening, and plyometric exercises [56]. If symptoms persist or reoccur at any point during the throwing program, surgical intervention can be considered.

In the era of biologic augmentation, the effectiveness of biologic agents in the treatment of patients with partial-thickness UCL injuries has been considered. One such biologic agent, platelet-rich plasma (PRP), has been extensively studied in the orthopedic literature with variable results depending on the pathology and anatomic site in question [57]. To date, a single study has evaluated the effectiveness of PRP in the treatment of partial-thickness UCL injury. In this study, Podesta and colleagues evaluated the effectiveness of PRP injections for throwers that had previously failed 2 months of nonoperative treatment, which included an interval throwing program. In their study, 88 % of athletes were able to return to throwing at an average of 12 weeks following PRP injection [58]. While these findings are promising, further studies specifically evaluating nonoperative management of partial-thickness injuries with or without biologic augmentation are necessary.

## Surgical Indications

Surgical management of UCL injury is reserved for throwing athletes with full-thickness UCL tears who wish to return to competition or individuals with partial-thickness tears that have persistent medial elbow pain or valgus laxity following an appropriate nonoperative treatment course.

## Surgical Techniques

Prior to Jobe's original description of UCL reconstruction [3], surgical intervention for UCL injury was limited to primary repair. While primary repair for acute avulsion injuries with suture anchor fixation or bone tunnels remains an option, the results for this technique are limited in the literature [59–61]. Early comparative studies revealed inferior results with repair as compared to reconstruction [2, 15], although those studies did not distinguish repair in acute injuries from repair in the more chronic setting where ligament attenuation is a known issue and reconstruction is preferable. In our experience, direct repair remains an option for acute proximal or distal avulsion injuries. Direct repair is particularly suitable for non-pitching athletes, such as baseball position players or non-throwing athletes that participate in football or wrestling. If repair is considered, it is important to carefully inspect the UCL at the time of surgery in order to rule out intrasubstance ligament injury or attenuation. If intrasubstance ligament injury or attenuation is noted, then a UCL reconstruction is performed. However, if the UCL injury appears to be a true avulsion injury, suture anchor methods have been described with good-to-excellent outcomes in young athletes [61].

The original UCL reconstruction as described by Jobe included a medial approach to the elbow with mobilization of the ulnar nerve for later transposition. Access to the UCL was gained by transecting the flexor–pronator mass off of the epicondyle, leaving a cuff of tendon attached to bone for later repair. With the flexor–pronator mass reflected distally, the UCL could be visualized from its origin at the medial epicondyle to its insertion on the sublime tubercle of the ulna. Tunnels were drilled at the sublime tubercle and medial epicondyle to allow passage of a palmaris autograft in a figure-of-eight fashion, which was then sutured again at its midpoint under appropriate tension. The mobilized ulnar nerve was then placed under the reflected flexor–pronator mass and the flexor–pronator mass repaired back to the cuff of tendon at medial epicondyle, resulting in a submuscular transposition of the ulnar nerve [3]. In the original series reported by Jobe et al. as well as the later comparative study by Conway et al. [2, 3], ulnar neuritis was a relatively common complication, contributing at least in part to low return to play numbers. In order to reduce this complication, the modified Jobe technique was described, which utilized a muscle splitting approach through the posterior aspect of the flexor–pronator mass in order to gain access to the underlying UCL [15, 62, 63]. Additionally, the humeral tunnels were oriented more anteriorly in order to prevent injury to the ulnar nerve [62]. While management of the ulnar nerve varied between authors, ranging from transposition with a flexor–pronator fascial sling to in situ decompression, the modified Jobe technique significantly reduced postoperative complications and allowed improved return to sport as compared to the original description [62].

In 2002, Rohrbough and colleagues described UCL reconstruction using the docking technique, which was the first major technique modification that addressed graft fixation, tensioning, and iatrogenic fracture concerns while also utilizing a flexor–pronator splitting approach [64]. Tunnels were created at the sublime tubercle and connected with a curette to maintain an approximately 1 cm bone bridge. A single dead-end humeral tunnel was made in the anterior portion of the medial epicondyle at the origin of the anterior band of the UCL, and two small holes were made with a dental drill or small burr to communicate with the humeral tunnel and allow suture passage. A palmaris or gracilis autograft was then passed through the ulnar tunnel and the sutured end of the graft pulled through one of the small communicating drill holes, effectively docking one limb of the graft. The free limb of the graft was then measured while maintaining the elbow in varus in order to estimate its length in the tunnel. A Krackow stitch was then placed in the remaining free limb of the graft and passed through the other small drill hole in the medial epicondyle to dock the free end in the humeral tunnel. With varus maintained at the elbow, the two free suture ends were tensioned and tied over the bone bridge at the medial epicondyle. Minor modification to the docking technique, including use of a doubled palmaris autograft, has also been described and referred to as the modified docking procedure [65]. The docking and modified docking technique provide greater control of graft tensioning while yielding equivalent or even improved biomechanical properties as compared to the Jobe technique [66–69].

More recent modifications to the Jobe and docking techniques have primarily focused on alternative or hybrid fixation at the ulna, humerus, or both. One popular modification is the eponymously named DANE TJ (David Altcheck, Neal ElAttrache, Tommy John) technique, which uses interference screw fixation at the UCL insertion on the ulna [70, 71]. As hypothesized by the authors, interference screw fixation better replicates the native anatomy of the UCL as it narrows at the ulnar footprint. Additionally, interference screw fixation eliminates the need for two bone tunnels, theoretically reducing the risk of iatrogenic fracture. Biomechanical comparisons of the different fixation techniques have been explored with variable results throughout the literature [66, 69, 72]. A clear limitation of these cadaveric biomechanical studies is that the in vivo dynamic stabilizers are rarely accounted for during testing and that healing is not considered, with each biomechanical study essentially serving as a time zero analysis of the construct strength.

As implant designs and fixation techniques continue to evolve, modifications to UCL reconstruction techniques will continue to be described. Suspensory and interference screw ulnar and humeral fixation using manufacturer-specific devices are frequently reported in the literature with little biomechanical superiority or inferiority noted with these subtle technique variations [73–76]. Similarly, a variety of graft choices have been described, including palmaris, gracilis, toe extensor, plantaris, and Achilles autograft as well as hamstring allograft [3, 77, 78], all of which have provided satisfying results in the literature when coupled with modern techniques. When carefully evaluating the literature, major technique advances since Jobe's original technique description include the use of the flexor–pronator splitting approach as well as patient-specific management of the ulnar nerve depending on preoperative symptoms and intraoperative evaluation. In general, these advances have reduced postoperative complications and led to lower rates of revision surgery despite the increased rate of primary reconstructions being performed [6].

## Postoperative Management

Patients are typically placed in a posterior splint for 1–2 weeks postoperatively with the elbow immobilized in 90° of flexion. Finger and wrist range of motion protocols vary while immobilized at the elbow, but with the flexor–pronator splitting approach, can typically be started as pain allows postoperatively as compared to the original Jobe description which took down the origin of the flexor–pronator mass [79]. After this short period of immobilization, patients are transitioned to a hinged elbow brace, with initial range of motion limited to 45–90° of motion, increasing range of motion by approximately 15° per week with the goal or reaching full passive range of motion by 6 weeks postoperatively. As elbow flexion contractures are common even in the throwing arm of uninjured athletes, gentle stretching exercises to reduce flexion contractures can be used but should be carefully guided by a patient's symptoms. At 6 weeks postoperatively, the hinged elbow brace can be discontinued and light strengthening exercises can commence. In addition to the elbow, shoulder and wrist strengthening and range of motion should also be addressed. At 12 weeks postoperatively, more vigorous strengthening exercises can begin, and an organized throwing program, such as the thrower's ten program [55], can begin at 14–16 weeks postoperatively. Progression through an organized throwing program should include careful monitoring of symptoms, including medial elbow pain. Throwing off a mound can be expected at 6–9 months postoperatively, with return to competition at 9–12 months in most throwing athletes. For non-throwing athletes, postoperative protocols are less well defined but similarly should focus on obtaining full range of motion by 6 weeks with gradual strengthening beginning at this time as well. More aggressive strengthening can begin at 12 weeks postoperatively, with the goal of achieving normal strength and pain free range of motion prior to returning to sport.

## Surgical Outcomes

Since the first published outcomes of UCL reconstruction using Jobe's original figure-of-eight technique were reported in 1986 [3], the technique, perioperative management, and outcome measures of interest for medial ulnar ligament reconstruction have continued to evolve. While initial outcomes focused simply on return to sport and complications with the use of a single technique, today's outcomes cover an array of techniques [80] with outcomes that extend beyond return to sport, focusing on the quality of return to sport in a variety of patients [2, 81–87]. Given the ongoing changes both technically and with outcomes reporting, direct comparisons between studies and comparative study designs are limited. However, careful analysis of the reported outcomes provides useful information for the practicing surgeon and patient following UCL reconstruction.

## Medial Ulnar Collateral Ligament Repair

Reporting of results for primary repair of UCL injuries is limited in the literature, and is primarily reserved for acute avulsion type injuries [34, 60] or in the setting of traumatic elbow dislocation with persistent instability [88]. Jobe and colleagues compared the results of primary UCL repair with their initial figure-of-eight reconstruction technique and found that 50 % of patients with direct repair returned to sport as opposed to 68 % of patients who had reconstruction. Results for repair were even less satisfying when evaluating professional baseball players as a subset [2]. Other comparative studies revealed similar results, with reconstruction providing superior results as compared to primary repair [15]. These early findings potentially set the stage for limited reporting of primary repair results. More recently, Richard and colleagues reported 90 % return to sport for collegiate athletes with acute UCL injuries. In their series, all three overhead athletes were able to return to sport [60]. Similarly, return to sport rates above 90 % have been reported for primary repair of acute, UCL injuries in patients younger than 22 years of age and in competitive female athletes [59, 61]. The more promising recent results for primary repair are likely secondary to improved indications, namely limiting repair to acute avulsion type injuries, whereas older studies likely included primary repair for more chronic injuries with attenuation of the ligament. In light of these findings and limited high level evidence, primary ligament repair may provide satisfactory surgical results in the appropriately indicated patient, although reconstruction remains the treatment of choice for the majority of throwing athletes or those who fail nonoperative treatment.

## Medial Ulnar Collateral Ligament Reconstruction

UCL reconstruction is typically reserved for overhead athletes with full-thickness tears or athletes with partial-thickness tears that have failed a period of nonoperative treatment due to persistent medial elbow pain. Since Jobe's original description [3], a variety of technique modifications have been made. Some of the technique changes altered the original approach, the so-called modified Jobe technique, which was performed through a flexor–pronator muscle-splitting approach [62], while others altered graft fixation at the sublime tubercle and medial epicondyle [64, 66, 70, 89]. Other changes to the original technique, including graft choice modifications, have also been described in the literature [65, 78]. With multiple technique descriptions, direct comparisons are limited. However, several general trends can be elucidated from the literature since the original technique descriptions.

Several recent systematic reviews have helped consolidate the results of the available Level 3 and 4 data with respect to UCL reconstruction [77, 80, 90]. The original outcomes reported by Jobe et al. noted a 62.5 % return to sport with nearly one-third of patients report ulnar nerve for at least some period of time postoperatively [3]. Over the next several decades, operative techniques were modified to improve upon these results. More recent studies have reported excellent results in over 90 % of patients with a return to sport rate of 90 % for docking and modified docking techniques [77, 80]. Additionally, while the most common complication postoperatively remained ulnar nerve neuritis or neuropraxia, the complication rate for this dropped to nearly 2 % for modern techniques using a muscle-splitting approach [80]. Other commonly reported complications included reconstruction failure, infection, tunnel fracture, and heterotopic ossification. Today, UCL reconstruction is most frequently performed through a muscle-splitting approach using either palmaris or gracilis autograft. While the aggregate numbers in the literature predominantly describe the modified Jobe technique, there has been a trend toward increased use of the docking or modified docking technique, which is the technique of choice for the senior author given its consistent ability to allow return to sport while avoiding significant complications.

While return to sport data has been consistently reported, other outcomes of interest have recently been investigated, particularly in high demand athletes, including collegiate and professional pitchers. Despite the optimistic return to sport results with new and improving techniques, there is some evidence to suggest that pitchers who underwent UCL reconstruction frequently return to the disabled list for ipsilateral throwing arm injuries with a decline in common pitching performance metrics compared to preinjury including earned run average, innings pitched, and average fastball velocity [84, 87]. Although less frequently reported, this information is important to convey to elite athletes as their goals often extend beyond simply returning to sport, but frequently include goals that allow them excel in a competitive environment.

## Revision Medial Ulnar Collateral Ligament Reconstruction

Despite the recent increased incidence of UCL reconstructions, the rate of reconstructions requiring revision has decreased, possibly secondary to improved surgical technique and postoperative rehabilitation efforts [6]. However, when reconstructions do fail and revision reconstruction is required, the return to sport rate for professional baseball pitchers is significantly lower than for primary reconstruction [91–93]. Additionally, complications are more frequently noted in revision surgery as compared to more recently described primary reconstruction techniques [93]. Revision reconstruction procedures pose several technical challenges, including difficulty with fixation depending on the location and mode of failure, as well as obvious limitations with graft choice depending on the primary surgical technique. Given these less than satisfactory results and notable technical challenges with revision reconstruction procedures, future efforts should aim to continue to improve upon primary reconstruction techniques in order to decrease the revision rate, while also aiming to improve upon revision reconstruction techniques and rehabilitation protocols given the increasing number of at risk patients with a history of UCL reconstruction.

## Authors Preferred Technique

While a variety of reconstruction options exist, the authors prefer the docking technique for UCL reconstruction. One of the first decisions to be made when considering reconstruction is to determine whether arthroscopic evaluation is warranted. Arthroscopic evaluation of the elbow allows for assessment and treatment of posteromedial impingement, osteochondral defects, or loose bodies that may be suspected based on preoperative imaging or physical exam. An arthroscopic valgus stress exam can also be performed during arthroscopic evaluation, demonstrating gapping across the medial ulnohumeral joint with significant UCL injury (Fig. 12.3). The authors do no routinely perform elbow arthroscopy prior to every UCL reconstruction. Rather, arthroscopy is done when intraarticular pathology is suspected or identified based on preoperative physical exam and imaging.

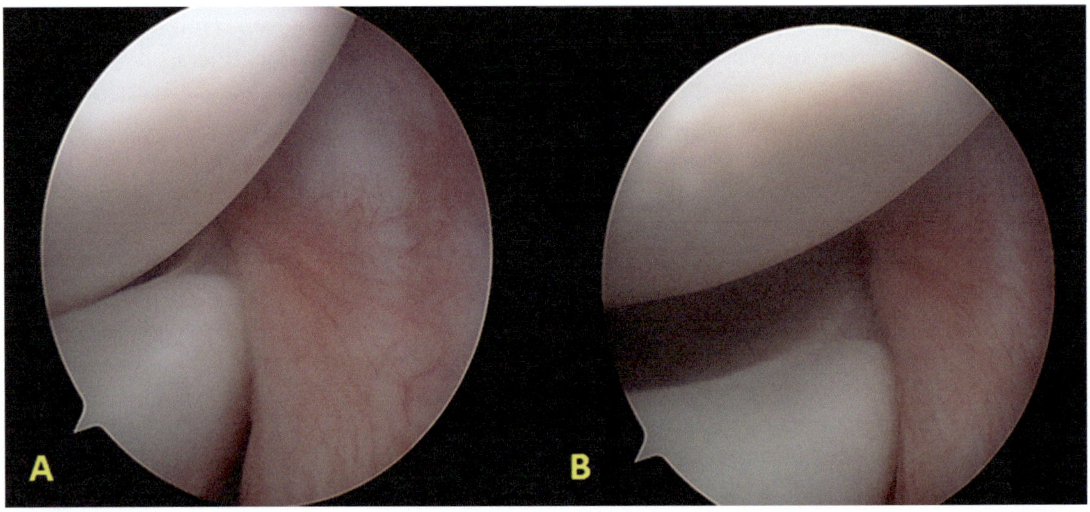


**Fig. 12.3** Elbow arthroscopy visualizing the medial ulnohumeral joint (**a**) without and (**b**) with valgus stress applied. Notable gapping with valgus stress is consistent with ulnar collateral ligament insufficiency

## Patient Positioning

Patient positioning is an important consideration and may be dictated by concomitant pathology requiring additional procedures at the time of UCL reconstruction. Supine positioning with an arm board and the shoulder externally rotated to allow access to the medial side of the elbow is frequently described. It is the authors' preference to perform surgery with the patient positioned prone with the arm placed in an arthroscopic arm holder. For one, this positioning allows easy transition if arthroscopic evaluation precedes UCL reconstruction. The arm can then be internally rotated at the shoulder with the forearm placed on a well-padded Mayo stand (Fig. 12.4). This position maintains the elbow in varus throughout the procedure while still allowing range of motion at the elbow.

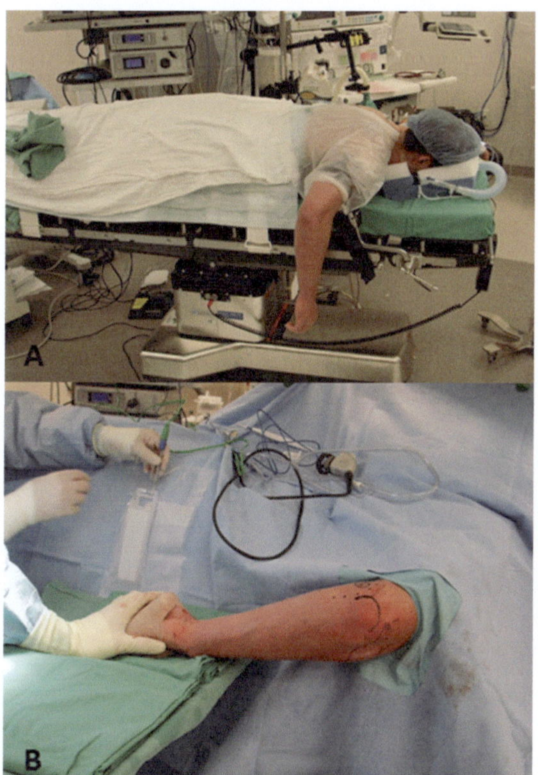


**Fig. 12.4** (**a**) The patient is positioned prone with the arm in an arm holder for arthroscopic evaluation. (**b**) Following arthroscopic evaluation, the shoulder is internally rotated and the forearm placed on a well-padded Mayo stand to access the medial elbow

## Surgical Technique

Several graft options exist for UCL reconstruction including autograft gracilis or palmaris as well as allograft. It is the author's preference to use ipsilateral palmaris autograft when present. The palmaris borders can be marked in the preoperative holding area while the patient is able to perform active thumb opposition to the small finger with wrist flexion for easy identification of the palmaris during surgery. We typically make a small, transverse incision at the flexion crease of the wrist over the identified palmaris tendon. The tendon is freed from any underlying adhesions, and a size 0 braided suture is placed in a Krackow fashion along the distal 15–20 mm of the tendon and any residual tendon amputated distal to the sutures. A small tendon harvester is then used to obtain the graft. Residual muscle belly is dissected of the proximal aspect of the harvested tendon in preparation for later graft passage.

The palpable landmarks at the medial elbow, including the medial epicondyle, medial intermuscular septum, proximal olecranon, and sublime tubercle of the ulna are marked. It also helps to carefully delineate the borders of the cubital tunnel using these landmarks. A 10–12 cm curvilinear incision is made over the medial epicondyle. Branches of the medial antebrachial cutaneous nerve can frequently be identified just superficial to the antebrachial fascia and should be identified and protected throughout the case. The fascia of the flexor–pronator mass is then identified as is the ulnar nerve within the cubital tunnel. In the absence of preoperative ulnar nerve symptoms or instability, the ulnar nerve is left alone. If there are noted ulnar nerve symptoms, instability of the ulnar nerve with elbow range of motion, or subluxation of the nerve onto the epicondyle, we proceed with subcutaneous ulnar nerve transposition. In this setting, the ulnar nerve is exposed and mobilized prior to UCL reconstruction. In addition, a strip of the medial intermuscular septum is prepared and used as a fascial sling to stabilize the nerve after transposition. The septum is amputated as proximal as possible and then a strip of septum is mobilized off the humerus from proximal to distal, keeping the most distal attachment at the epicondyle intact.

After the ulnar nerve is identified, the fascia overlying the flexor–pronator mass is split in line with the underlying muscle fibers at the junction of the anterior two-thirds and posterior one-third of the flexor–pronator mass (Fig. 12.5). The muscle fibers of the underlying flexor carpi ulnaris can then be bluntly split and blunt, deep retractors placed to visualize the UCL. In the majority of cases, the UCL is significantly attenuated. The anterior band of the UCL is identified deep to the muscular layer and is split longitudinally, allowing visualization of the ulnohumeral joint, which aids with ulnar tunnel placement.

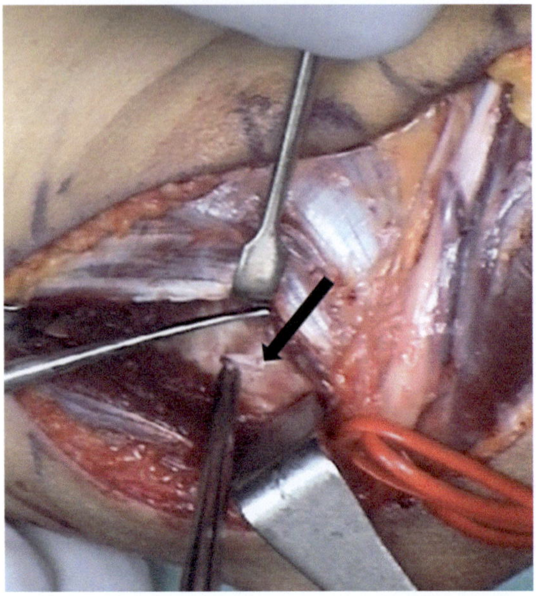

**Fig. 12.5** The flexor–pronator fascia and flexor carpi ulnar muscle belly are split an retracted, allowing visualization of the underling medial ulnar collateral ligament (*arrow*)

We begin with preparation of the ulnar tunnels at the sublime tubercle. With the sublime tubercle identified, approximately 10–15 mm distal to the ulnohumeral joint line, a 3.2 or 3.5 mm drill is used to make anterior and posterior converging drill holes, maintaining a 1 cm bone bridge between the tunnels. This can be done freehand or using a commercially available converging drill guide. A small curette is used to further prepare and connect the converging tunnels. With the tunnels connected, a shuttling suture or suture passing device is passed in preparation for graft passage (Fig. 12.6). Using the shuttling suture, the graft is shuttled through the ulnar tunnels from posterior to anterior.

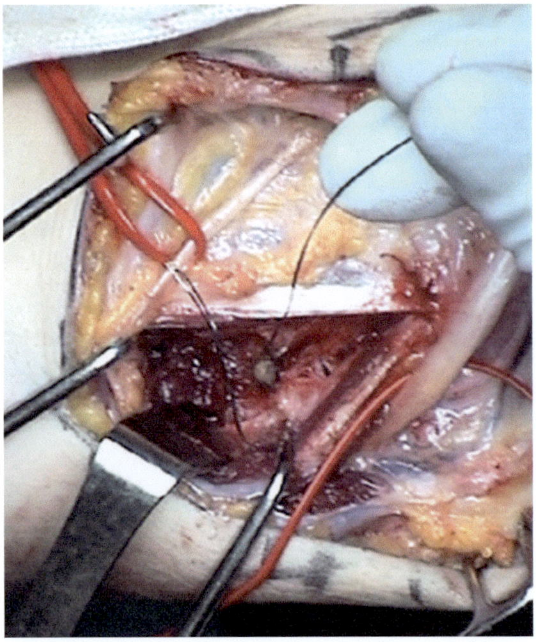

**Fig. 12.6** Shuttling wire placed through the ulnar tunnels at the sublime tubercle in preparation for graft passage. A branch of the medial antebrachial cutaneous nerve and ulnar nerve are protected with vessel loops

Attention is then turned to the medial epicondyle and the humeral tunnel. With the medial epicondyle exposed, a 4.5–5.0 mm drill or burr is used to make a tunnel at the origin of the anterior band of the UCL. The origin of the anterior band sits just anterior to the distal most point of the epicondyle in the axial plane. The tunnel is aimed directly proximal, roughly in line with the shaft of the humerus, with an ideal tunnel length measuring 15–20 mm. In order to obtain adequate tunnel length, the tunnel can be angled slightly posterior and lateral compared to the anatomic axis of the medial epicondyle [94]. Commercial guides are available to assist with humeral tunnel drilling as well. The proximal and posterior cortex of the epicondyle should be left intact. Near the proximal aspect of the tunnel, a 1.8–2.0 mm drill is used to drill two tunnels that connect to the 4.5 mm tunnel, leaving a stable bone bridge on the proximal epicondyle between the two small drill holes, which allows for suture passage. Alternatively, several commercial drill guides exist that allow for targeting of these small suture passage tunnels to the 4.5 mm tunnel. The exit location of these suture tunnels is somewhat dependent on any concurrent ulnar nerve surgery. If the ulnar nerve is transposed, we prefer to place one tunnel anterior to the supracondylar ridge and the other posterior. If the ulnar nerve is left in situ, then we aim to place both suture tunnels anterior to the supracondylar ridge in order to prevent irritation of the ulnar nerve within the cubital tunnel. Using a shuttling suture or device through the more anterior suture passage tunnel, the anterior limb of the prepared graft is pulled into the humeral tunnel. Maintaining the arm in varus, the posterior limb of the graft is pulled into position and measured in order to ensure that there is enough graft length to fill the humeral tunnel without bottoming out within the tunnel, which would prevent tensioning. Typically, we aim to have 10–15 mm of each limb of graft within the humeral tunnel. Using this measurement, the posterior limb is prepared with a braided size 0 Krackow stitch. Final graft length is confirmed and then excess graft is removed. Prior to final graft docking and tensioning, the longitudinal split in the native UCL is repaired using size 0 suture in a running fashion from distal to proximal. Then, using the more posterior suture passage tunnel, the posterior limb of the graft is pulled into the humeral tunnel (Fig. 12.7). Graft tension is checked to ensure that it is appropriate through a full range of motion. The arm is maintained in varus with the forearm supinated and elbow positioned at approximately 45–60° of flexion and the sutures are tied over the bone bridge at the proximal epicondyle (see Video 12.1). With the graft in place, we routinely close the split in the flexor–pronator fascia with a running absorbable size 0 suture. The ulnar nerve is addressed with final transposition using soft-tissue sling stabilization, if warranted, prior to skin closure.

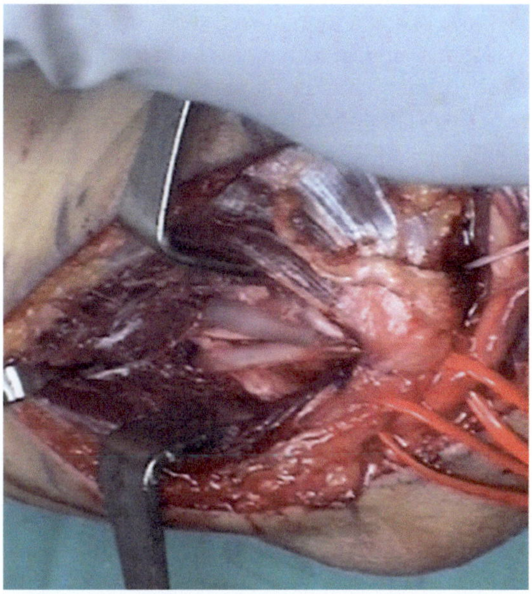

**Fig. 12.7** Both limbs of the graft are pulled into the humeral tunnel and docked prior to positioning in varus, manual tensioning, and tying suture over the humeral bone bridge

### Postoperative Management

The patient is placed in a hinged elbow brace to allow range of motion between 60° and 90° for the first 10–14 days postoperatively. After 2 weeks, the brace is opened to allow range of motion from 45° to 90°, thereafter increasing both flexion and extension over the next 4 weeks with the goal of achieving full elbow range of motion at 6 weeks after surgery. The elbow brace is discontinued at 6 weeks at which time shoulder range of motion and strengthening is emphasized. At 12 weeks, vigorous elbow and shoulder strengthening exercises commence. In throwing athletes, a throwing program is typically initiated at 14–16 weeks postoperatively. Position players are typically finished with their throwing rehabilitation program by 6–8 months postoperatively, while pitchers are typically fully rehabilitated by 9–14 months postoperatively and can return to competition.

## Conclusions

Since its first description over four decades ago, the management of UCL injuries and UCL reconstruction procedures has continued to evolve. UCL reconstruction has provided consistent outcomes for overhead athletes who have failed a trial of conservative management, which typically includes rest and a graduated throwing program. While our surgical techniques and outcomes continue to improve, there remains significant concern with the increasing incidence of elbow injuries in adolescent athletes which has been accompanied by an increase in UCL reconstruction procedures in this age group. Injury prevention remains the greatest area for improvement when it comes to UCL injuries, and future studies that investigate the efficacy and adherence to specific throwing guidelines, including pitch counts and rest, are warranted as many of our current guidelines and recommendations are based on anecdotal evidence and expert opinion. While injury prevention requires a collaborative effort from surgeons, coaches, parents, and players, it provides the best opportunity to reverse the concerning trends seen in recent years.

## References


1. Waris W. Elbow injuries in javelin throwers. Acta Chir Scand. 1946;93:563–75.
2. Conway J, Jobe FW, Glousman R, Pink M. Medial instability of the elbow in throwing athletes. Treatment by repair or reconstruction of the ulnar collateral ligament. J Bone Joint Surg Am. 1992;74:67–83.
3. Jobe FW, Stark H, Lombardo S. Reconstruction of the ulnar collateral ligament in athletes. J Bone Joint Surg Am. 1986;68:1158–63.
4. Erickson BJ, Nwachukwu BU, Rosas S, Schairer WW, McCormick FM, Bach BR, et al. Trends in medial ulnar collateral ligament reconstruction in the United States: a retrospective review of a large private-payer database from 2007 to 2011. Am J Sports Med. 2015;43:1770–4.
5. Conte SA, Fleisig GS, Dines JS, Wilk KE, Aune KT, Patterson-Flynn N, et al. Prevalence of ulnar collateral ligament surgery in professional baseball players. Am J Sports Med. 2015;43:1764–9.
6. Wilson AT, Pidgeon TS, Morrell NT, DaSilva MF. Trends in revision elbow ulnar collateral ligament reconstruction in professional baseball pitchers. J Hand Surg Am. 2015;40:2249–54.
7. Fleisig GS, Andrews JR. Prevention of elbow injuries in youth baseball pitchers. Sports Health. 2012;4:419–24.
8. Fuss FK. The ulnar collateral ligament of the human elbow joint. Anatomy, function and biomechanics. J Anat. 1991;175:203–12.
9. Farrow LD, Mahoney AJ, Stefancin JJ, Taljanovic MS, Sheppard JE, Schickendantz MS. Quantitative analysis of the medial ulnar collateral ligament ulnar footprint and its relationship to the ulnar sublime tubercle. Am J Sports Med. 2011;39:1936–41.
10. Morrey BF, An KN. Functional anatomy of the ligaments of the elbow. Clin Orthop Relat Res. 1985;(201):84–90.
11. Hotchkiss RN, Weiland AJ. Valgus stability of the elbow. J Orthop Res. 1987;5:372–7.
12. Søjbjerg JO, Ovesen J, Nielsen S. Experimental elbow instability after transection of the medial collateral ligament. Clin Orthop Relat Res. 1987;(218):186–90.
13. Floris S, Olsen BS, Dalstra M, Søjbjerg JO, Sneppen O. The medial collateral ligament of the elbow joint: anatomy and kinematics. J Shoulder Elbow Surg. 1998;7(4):345–51.
14. Dugas JR, Ostrander RV, Cain EL, Kingsley D, Andrews JR. Anatomy of the anterior bundle of the ulnar collateral ligament. J Shoulder Elbow Surg. 2007;16:657–60.
15. Azar FM, Andrews JR, Wilk KE, Groh D. Operative treatment of ulnar collateral ligament injuries of the elbow in athletes. Am J Sports Med. 2000;28:16–23.
16. Fleisig GS, Andrews JR, Dillman CJ, Escamilla RF. Kinetics of baseball pitching with implications about injury mechanisms. Am J Sports Med. 1995;23:233–9.
17. Dugas JR. Valgus extension overload: diagnosis and treatment. Clin Sports Med. 2010;29:645–54.
18. Harris JD, Lintner DM. Nerve injuries about the elbow in the athlete. Sports Med Arthrosc. 2014;22:e7–15.
19. Furushima K, Itoh Y, Iwabu S, Yamamoto Y, Koga R, Shimizu M. Classification of olecranon stress fractures in baseball players. Am J Sports Med. 2014;42:1343–51.
20. Dugas JR, Weiland AJ. Vascular pathology in the throwing athlete. Hand Clin. 2000;16:477–85.
21. Morrey BF. Applied anatomy and biomechanics of the elbow joint. Instr Course Lect. 1985;35:59–68.
22. Beals RK. The normal carrying angle of the elbow. A radiographic study of 422 patients. Clin Orthop Relat Res. 1976;(119):194–6.
23. King JW, Brelsford HJ, Tullos HS. Analysis of the pitching arm of the professional baseball pitcher. Clin Orthop Relat Res. 1969;(67):116–23.
24. Patel RM, Lynch TS, Amin NH, Calabrese G, Gryzlo SM, Schickendantz MS. The thrower's elbow. Orthop Clin North Am. 2014;45:355–76.
25. Timmerman LA, Schwartz ML, Andrews JR. Preoperative evaluation of the ulnar collateral ligament by magnetic resonance imaging and computed tomography arthrography evaluation in 25 baseball players with surgical confirmation. Am J Sports Med. 1994;22:26–32.
26. Safran MR, McGarry MH, Shin S, Han S, Lee TQ. Effects of elbow flexion and forearm rotation on valgus laxity of the elbow. J Bone Joint Surg Am. 2005;87:2065–74.
27. Bruce JR, Hess R, Joyner P, Andrews JR. How much valgus instability can be expected with ulnar collateral ligament (UCL) injuries? A review of 273 baseball players with UCL injuries. J Shoulder Elbow Surg. 2014;23:1521–6.
28. Callaway G, Field L, Deng X-H, Torzilli P, O'Brien S, Altchek D, et al. Biomechanical evaluation of the

medial collateral ligament of the elbow. J Bone Joint Surg Am. 1997;79:1223–31.

29. Ciccotti MG, Atanda A, Nazarian LN, Dodson CC, Holmes L, Cohen SB. Stress sonography of the ulnar collateral ligament of the elbow in professional baseball pitchers: a 10-year study. Am J Sports Med. 2014;42:544–51.
30. Safran MR. Ulnar collateral ligament injury in the overhead athlete: diagnosis and treatment. Clin Sports Med. 2004;23:643–63.
31. O'Driscoll SW, Lawton RL, Smith AM. The "moving valgus stress test" for medial collateral ligament tears of the elbow. Am J Sports Med. 2005;33:231–9.
32. Myers JB, Laudner KG, Pasquale MR, Bradley JP, Lephart SM. Glenohumeral range of motion deficits and posterior shoulder tightness in throwers with pathologic internal impingement. Am J Sports Med. 2006;34:385–91.
33. Crockett HC, Gross LB, Wilk KE, Schwartz ML, Reed J, O'Mara J, et al. Osseous adaptation and range of motion at the glenohumeral joint in professional baseball pitchers. Am J Sports Med. 2002;30:20–6.
34. Salvo JP, Rizio L, Zvijac JE, Uribe JW, Hechtman KS. Avulsion fracture of the ulnar sublime tubercle in overhead throwing athletes. Am J Sports Med. 2002;30:426–31.
35. Mulligan SA, Schwartz ML, Broussard MF, Andrews JR. Heterotopic calcification and tears of the ulnar collateral ligament: radiographic and MR imaging findings. AJR Am J Roentgenol. 2000;175:1099–102.
36. Ellenbecker TS, Mattalino AJ, Elam EA, Caplinger RA. Medial elbow joint laxity in professional baseball pitchers a bilateral comparison using stress radiography. Am J Sports Med. 1998;26:420–4.
37. Rijke AM, Goitz HT, McCue FC, Andrews JR, Berr SS. Stress radiography of the medial elbow ligaments. Radiology. 1994;191:213–6.
38. Carrino JA, Morrison WB, Zou KH, Steffen RT, Snearly WN, Murray PM. Noncontrast MR imaging and MR arthrography of the ulnar collateral ligament of the elbow: prospective evaluation of two-dimensional pulse sequences for detection of complete tears. Skeletal Radiol. 2001;30:625–32.
39. Murphy B. MR imaging of the elbow. Radiology. 1992;184:525–9.
40. Tuite MJ, Kijowski R. Sports-related injuries of the elbow: an approach to MRI interpretation. Clin Sports Med. 2006;25:387–408.
41. Steinbach LS, Fritz RC, Tirman PF, Uffman M. Magnetic resonance imaging of the elbow. Eur J Radiol. 1997;25:223–41.
42. Atanda A, Buckley PS, Hammoud S, Cohen SB, Nazarian LN, Ciccotti MG. Early anatomic changes of the ulnar collateral ligament identified by stress ultrasound of the elbow in young professional baseball pitchers. Am J Sports Med. 2015;43:2943–9.
43. Sasaki J, Takahara M, Ogino T, Kashiwa H, Ishigaki D, Kanauchi Y. Ultrasonographic assessment of the ulnar collateral ligament and medial elbow laxity in college baseball players. J Bone Joint Surg Am. 2002;84:525–31.
44. Olsen SJ, Fleisig GS, Dun S, Loftice J, Andrews JR. Risk factors for shoulder and elbow injuries in adolescent baseball pitchers. Am J Sports Med. 2006;34:905–12.
45. Yang J, Mann BJ, Guettler JH, Dugas JR, Irrgang JJ, Fleisig GS, et al. Risk-prone pitching activities and injuries in youth baseball findings from a national sample. Am J Sports Med. 2014;42:1456–63.
46. Grantham WJ, Byram IR, Meadows MC, Ahmad CS. The impact of fatigue on the kinematics of collegiate baseball pitchers. Orthop J Sports Med. 2014;2:2325967114537032.
47. Bohne C, George SZ, Zeppieri Jr G. Knowledge of injury prevention and prevalence of risk factors for throwing injuries in a sample of youth baseball players. Int J Sports Phys Ther. 2015;10:464–75.
48. Fazarale JJ, Magnussen RA, Pedroza AD, Kaeding CC. Knowledge of and compliance with pitch count recommendations: a survey of youth baseball coaches. Sports Health. 2012;4:202–4.
49. Fleisig GS, Andrews JR, Cutter GR, Weber A, Loftice J, McMichael C, et al. Risk of serious injury for young baseball pitchers a 10-year prospective study. Am J Sports Med. 2011;39:253–7.
50. USA Baseball. Guidelines for youth and adolescent pitchers. Accessed May 21, 2016. Available from: http://m.mlb.com/pitchsmart/pitching-guidelines/.
51. Little League Baseball. Regular season pitching rules - Baseball. Accessed May 21, 2016. Available from: http://www.littleleague.org/learn/rules/pitch-count.htm.
52. Dines JS, Frank JB, Akerman M, Yocum LA. Glenohumeral internal rotation deficits in baseball players with ulnar collateral ligament insufficiency. Am J Sports Med. 2009;37:566–70.
53. Dodson CC, Slenker N, Cohen SB, Ciccotti MG, DeLuca P. Ulnar collateral ligament injuries of the elbow in professional football quarterbacks. J Shoulder Elbow Surg. 2010;19:1276–80.
54. Rettig AC, Sherrill C, Snead DS, Mendler JC, Mieling P. Nonoperative treatment of ulnar collateral ligament injuries in throwing athletes. Am J Sports Med. 2001;29:15–7.
55. Wilk KE, Yenchak A, Arrigo CA, Andrews JR. The advanced throwers ten exercise program: a new exercise series for enhanced dynamic shoulder control in the overhead throwing athlete. Phys Sportsmed. 2011;39:90–7.
56. Wilk KE, Macrina LC, Cain EL, Dugas JR, Andrews JR. Rehabilitation of the overhead athlete's elbow. Sports Health. 2012;4:404–14.
57. Moraes VY, Lenza M, Tamaoki MJ, Faloppa F, Belloti JC. Platelet-rich therapies for musculoskeletal soft tissue injuries. Cochrane Database Syst Rev. 2014;(4):CD010071.
58. Podesta L, Crow SA, Volkmer D, Bert T, Yocum LA. Treatment of partial ulnar collateral ligament

tears in the elbow with platelet-rich plasma. Am J Sports Med. 2013;41:1689–94.
59. Argo D, Trenhaile SW, Savoie FH, Field LD. Operative treatment of ulnar collateral ligament insufficiency of the elbow in female athletes. Am J Sports Med. 2006;34:431–7.
60. Richard MJ, Aldridge 3rd JM, Wiesler ER, Ruch DS. Traumatic valgus instability of the elbow: pathoanatomy and results of direct repair. Surgical technique. J Bone Joint Surg Am. 2009;91:191–9.
61. Savoie FH, Trenhaile SW, Roberts J, Field LD, Ramsey JR. Primary repair of ulnar collateral ligament injuries of the elbow in young athletes: a case series of injuries to the proximal and distal ends of the ligament. Am J Sports Med. 2008;36:1066–72.
62. Thompson WH, Jobe FW, Yocum LA, Pink MM. Ulnar collateral ligament reconstruction in athletes: muscle-splitting approach without transposition of the ulnar nerve. J Shoulder Elbow Surg. 2001;10:152–7.
63. Smith GR, Altchek DW, Pagnani MJ, Keeley JR. A muscle-splitting approach to the ulnar collateral ligament of the elbow. Neuroanatomy and operative technique. Am J Sports Med. 1996;24(5):575–80.
64. Rohrbough JT, Altchek DW, Hyman J, Williams RJ, Botts JD. Medial collateral ligament reconstruction of the elbow using the docking technique. Am J Sports Med. 2002;30:541–8.
65. Paletta GA, Wright RW. The modified docking procedure for elbow ulnar collateral ligament reconstruction: 2-year follow-up in elite throwers. Am J Sports Med. 2006;34:1594–8.
66. Armstrong A, Dunning C, Ferreira L, Faber K, Johnson J, King G. A biomechanical comparison of four reconstruction techniques for the medial collateral ligament-deficient elbow. J Shoulder Elbow Surg. 2005;14:207–15.
67. Ciccotti MG, Siegler S, Kuri JA, Thinnes JH, Murphy DJ. Comparison of the biomechanical profile of the intact ulnar collateral ligament with the modified jobe and the docking reconstructed elbow: an in vitro study. Am J Sports Med. 2009;37:974–81.
68. Paletta GA, Klepps SJ, Difelice GS, Allen T, Brodt MD, Burns ME, et al. Biomechanical evaluation of 2 techniques for ulnar collateral ligament reconstruction of the elbow. Am J Sports Med. 2006;34:1599–603.
69. Shah RP, Lindsey DP, Sungar GW, McAdams TR. An analysis of four ulnar collateral ligament reconstruction procedures with cyclic valgus loading. J Shoulder Elbow Surg. 2009;18:58–63.
70. Dines JS, ElAttrache NS, Conway JE, Smith W, Ahmad CS. Clinical outcomes of the DANE TJ technique to treat ulnar collateral ligament insufficiency of the elbow. Am J Sports Med. 2007;35:2039–44.
71. Conway JE. The DANE TJ procedure for elbow medial ulnar collateral ligament insufficiency. Tech Shoulder Elbow Surg. 2006;7:36–43.
72. Ahmad CS, Lee TQ, ElAttrache NS. Biomechanical evaluation of a new ulnar collateral ligament reconstruction technique with interference screw fixation. Am J Sports Med. 2003;31:332–7.
73. Hurbanek JG, Anderson K, Crabtree S, Karnes GJ. Biomechanical comparison of the docking technique with and without humeral bioabsorbable interference screw fixation. Am J Sports Med. 2009;37:526–33.
74. Jackson TJ, Adamson GJ, Peterson A, Patton J, McGarry MH, Lee TQ. Ulnar collateral ligament reconstruction using bisuspensory fixation: a biomechanical comparison with the docking technique. Am J Sports Med. 2013;41:1158–64.
75. Lynch JL, Maerz T, Kurdziel MD, Davidson AA, Baker KC, Anderson K. Biomechanical evaluation of the tightrope versus traditional docking ulnar collateral ligament reconstruction technique kinematic and failure testing. Am J Sports Med. 2013;41:1165–73.
76. Lynch JL, Pifer MA, Maerz T, Kurdziel MD, Davidson AA, Baker KC, et al. The graftlink ulnar collateral ligament reconstruction biomechanical comparison with the docking technique in both kinematics and failure tests. Am J Sports Med. 2013;41:2278–87.
77. Vitale MA, Ahmad CS. The outcome of elbow ulnar collateral ligament reconstruction in overhead athletes a systematic review. Am J Sports Med. 2008;36(6):1193–205.
78. Savoie FH, Morgan C, Yaste J, Hurt J, Field L. Medial ulnar collateral ligament reconstruction using hamstring allograft in overhead throwing athletes. J Bone Joint Surg Am. 2013;95:1062–6.
79. Ellenbecker TS, Wilk KE, Altchek DW, Andrews JR. Current concepts in rehabilitation following ulnar collateral ligament reconstruction. Sports Health. 2009;1:301–13.
80. Watson JN, McQueen P, Hutchinson MR. A systematic review of ulnar collateral ligament reconstruction techniques. Am J Sports Med. 2014;42:2510–6.
81. Lansdown DA, Feeley BT. The effect of ulnar collateral ligament reconstruction on pitch velocity in major league baseball pitchers. Orthop J Sports Med. 2014;2:2325967114522592.
82. Fleisig GS, Leddon CE, Laughlin WA, Ciccotti MG, Mandelbaum BR, Aune KT, et al. Biomechanical performance of baseball pitchers with a history of ulnar collateral ligament reconstruction. Am J Sports Med. 2015;43:1045.
83. Dines JS, Jones KJ, Kahlenberg C, Rosenbaum A, Osbahr DC, Altchek DW. Elbow ulnar collateral ligament reconstruction in javelin throwers at a minimum 2-year follow-up. Am J Sports Med. 2012;40:148–51.
84. Makhni EC, Lee RW, Morrow ZS, Gualtieri AP, Gorroochurn P, Ahmad CS. Performance, return to competition, and reinjury after tommy john surgery in major league baseball pitchers: a review of 147 cases. Am J Sports Med. 2014;42:1323–32.
85. Domb BG, Davis J, Alberta FG, Mohr KJ, Brooks AG, ElAttrache NS, et al. Clinical follow-up of professional baseball players undergoing ulnar collateral ligament reconstruction using the new Kerlan-Jobe Orthopaedic Clinic overhead athlete shoulder and elbow score (KJOC Score). Am J Sports Med. 2010;38:1558–63.

86. Jiang JJ, Leland JM. Analysis of pitching velocity in Major League Baseball play before and after ulnar collateral ligament reconstruction. Am J Sports Med. 2014;42:880–5.
87. Keller RA, Steffes MJ, Zhuo D, Bey MJ, Moutzouros V. The effects of medial ulnar collateral ligament reconstruction on Major League pitching performance. J Shoulder Elbow Surg. 2014;23:1591–8.
88. Mathew PK, Athwal GS, King GJ. Terrible triad injury of the elbow: current concepts. J Am Acad Orthop Surg. 2009;17:137–51.
89. Large TM, Coley ER, Peindl RD, Fleischli JE. A biomechanical comparison of 2 ulnar collateral ligament reconstruction techniques. Arthroscopy. 2007;23:141–50.
90. Purcell DB, Matava MJ, Wright RW. Ulnar collateral ligament reconstruction: a systematic review. Clin Orthop Relat Res. 2007;(455):72–7.
91. Marshall NE, Keller RA, Lynch JR, Bey MJ, Moutzouros V. Pitching performance and longevity after revision ulnar collateral ligament reconstruction in major league baseball pitchers. Am J Sports Med. 2015;43:1051–6.
92. Jones KJ, Conte S, Patterson N, ElAttrache NS, Dines JS. Functional outcomes following revision ulnar collateral ligament reconstruction in Major League Baseball pitchers. J Shoulder Elbow Surg. 2013;22:642–6.
93. Dines JS, Yocum LA, Frank JB, ElAttrache NS, Gambardella RA, Jobe FW. Revision surgery for failed elbow medial collateral ligament reconstruction. Am J Sports Med. 2008;36:1061–5.
94. Byram IR, Khanna K, Gardner TR, Ahmad CS. Characterizing bone tunnel placement in medial ulnar collateral ligament reconstruction using patient-specific 3-dimensional computed tomography modeling. Am J Sports Med. 2013;41:894–902.

# Treatment of Combined Medial and Lateral Collateral Ligament Insufficiency

# 13

Lawrence Camarda and Gregory I. Bain

## Background

The most common mechanism of elbow ligament injuries occurs with a dislocation. The most common types of elbow dislocations are those that occur posteriorly (simple dislocations) involving only soft-tissue injuries, whereas complex dislocations have associated fractures. In these specific cases, medial and lateral ligament insufficiency could be observed, despite osteosynthesis of the skeletal injury. Further, outcome studies demonstrate that injuries resulting in significant ligamentous disruption have worse results than isolated fractures [1, 2]. Key aspects such as instability patterns, pathoanatomy, diagnosis, and treatment options of elbow ligament insufficiency are reviewed.

L. Camarda, MD, PhD
Department of Orthopedic Surgery, Univerità degli Studi di Palermo, Via del Vespro, Palermo 90100, Italy
e-mail: lawrence.camarda@unipa.it

G.I. Bain, MBBS, FRACS, PhD (✉)
Department of Orthopedic Surgery, Flinders University of South Australia, Adelaide, Australia
e-mail: greg@gregbain.com.au

## Instability Classification

### Lateral Instability

(a) *Posterolateral rotatory instability (PLRI)*—Described by O'Driscoll, it is considered to be the most common pattern of symptomatic chronic instability of the elbow [3]. Most commonly it results from a simple elbow dislocation [4, 5]. The primary cause of PLRI involves the disruption of the LCL complex, more specifically the LUCL. However, MCL and overlying flexor–pronator muscle group rupture could also be observed, depending on the degree of the trauma progression.

(b) *Varus*—This is caused by disruption of the LCL complex. It is seen in acute elbow dislocations and in severe cases where the LCL has failed to heal. The physiological forces across the elbow are principally valgus because of the anatomical alignment, and therefore this pattern of instability may not be clinically obvious. PLRI is a more likely clinical problem with disruption of the LCL complex [6]. Chronic attenuation of the lateral ligament complex may also be secondary to overuse, such as in patients who use their arms as weight-bearing extremities (e.g., polio with crutch-walking) [6].

© Springer International Publishing Switzerland 2017

R.Z. Tashjian (ed.), *The Unstable Elbow*, DOI 10.1007/978-3-319-46019-2_13

## Medial Instability

(a) *Posteromedial varus instability*)—This is a rare instability pattern and it is associated with anteromedial facet fractures of the coronoid secondary to varus/posteromedial injuries of the elbow with axial loading. They almost always present with an associated injury to the LCL. Generally, the posterior band of the MCL is ruptured while the anterior band is intact and attached to the anteromedial coronoid facet. The lateral joint space is usually widened and there is no radial head or neck fracture.

(b) *Valgus*—This instability pattern involves disruption of the MCL complex. It is uncommon in the general population and it is often seen in most athletes (throwing athletes) as a result of repetitive micro-trauma and chronic overload. However, it could be observed following an acute trauma such as a dislocation. In these patients, MCL insufficiency is usually associated with radial head fractures and possibly disruption of the common flexor origin.

## Anterior Instability

This is typically seen in association with olecranon fractures [6]. Because of good outcomes of treatment of olecranon fractures, chronic anterior instability is rarely encountered.

## Global Instability

This is a rare condition and it is characterized by a severe multidirectional instability of the elbow. It usually follows severe trauma such as fracture-dislocation. It is associated with rupture of both collateral ligament complexes and circumferential capsular stripping of the elbow.

## Pathoanatomy

### PLRI

Posterolateral rotatory instability [3] classically refers to an injury to the lateral ulnar collateral ligament (LUCL) that results in external rotatory subluxation of the ulna on the humerus, with posterior and valgus displacement. Specifically, the radial head rotates away from the capitellum, and the ulna essentially "pivots" on the MCL rotating off the lateral trochlea.

The LCL complex most commonly fails by avulsing the capsule and common extensor origin from the lateral epicondyle [7]. LCL injury is most commonly the result of trauma such as a fall on an outstretched hand or any other mechanism that imparts axial compression, valgus force and supination. Other causes of injury to the LCL complex include chronic cubitus varus, multiple steroid injections for lateral epicondylitis, and/or connective tissue disease [8–10]. Iatrogenic causes can include an open or arthroscopic procedure to the lateral side of the elbow with inadequate repair/reconstruction of the lateral ligaments or of the common extensor, providing some dynamic stability [8, 11]. Resection of the radial head, even in the presence of intact ligament, has also been shown to be a risk factor for the development of PLRI [12]. A staging system (Table 13.1) developed

**Table 13.1** Staging of posterolateral rotatory instability

| Stages | Degrees of capsuloligamentous disruption |
|---|---|
| 1 | Subluxation of the elbow in a posterolateral direction |
| 2 | Subluxation of the elbow joint with the coronoid perched underneath the trochlea |
| 3 | Complete dislocation with the coronoid resting behind the trochlea |
| 3A | Includes the posterior band of the medial collateral ligament tear |
| 3B | Includes the anterior and posterior bands of the medial collateral ligament tear |

for PLRI has been described by O'Driscoll [3] and may influence a patient's history, clinical examination and choice of treatment. Disruption of the LCL complex (particularly the LUCL) results in posterolateral rotatory subluxation of the elbow. With further injury, there is a disruption of the anterior and posterior capsules, and finally the MCL. When the lateral and medial soft tissues are disrupted, the joint can dislocate even with immobilization of the elbow in 90° of flexion. This progression of injury is also referred to as the Circle of Horii [12].

## Medial Instability

MCL complex injury occurs when the elbow is subjected to a valgus force, which disrupts the medial side of the elbow, exceeding the tensile properties of the MCL. The chronic injury is more commonly seen in athletes, in particular overhead athletes, such as pitchers, javelin throwers, tennis, and water polo players. Acute disruption of the MCL can occur following a significant traumatic event.

Like the LCL, the MCL most commonly avulses from the humeral origin [13]. Cadaveric studies indicate that 100 % of the anterior bundle of the MCL must be sectioned before demonstrating significant valgus or rotatory elbow instability [14]. In the presence of an associated coronoid process fracture, the MCL complex may fail in a "Z" configuration where the anterior band of the MCL remains intact at its distal insertion on the coronoid fragment while the posterior band avulses from the proximal origin on the humerus. If there is no fracture of the coronoid process, then there is a rent in the anterior capsule that extends to the medial epicondyle, and the entire MCL complex is then avulsed from the medial epicondyle [13].

## Evaluation

The first step in assessment is acquiring a good history and examination. A detailed history of the event must be obtained, including the mechanism of injury and the position of the arm at the time of the trauma. Beginning with inspection, clinicians may observe an effusion or ecchymosis over the elbow. Elbow deformity and swelling on the medial or lateral side of the elbow suggest injury to the underlying soft tissue and bony structures. A neuromuscular examination should be performed. Two-dimensional X-ray images should be taken before and after repositioning maneuvers and should include evaluation of the radial head and the olecranon. On a true lateral radiograph, lateral ligament instability may be identified by subtle opening of the trochlea–trochlear notch interval, and is referred to as the "drop sign"[15]. Furthermore, fluoroscopy represents an additional valuable tool to assess instability. It allows the surgeon to observe medial or lateral joint space widening, while a varus or valgus force is applied to the elbow. When the level of suspicion is high and radiograph results are normal, magnetic resonance imaging (MRI) could be performed. While the utility of MRI is still controversial [16–18], damage of the LCL complex can be typically seen in the presence of a significant injury.

Arthroscopic evaluation can be used for direct visualization of the elbow joint and its surrounding structures as an adjunct procedure to reconstruction. The primary advantage includes the evaluation of the joint space opening of the ulnohumeral joint during rotational, varus, and valgus stresses to the elbow [14]. This can allow for accurate clinical staging and appropriate corrective surgery. Further, arthroscopy may also help to identify elbow joint arthritis and loose fragments associated joint injuries [19].

## PLRI Assessment

Diagnosis can be made historically based upon presentation of painful, recurrent clicking, snapping, or locking of elbow with pain located posterior to the proximal radioulnar joint as the elbow moves into supination and extension. Patients often report their elbow feels loose or like it is sliding out of place. On physical exam, patients often have normal upper extremity strength and elbow range of motion. Often the only abnormality in the examination is a positive pivot shift test. During this test the radial head is subluxed with a combination of full supination, axial compression, and valgus load as the elbow is placed in 40° flexion. The patient would have apprehension when performing this maneuver, which may mask the instability and make the assessment difficult. Discomfort and the sensation of instability can be reduced with local anesthetic, and fluoroscopy can identify subtle forms of instability. Surgery is indicated in patients with symptomatic instability and involves a LCL repair in the acute setting or a reconstruction in those cases without adequate ligamentous tissues.

## Medial Instability Assessment

Patients with medial instability usually report medial elbow pain and decreased strength during overhead activity. Further, patients may complain about ulnar neuropathy, generally owing to a valgus stretching of the nerve. In case of an isolated MCL injury, patients can present with tenderness 2 cm distal to the medial epicondyle. Valgus instability is tested with the patients' elbow flexed between 20° and 30° to unlock the olecranon from its fossa as valgus stress is applied. The test is positive if there is a loss of a firm end point and increased medial side joint opening, comparing with the contralateral upper extremity. The test produces pain in approximately 50 % of patients with a torn MCL, and it has a sensitivity and specificity of 66 % and 60 % respectively [20, 21]. The "milking maneuver" is performed by either the patient or the examiner pulling on the patient's thumb to create valgus stress with the patients' forearm supinated and elbow flexed beyond 90° [22]. The "moving valgus stress test" is a modification of the milking maneuver where valgus stress is applied constantly, while the elbow is moved through an arc of flexion and extension [23]. For both tests, the subjective feeling of apprehension, instability, or localized pain to the MCL indicates MCL injury.

## Nonoperative Treatment

In acute setting, simple elbow dislocations without associate fractures should be managed with closed reduction. It can be completed with or without sedation [24]. The reduction is performed by flexing the elbow to approximately 25° while applying longitudinal traction combined with supination at the forearm and countertraction at the upper arm provided by an assistant [25, 26]. Complete range of motion of the elbow should be evaluated as well as the joint stability. Crepitus during joint motion suggests a fracture or an osteochondral fragment trapped in the joint. If the elbow is unstable, the point of instability should be noted. Specifically, valgus and varus instability should be assessed with the elbow in 30° of flexion and full extension. If dislocation occurs during extension, the elbow should be reassessed with the forearm in pronation. If greater than 45° of pronation is required to maintain the reduction, operative intervention is indicated [6, 25, 26]. For stable elbows, short-term immobilization should be followed by early ROM exercises. For unstable elbows, initial management includes immobilization for approximately 2–3 weeks, followed by flexion and extension in a hinged split for 4 weeks. Afterwards, complete ROM may be allowed. Lateral injuries should be treated by placing the forearm in pronation with the elbow flexed at 90° for 1–2 weeks, followed by use of an elbow brace. For incomplete injuries that involve disruption of the MCL complex, the forearm should be placed in supination for 2–3 weeks. However, after elbow immobilization care should be taken to avoid excessive valgus load.

In asymptomatic patients, chronic instability could be managed nonoperatively with avoidance of instability-causing activities, elbow bracing to limit supination and valgus loading, application of a sugar tong cast, pain control, and/or physical therapy [8, 27]. If symptoms or instability persist, operative intervention is then indicated.

## Surgical Management

### Approach to the Elbow

The patient is placed in the lateral decubitus position with the arm supported over a bolster. The lateral structures are approached through the Kocher interval between anconeus and extensor carpi ulnaris. The anconeus is reflected exposing the LCL complex remnants. Typically, in acute trauma, this procedure reveals an avulsion of the majority of the soft tissue off the lateral epicondyle in one soft tissue sleeve, exposing the joint. In chronic situations, the avulsion ligament may be partly healed or attenuated.

A number of methods to access the MCL complex have been described. In cases of acute injuries, there is usually a rent in the common flexor muscles that leads to the joint. In the chronic case the muscle rent will be healed and a muscle-splitting approach through the common flexor muscles could be performed [28]. Independently from the approach used, the ulnar nerve should be identified and protected throughout the entire procedure. It is important to not leave the nerve unstable or in a hostile bed, in which case an ulnar nerve transposition is required.

### Acute Injuries

#### LCL and MCL Repair

In the acute setting a repair is performed. Acute primary repair of the LCL and MCL can be performed within the first few weeks following the injury. Anatomic repair of soft-tissue avulsions from bone can be performed with transosseous suture or suture anchors. Our preferred technique of LCL repair is an anatomical repair using grasping sutures and tensionable suture anchors [29]. In the sub-acute setting the ligaments are soft and do not hold sutures well. In chronic cases there may be significant scar tissue and the ligaments may be retracted so that they cannot be delivered onto the epicondyle.

The advantages of using tensionable anchors are as follows:

1. Tensioning of the ligaments can be performed in a controlled manner.
2. Sequential tensioning of the MCL and LCL may be performed.
3. They allow cycling of the elbow and on-table clinical assessment of stability and balance before final tensioning.
4. They allow locking of the repair at the desired tension.

Once having identified the lateral capsule complex, grasping sutures (e.g., Bunnell or Krackow) are placed in the avulsed LCL complex. The suture ends are then loaded into the eyelet of the tensionable anchor. The anchor is then placed into the lateral epicondyle at the anatomical insertion site of the LCL. At this point, the sutures remain unlocked and un-tensioned in the anchor. We term this “prefabrication” where all anchors and sutures are initially placed, before final tensioning. The elbow is examined for the full ROM and a gentle assessment of stability is performed. If there is any persistent instability, then further stabilization is required. This may include stabilization of the medial structures.

Once having identified the MCL instability, grasping sutures are placed in the avulsed ligament. The anchors are then deployed into the anatomical MCL footprint before any tensioning is performed. That is the mid-position of the sharp distal surface of the medial epicondyle. If both the MCL and LCL are being repaired, the authors recommend tensioning each side alternatively. During a combined repair, the MCL is tensioned first with the elbow in flexion and the forearm in supination. The LCL is then tensioned with the forearm in pronation. The surgeon should perform repeated reassessments of elbow stability and range during tensioning. It is important not to over tension one side as this may lead to an inability to reduce the opposite side [29]. During MCL repair, the ulnar nerve should be protected without transposition.

## Chronic Injuries

### LCL Reconstruction

Open ligament reconstruction is indicated in patients with poor ligamentous tissue quality, when a prior repair has failed, or in the presence of chronic recurrent instability. Ligament reconstruction using graft tissue can offer an isometric, extracapsular and anatomic solution [30] Many techniques and choices of graft have been described, including advancement and imbrication of the LCL, autologous palmaris longs tendon, a strip of the triceps tendon, plantaris tendon, and synthetic ligament augmentation [30–32].

***Surgeons preferred technique***: The technique we use is different from the Nestor or docking technique [30]. We know that the site of primary failure of the acute instabilities is usually from the humerus. We therefore use a technique that "wraps around the lateral condyle" so that it is intrinsically stable, so that the weakest point is distal. The final construct obtained is extremely stable on the table (Fig. 13.1).

*Graft selection*: The authors prefer to use an autogenous hamstring graft, which is robust and gives the required length (15–20 cm) needed for the technique. However if allograft is available, it is a reasonable alternative with comparable outcomes in the literature.

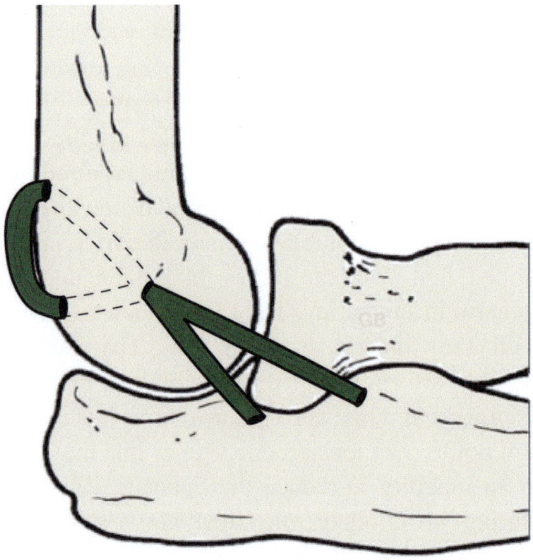

**Fig. 13.1** Lateral view of the elbow demonstrating the LCL reconstruction. © Gregory I. Bain

*Ulna drill holes*: Two full 4.5-mm drill holes are created in the insertion point of the LUCL on the supinator crest of the ulna. We place them just proximal and just distal to the ulnar insertion of the LUCL, just distal to the capsular attachment. The exit sites of the drill holes are identified on the medial side of the ulna.

*Humeral drill holes*: The isometric point of the origin of the LCL complex is identified, on the lateral epicondyle, at the center of the capitellum as seen from the lateral side. A position 2 mm proximal is identified and a 4.5 mm drill is advanced through this point. The drill is directed from anterior to posterior, and exits posterosuperiorly. The drill is then removed and advanced again through the isometric point to create a second drill hole that exits posteroinferiorly.

We smooth the entrance of the hole with a curette, so the tendon graft can easily pass through the drill holes. If the ulnar cortex is particularly hard, we will "tap" the hole so that the screw does not cut the graft.

*Tendon passage*: Both free ends of the tendon graft are sutured with a nonabsorbable suture allowing graft hole transfer and tensioning. One free end of the graft is passed through the posterior inferior hole and exits the anterior hole. The other through the posterior superior hole and exits the anterior hole. This creates a loop of tendon around the posterior condyle.

Each end of the graft is then advanced through the drill holes in the ulna from lateral to medial. At this point, the graft is tensioned while the elbow is cycled through a range of motion and the stability is assessed.

*Graft fixation*: The graft is secured into the drill holes with interference screws. The first screw is inserted into the anterior humeral drill hole. The graft is again tensioned and cyclic loading is performed. Interference fit screws are then inserted into the ulna drill holes. We usually use the 5.5 mm screws in the humerus and either 4.0 or 5.5 mm screws in the ulna. Any redundant capsule is then plicated.

We use the above principles of osseous preparation, graft preparation and fixation for all of the ligamentous elbow reconstructions described in this manuscript.

### MCL Reconstruction

MCL Reconstructive surgery is indicated in patients in which conservative therapy fails, in patients with delayed presentation of acute traumatic ruptures, or in chronic dislocations where it is not possible to perform a primary repair. Further, it has been shown that in competitive throwing athletes, MCL reconstruction using a free tendon graft yields better results over direct repair of the tendon.

Jobe developed the original MCL reconstruction and described the technique with initial results [33]. The technique used a tendinous detachment and reflection of the flexor-pronator muscle group, sub muscular transposition of the ulnar nerve, and creation of humeral tunnels that penetrated the posterior humeral cortex. Since then different modifications of the original technique have been described.

#### Surgeons Preferred Technique

*Ulna drill holes*: Two full 4.5-mm drill holes are created in the ulna and placed in the site of the anatomic origin of the anterior and posterior bundles of MCL. Specifically, one drill hole is made adjacent to the sublime tubercle and another at the medial margin of the greater sigmoid notch.

*Humeral drill holes*: On the humeral side, the medial epicondyle is drilled in a "V" fashion creating two proximal divergent tunnels. The base of the "V" is at the origin of the MCL on the anteroinferior aspect of the medial epicondyle and the limbs diverge proximally in a posterior and posterosuperior direction. In this fashion, two separated tunnels that connected to the primary humeral tunnel at the origin of the MCL are created.

*Tendon passage*: At this point, the hamstring graft is passed through the drill holes in the medial epicondyle, with the two limbs of the graft passed then through the drill holes in the ulna side. Finally, graft is tensioned with the elbow in varus and supination and fixed with interference screws both in the ulna and in the medial epicondyle.

*Graft fixation*: We use the same size screws as used for the lateral side reconstruction. The elbow is brought to full range of motion, and care is taken to smooth any rough edges that might abrade the graft. Any part of the native MCL remaining is sutured and incorporated into the bone tunnel to reinforce stability.

## Complications

Good or excellent results following surgery have been reported for isolated MCL and LCL surgery. However, despite an accurate repair or reconstruction up to 11 % of patients may have complications [31, 34]. Specifically, instability can still occur after ligament reconstruction. Other reported complications include infection, bony bridge fracture, ulnar neuropathy, cutaneous nerve injury, and arthrofibrosis resulting in flexion contracture. Primary ligament repair combined with early postoperative exercise have been reported to produce satisfactory outcomes in unstable elbow dislocation, with low rate of residual instability [35–37]. Jones et al. reported residual instability in eight patients (25 %) treated for PLRI with the docking technique at a mean of 7 years. Nestor et al. described results on 11 patients (three repairs and eight reconstructions) who underwent surgery for PLRI reporting excellent outcomes in patients that underwent ligaments repairs. Further, four patients that underwent ligament reconstruction noted fair and poor outcomes. Sanchez-Sotelo et al. reported their outcomes in 44 patients (12 repairs and 22 reconstructions) that underwent surgery for PLRI. Five patients (11 %) noted further instability, and 27 % of patients described fair or poor results [31].

## Combined LCL and MCL Reconstruction for Global Instability

In some cases, the soft-tissue injury is not limited to the medial or lateral aspect of the joint, but rather presents as multidirectional elbow instability with insufficiency of the entire collateral ligament complex. For these patients, the authors have developed a less invasive reconstruction technique using a single circumferential tendon graft technique that addresses both the medial and lateral instability with a single tendon graft [38]. This technique may also be used in patients with complex fracture dislocations or terrible triad injuries, when there is residual instability following fixation of fractures. This may also be used as an alternative to dynamic or static external fixation when fracture fixation and ligament repairs have failed to restore stability [38]. Finally, it may also be considered in cases of severe elbow stiffness where heterotopic ossification involves the ligaments and needs removal in order to restore motion but in doing so will compromise the function of the ligaments.

Limited data is reported on the results of a double ligament reconstruction. Van Riet et al. originally reported on the surgical technique of simultaneous medial and lateral collateral ligament reconstruction utilizing a single or double loop technique [38]. More recently, Finkbone et al. has reported on a similar technique of reconstruction [39]. The authors described this as a "box-loop" reconstruction where a donor tendon is passed through a humeral tunnel along its flexion-extension axis and an ulnar tunnel connecting the sublime tubercle and supinator crest. The graft is then tied back on itself creating one continuous graft. The technique was performed on 14 patients with an average follow-up of 64 months. The authors reported an average ASES score of 81. The average Quick DASH was 13 and the average MEPS was 88. Radiographs showed all ulnohumeral joints were congruent without signs of instability and no patients required additional surgery for instability, range of motion or arthritis.

## Surgeons Preferred Technique

A midline posterior skin incision is preferred because it allows access to medial and lateral structures [40]. Full-thickness fasciocutaneous flaps are created and elevated to expose the medial or lateral aspect of the elbow. Laterally, structures are approached through the Kocher interval between anconeus and extensor carpi ulnaris. On the medial side, a muscle-splitting approach through the common flexor muscles could be performed. Following the circumferential tendon graft technique, a single-loop or a double-loop technique could be performed depending on the severity of the elbow instability. The single-loop technique provides a reconstruction of the anterior band of the MCL and the LUCL, while the double-loop technique reconstructs all four ligament units (LUCL, posterolateral capsule, and anterior and posterior bands of the MCL).

### Circumferential Single-Loop Technique

*Humeral drill holes*: A 2-mm guidewire is drilled through the lateral epicondyle to the anteroinferior aspect of the medial epicondyle, which is the isometric points that make up the axis of rotation. A 4.5-mm drill hole is reamed through the humerus over this guidewire.

*Ulna drill holes*: A 4.5-mm drill hole is created passing from the sublime tubercle on the medial side to the supinator crest on the lateral side.

*Tendon passage and fixation*: The hamstring tendon graft is passed through the humeral tunnel and secured with 5.5 mm interference screws on the medial and lateral sides. Each tendon end is then passed through the ulnar tunnel and also secured with a single 4.0 mm interference screw (Fig. 13.2). The flexor-pronator mass is repaired back to the medial epicondyle, and the Kocher interval is closed.

### Circumferential Double-Loop Technique

This is similar to the single-loop technique but also reconstructs the posterior band of the MCL and the posterolateral capsule. This is accom-

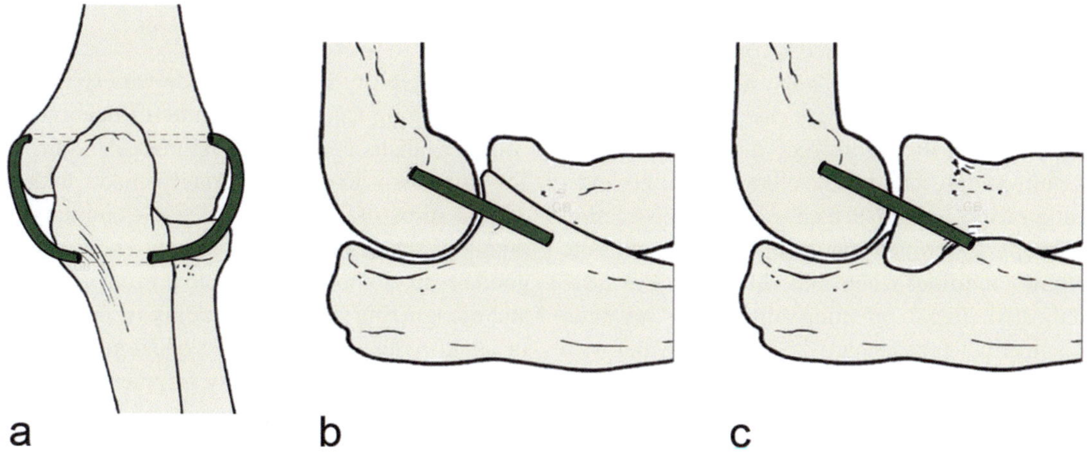


**Fig. 13.2** AP (**a**), medial (**b**), and lateral view (**c**) of the elbow demonstrating the single-loop circumferential graft reconstruction. © Gregory I. Bain

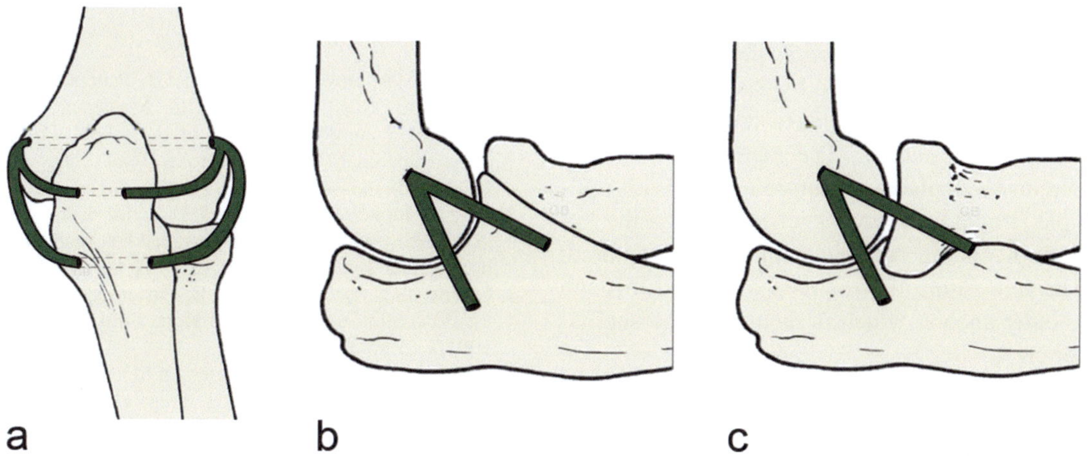


**Fig. 13.3** AP (**a**), medial (**b**), and lateral view (**c**) of the elbow demonstrating the double-loop circumferential graft reconstruction. © Gregory I. Bain

plished by creating a second ulnar drill hole from the posterior supinator crest laterally to the posteromedial olecranon facet at the attachment of the posterior band of the MCL. The humeral side is the same as the single loop technique.

*Tendon passage and fixation*: The free ends of the graft, exiting the humerus, are then split longitudinally to create two free tails of equal size. One tail from each side is passed through the posterior ulnar drill hole, and the other tails through the anterior drill hole. The graft is tensioned and secured with interference screws (Fig. 13.3).

## External Fixation

We have previously used many external fixators, but now only use them in very selected cases. Some surgeons will manage a terrible triad injury with stabilization of the radial head and an external fixator. Our preference would be to surgically stabilize the radial head, coronoid process and the associated ligmentous injuries.

We reserve the use of external fixation in complex cases where we can't obtain stability with a repair or reconstruction. Therefore we use them as a primary stabilizer most commonly in open elbow dislocations with bone and or soft tissue loss. However even in these cases, we would prefer to primarily reconstruct the tissues and if required apply a flap to the elbow. The other indication for an external fixator is with distraction arthroplasty, which we use only for chronic elbow conditions where an arthroplasty is contraindicated (e.g., infection or higher demand younger patient such as a 45 year old farmer with post-traumatic arthritis).

## Internal Fixation

Although we rarely use external fixators, we are now using internal fixators. There are two types. The plate fixation method as proposed by Jorge Orbay and manufactured by Skeletal Dynamics [41]. The other option is to create an internal fixator, with sutures. The method the authors use involves placing a suture anchor with multiple strands into the isometric point on the lateral epicondyle. Any ligament tears are repaired. The free suture limb is then advanced through another anchor, which is secures to the supinator crest.

## Post-operative Protocol

At the completion of the procedure the stability is assessed. If good stability has been obtained we often apply a plaster slab for 1 week at 90° of flexion. The arm is positioned in pronation or supination to protect the stabilization. A hinged brace is then worn for 2–4 weeks depending upon complexity of the case. An extension block at 30° is used for complex cases, and reduced every few weeks, aiming for full extension by 3–6 weeks The patient can return to light work activities at 6 weeks and heavy work activities at 3–6 months postoperatively.

## Conclusions

Elbow instability includes a wide variety of disorders ranging from simple acute dislocations to complex dislocation with additional injuries. The diagnosis can be accurately made with a combination of history, physical examination, imaging, and arthroscopic surgery. The key to a good result is knowledge of the normal anatomy and recognizing the pathoanatomy of the injury. In acute cases, the principles of surgery are to repair the soft tissue and bony fragments to yield stability. In chronic recurrent instability, reconstruction of the collateral ligament complexes is mandatory.

## References

1. McKee MD, Bowden SH, King GJ, Patterson SD, Jupiter JB, Bamberger HB, et al. Management of recurrent, complex instability of the elbow with a hinged external fixator. J Bone Joint Surg Br. 1998;80(6):1031–6.
2. Ring D, Jupiter JB, Zilberfarb J. Posterior dislocation of the elbow with fractures of the radial head and coronoid. J Bone Joint Surg Am. 2002;84-A(4):547–51.
3. O'Driscoll S, Bell D, Morrey B. Posterolateral rotatory instability of the elbow. J Bone Joint Surg Am. 1991;73(3):440–6.
4. Dunning CE, Zarzour ZD, Patterson SD, Johnson JA, King GJ. Ligamentous stabilizers against posterolateral rotatory instability of the elbow. J Bone Joint Surg Am. 2001;83-A(12):1823–8.
5. Seki A, Olsen BS, Jensen SL, Eygendaal D, Sojbjerg JO. Functional anatomy of the lateral collateral ligament complex of the elbow: configuration of Y and its role. J Shoulder Elbow Surg. 2002;11(1):53–9.
6. O'Driscoll SW. Classification and evaluation of recurrent instability of the elbow. Clin Orthop Relat Res 2000;(370):34–43.
7. McKee MD, Schemitsch EH, Sala MJ, O'driscoll SW. The pathoanatomy of lateral ligamentous disruption in complex elbow instability. J Shoulder Elbow Surg. 2003;12(4):391–6.
8. Charalambous CP, Stanley JK. Posterolateral rotatory instability of the elbow. J Bone Joint Surg Br. 2008;90(3):272–9.
9. Cheung EV, Sperling JW. Management of proximal humeral nonunions and malunions. Orthop Clin North Am. 2008;39(4):475–82.

10. Kalainov DM, Cohen MS. Posterolateral rotatory instability of the elbow in association with lateral epicondylitis. A report of three cases. J Bone Joint Surg Am. 2005;87(5):1120–5.
11. Cohen MS, Hastings 2nd H. Rotatory instability of the elbow. The anatomy and role of the lateral stabilizers. J Bone Joint Surg Am. 1997;79(2):225–33.
12. Hall JA, McKee MD. Posterolateral rotatory instability of the elbow following radial head resection. J Bone Joint Surg Am. 2005;87(7):1571–9.
13. Mehta JA, Bain GI. Elbow dislocations in adults and children. Clin Sports Med. 2004;23(4):609–27.
14. Field LD, Altchek DW. Evaluation of the arthroscopic valgus instability test of the elbow. Am J Sports Med. 1996;24(2):177–81.
15. Watts A, Bain G. New techniques in elbow arthroscopy. In: Savoie FH, Field LD, editors. AANA advanced arthroscopy: the elbow and wrist. Philadelphia, PA: Saunders-Elsevier; 2010. p. 124–31.
16. Carrino JA, Morrison WB, Zou KH, Steffen RT, Snearly WN, Murray PM. Lateral ulnar collateral ligament of the elbow: optimization of evaluation with two-dimensional MR imaging. Radiology. 2001;218(1):118–25.
17. Grafe MW, McAdams TR, Beaulieu CF, Ladd AL. Magnetic resonance imaging in diagnosis of chronic posterolateral rotatory instability of the elbow. Am J Orthop (Belle Mead NJ). 2003;32(10):501–3.
18. Potter HG, Weiland AJ, Schatz JA, Paletta GA, Hotchkiss RN. Posterolateral rotatory instability of the elbow: usefulness of MR imaging in diagnosis. Radiology. 1997;204(1):185–9.
19. Mehta JA, Bain GI. Posterolateral rotatory instability of the elbow. J Am Acad Orthop Surg. 2004;12(6): 405–15.
20. Thompson WH, Jobe FW, Yocum LA, Pink MM. Ulnar collateral ligament reconstruction in athletes: muscle-splitting approach without transposition of the ulnar nerve. J Shoulder Elbow Surg. 2001;10(2):152–7.
21. Timmerman LA, Schwartz ML, Andrews JR. Preoperative evaluation of the ulnar collateral ligament by magnetic resonance imaging and computed tomography arthrography. Evaluation in 25 baseball players with surgical confirmation. Am J Sports Med. 1994;22(1):26–31.
22. Safran MR. Ulnar collateral ligament injury in the overhead athlete: diagnosis and treatment. Clin Sports Med. 2004;23(4):643–63.
23. O'Driscoll SW, Lawton RL, Smith AM. The "moving valgus stress test" for medial collateral ligament tears of the elbow. Am J Sports Med. 2005;33(2):231–9.
24. Modi CS, Lawrence E, Lawrence TM. (iv) Elbow instability. Orthop Trauma. 2012;26(5):316–27.
25. Kuhn MA, Ross G. Acute elbow dislocations. Orthop Clin North Am. 2008;39(2):155–61. v.
26. Bell S. Elbow instability, mechanism and management. Curr Orthop. 2008;22(2):90–103.
27. Kent M, Brown D, Brownson P. Posterolateral rotatory instability of the elbow: a new use for the sugar tong cast. Injury Extra. 2006;37:264–6.
28. Smith GR, Altchek DW, Pagnani MJ, Keeley JR. A muscle-splitting approach to the ulnar collateral ligament of the elbow. Neuroanatomy and operative technique. Am J Sports Med. 1996;24(5):575–80.
29. Lee YC, Eng K, Keogh A, McLean JM, Bain GI. Repair of the acutely unstable elbow: use of tensionable anchors. Tech Hand Up Extrem Surg. 2012; 16(4):225–9.
30. Nestor BJ, O'Driscoll SW, Morrey BF. Ligamentous reconstruction for posterolateral rotatory instability of the elbow. J Bone Joint Surg Am. 1992;74(8): 1235–41.
31. Sanchez-Sotelo J, Morrey BF, O'Driscoll SW. Ligamentous repair and reconstruction for posterolateral rotatory instability of the elbow. J Bone Joint Surg Br. 2005;87(1):54–61.
32. Eygendaal D. Ligamentous reconstruction around the elbow using triceps tendon. Acta Orthop Scand. 2004;75(5):516–23.
33. Jobe FW, Stark H, Lombardo SJ. Reconstruction of the ulnar collateral ligament in athletes. J Bone Joint Surg Am. 1986;68(8):1158–63.
34. Vitale MA, Ahmad CS. The outcome of elbow ulnar collateral ligament reconstruction in overhead athletes. A systematic review. Am J Sport Med. 2008;36:1193–205.
35. Micic I, Kim S, Park I, Kim P, Jeon I. Surgical management of unstable elbow dislocation without intraarticular fracture. Int Orthop. 2009;33(4):1141–7.
36. Heo YM, Yi JW, Lee JB, Lee DH, Park WK, Kim SJ. Unstable simple elbow dislocation treated with the repair of lateral collateral ligament complex. Clin Orthop Surg. 2015;7(2):241–7.
37. Jeon I, Kim S, Kim P. Primary ligament repair for elbow dislocation. Keio J Med. 2008;57(2): 99–104.
38. van Riet RP, Bain GI, Baird R, Lim YW. Simultaneous reconstruction of medial and lateral elbow ligaments for instability using a circumferential graft. Tech Hand Up Extrem Surg. 2006;10(4):239–44.
39. Finkbone PR, O'Driscoll SW. Box-loop ligament reconstruction of the elbow for medial and lateral instability. J Shoulder Elbow Surg. 2015;24: 647–54.
40. Patterson SD, Bain GI, Mehta JA. Surgical approaches to the elbow. Clin Orthop Relat Res 2000;(370): 19–33.
41. Orbay JL, Mijares MR. The management of elbow instability using an internal joint stabilizer: preliminary results. Clin Orthop Relat Res 2014;(472): 2049–60.

# Treatment of the Chronically Subluxated Elbow (Persistent Elbow Instability)

14

Carlos Kalbakdij, James M. Saucedo, Raul Barco, and Samuel A. Antuña

## Background

Despite our growing understanding of elbow biomechanics and the various patterns of instability, there still remain unanswered questions. One such challenge for the elbow surgeon is persistent elbow instability after a complex dislocation, which has been defined by Papandrea [1] as evidence of continuous dislocation or subluxation after initial treatment for the elbow dislocation with a coronoid fracture. The time period included in this definition is not well established, but most authors agree that 8–12 weeks from the injury might be the minimum time limit to consider an elbow chronically unstable.

At the end of this chapter, the authors hope to improve the reader's understanding of the various causes of persistent instability, develop a systematic and comprehensive approach to diagnosis, and a treatment algorithm to guide the surgeon's decision making process.

C. Kalbakdij, MD • R. Barco, MD, PhD, FEBOT
Department of Orthopedic surgery, Hospital Universitario La Paz, Paseo La Castellana 261, Madrid 28046, Spain
e-mail: carloskalbakdij@hotmail.com; raulbarco@hotmail.com

J.M. Saucedo, MD, MBA
Department of Orthopedics, The Hand Center of San Antonio, University of Texas Health Sciences Center of San Antonio, San Antonio, TX, USA
e-mail: saucedojames@gmail.com

S.A. Antuña, MD, PhD, FEBOT (✉)
Shoulder and Elbow Unit, Department of Orthopedics, Hospital Universitario La Paz, Madrid, Spain
e-mail: santuna@asturias.com

## Evaluation

In the initial evaluation of persistent elbow instability, it is necessary to identify and analyze each structure that provides primary or secondary stability. Evaluation begins with the history and physical examination of the elbow. One should note the mechanism of the original injury, symptoms that the patient is currently experiencing and what treatment has already been provided, including previous operative reports and progress notes. Physical examination of the elbow should be systematic, starting with inspection (Is there swelling or deformity? Where are the previous surgical scars?), palpation (Is there point tenderness?), range of motion (Is it painful? Is the elbow stiff? Is there clicking, popping, or crepitance?), and finally, appropriate provocative maneuvers (such as varus and valgus stress and the elbow pivot shift test). It is important to understand that the majority of patients presenting with persistent instability complain of stiffness and pain, and have already a variable degree of cartilage damage in the joint.

Imaging is truly part of the physical exam and should start with plain X-rays with multiple

© Springer International Publishing Switzerland 2017
R.Z. Tashjian (ed.), *The Unstable Elbow*, DOI 10.1007/978-3-319-46019-2_14

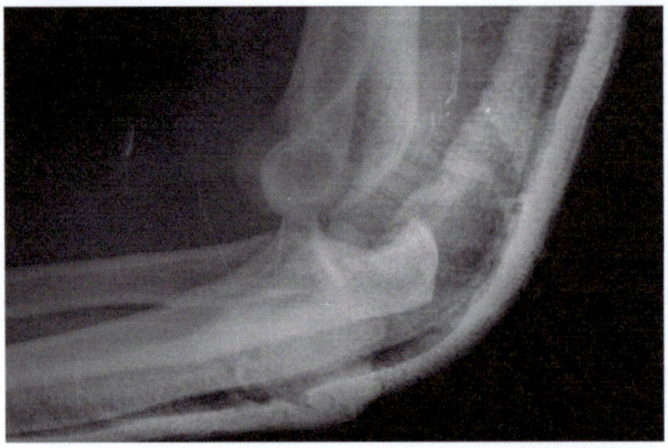

**Fig. 14.1** Lateral X-ray of a 71-year-old patient 3 weeks alter a radial head fracture dislocation of the elbow treated with cast immobilization. There is obvious subluxation of the joint the joint

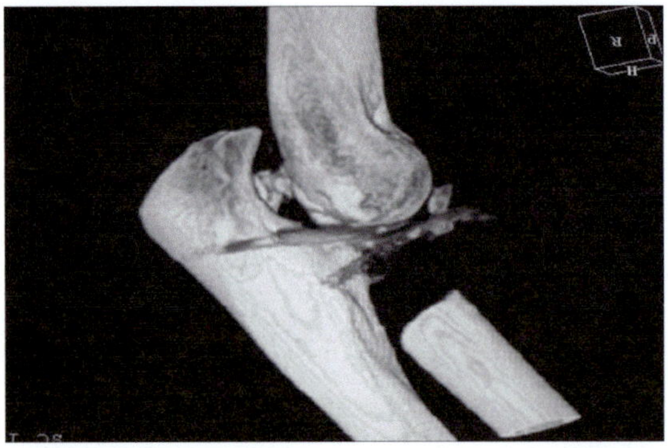

**Fig. 14.2** CT scan of a patient presenting with persistent instability after an attempt to reconstruct the coronoid and resection of the radial head

views, including AP, true lateral, radiocapitellar lateral (also known as Greenspan view) and oblique views (Fig. 14.1). Acute injury radiographs should be reviewed in addition to current films. Finally, computed tomography (CT) with three-dimensional reconstructions can provide important details about the injury pattern and inform preoperative planning (Fig. 14.2).

A critical feature of elbow stability is the ulnohumeral congruence. The congruent reduction is maintained by various structures: the bony articulation (olecranon and coronoid), the articular capsule, the lateral ulnar and medial collateral ligaments (LUCL and MCL, respectively) and the muscles crossing the elbow. Morrey et al. [2] experimentally demonstrated that the load carried by the radial head under a valgus force is minimal when the medial collateral ligament is intact, suggesting that stability is not significantly compromised after radial head excision with a functionally intact MCL. However, it provided secondary stabilization when the medial collateral ligament was insufficient. Due to the complexity of these injuries and extent of concomitant soft tissue damage, we believe that the standard of care in the acute setting should be to either fix the radial head fracture or replace it when it is irreparable, in order to restore its role as a secondary stabilizer.

Other experimental studies have shown that the instability is directly proportional to the percentage of bony deficiency affecting the ulnohumeral joint; it is necessary that at least 30 % of the olecranon [2, 3] and at least 50 % of the coronoid [4] be preserved in order to maintain articular reduction and stability. It is useful to remember these values when planning surgical treatment.

Understanding the pathology of a persistent unstable elbow involves evaluation of all potential causes and consequences of joint incongruence: coronoid deficiency, ligament insufficiency, absence or malunion of the radial head, cartilage damage, nerve involvement and capsular contracture. A global view of the problem and a clear plan to restore ulnohumeral congruence and stability is necessary to pursue a good clinical outcome.

## Treatment

A common problem in the chronically subluxated elbow is the coexistence of stiffness and instability; in those cases, treatment should prioritize correcting incongruence and restoring stability to avoid the development of potentially debilitating ulnohumeral osteoarthritis.

Treatment ranges from nonoperative strategies with physical therapy regimens to a wide spectrum of surgical options. The first step is to recognize the injury pattern and remember the objective: restore ulnohumeral congruence, reduce the radiocapitellar joint and restore elbow stability. While a functional range of motion is desired (Morrey et al. [5] established 30–130° as a functional range of motion), stability is of primary significance and should take priority. A stiff elbow is easier to manage than a chronically unstable one.

## Nonoperative Strategies and Therapy Protocols

In select cases of residual elbow subluxation, nonoperative treatment with exercises that focus on strengthening the dynamic stabilizers and avoidance of varus stress is a reasonable alternative. In 2008, Duckworth [6] suggested that this strategy be employed only in those cases of slight subluxation, defined by an ulnohumeral joint space between 4 and 7 mm, and only in cooperative patients. They studied 23 patients with 20 fracture-dislocations and three simple dislocations. Five were initially treated nonoperatively and the rest underwent surgery. The mean age was 43 years old, and average follow up was 24 months. All patients achieved stability. The mean ROM was 113°. All had concentric reductions at final follow up except one, who was reportedly asymptomatic. The mean Broberg-Morrey elbow score was 90 points. Four patients ultimately underwent surgery: two ulnar nerve transpositions, two heterotopic ossification excisions, one elbow contracture release, one skin graft, and one compartment syndrome. In general, nonoperative management should be reserved only for those patients with minimal instability and minimal loss of congruence.

## Surgical Management

Surgical planning of a persistent subluxed elbow includes assessment of all osseous and ligamentous structures around the elbow. All efforts should be aimed to restore as many stabilizers as possible.

### Radial Head Fracture

The Mason Classification for radial head fractures may be the most widely used [7]. Type 1 fractures are nondisplaced marginal fractures. Type 2 fractures are marginal fractures with displacement and type 3 fractures are comminuted fractures of the entire head [7]. In his original paper, Mason proposed nonoperative treatment for type 1 fractures and operative treatment for type 3 fractures [7]. Recent studies have validated that nonoperative treatment of isolated type 1 radial head fractures is reasonable, with 95 % of patients in one large series obtaining excellent or good outcomes [8]. In the setting of elbow instability with a type 1 fracture, nonoperative treatment may still be considered as long as there is a concentric reduction and a stable range of motion with no evidence of subluxation with flexion and extension. Type 3 fractures continue to be treated operatively with general consensus. The optimal treatment of type 2 fractures remains controversial. Some authors have reported excellent results after nonoperative treatment of certain isolated type 2 fractures [8] while others have reported very good results with operative treatment [9]. In the setting of complex dislocations, operative repair of type 2 fractures should be performed to maintain its role as a secondary stabilizer in the setting of an injured MCL.

In type 3 fractures, radial head arthroplasty offers better outcomes when it is made in the acute phase. Morrey [10] reported 92 % good outcome in the acute phase and 48 % good outcome when it is made in chronic phase. The worst result is seen in cases of delayed radial head arthroplasty. The use of allograft for reconstruction is unpredictable and in our opinion, should be avoided.

If the radial head is absent in the subacute setting due to a prior resection, it commonly needs to be replaced in order to help maintaining posterolateral and valgus stability in cases of chronic subluxation or instability. It is unclear which type of radial head arthroplasty is superior. However, the surgeon should not believe that radial head replacement alone solves the problem of an unstable elbow if the rest of anatomical structures involved are not addressed (Fig. 14.3).

### Ligamentous Injury

In a concentrically reduced ulnohumeral joint, one can expect ligamentous healing. In acute ligamentous injury with associated complex instability, primary repair is often feasible. However, in delayed cases, the surgeon should prepare for ligament reconstruction. Repair and

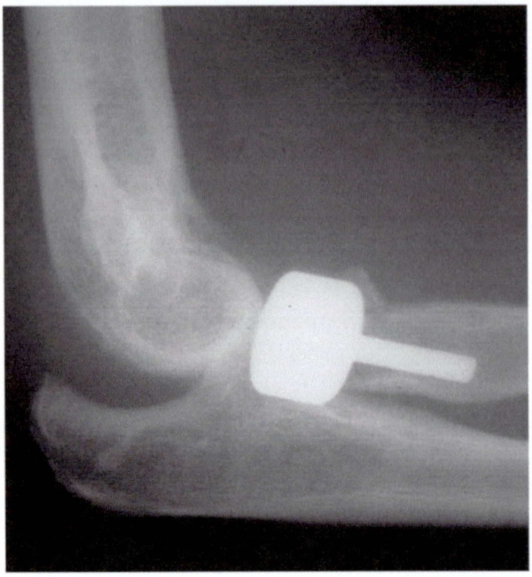

**Fig. 14.3** Patient with persistent instability after a radial head fracture associated with elbow instability in whom the radial head was replaced but the rest of stabilizers were not adequately addressed

reconstruction techniques are described in previous chapters, and we encourage the reader to review them. Occasionally, especially when there has been an associated neurologic injury, one may find significant heterotopic ossification that needs to be removed and compels the surgeon to undergo a ligament reconstruction (Fig. 14.4).

## Coronoid Fracture

Regan and Morrey [11] described three types of coronoid fracture. Type I fractures involve the tip of the coronoid, type II fractures involve more than the tip and less than 50 % of the coronoid, and type III fractures involve greater than 50 %. O'Driscoll et al. [4] described an alternative classification system involving three fracture types. Type 1 is a tip fracture, type 2 is an anteromedial facet fracture, and type 3 is a fracture through the

a

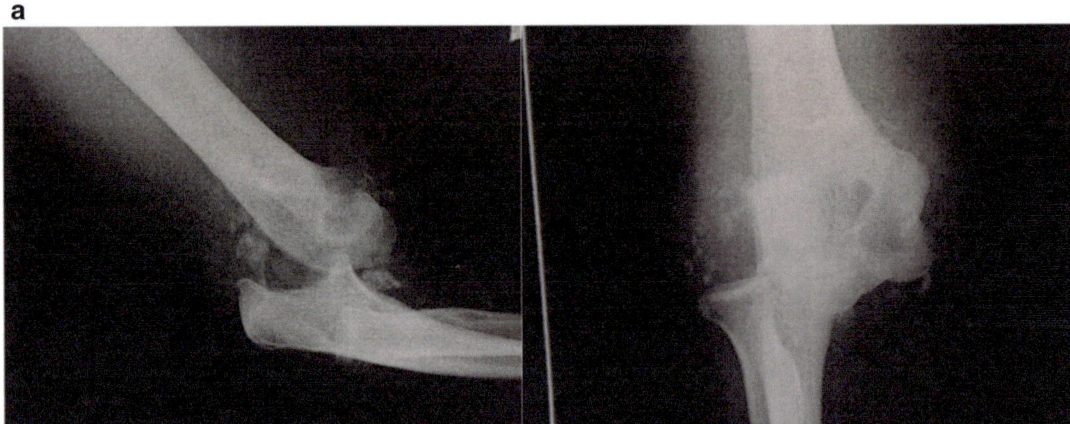

b

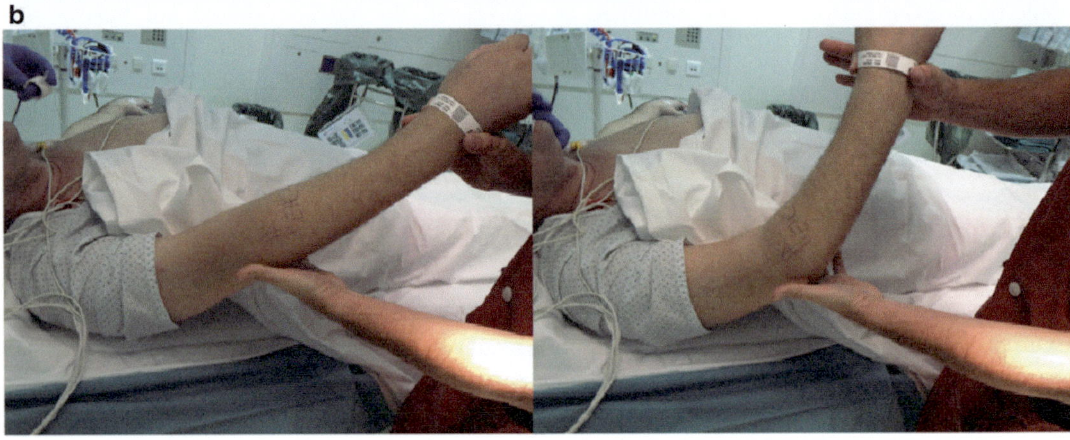

**Fig. 14.4** (**a**) Radiographs of a patient with a persistent elbow dislocation 6 weeks after high-energy trauma with central neurological injury. There is significant heterotopic ossification. (**b**) The elbow presents with severe stiffness

base of the coronoid process. This classification stresses the importance of identifying fractures of the anteromedial facet of the coronoid caused by a varus force, leading to posteromedial rotatory instability.

Classical recommendations have been to fix all Regan-Morrey type II and III coronoid fractures as well as any type I fractures associated with instability. In type I fractures, many authors feel that there is not enough evidence of instability associated with this particular fracture type. Therefore, some authors do not feel there is enough evidence supporting the importance of their repair of this fracture type. The coronoid process has three significant soft tissue insertions: the anterior joint capsule, the brachialis muscle and the ulnar collateral ligament. Anatomic evidence demonstrates that the capsule usually attaches below the tip of the coronoid process and the anterior band of the MCL attaches more distal [12, 13]. Repair of fractures, depending on size, will also incorporate some or all of these soft tissue insertions playing an important role in elbow stability.

Josefsson [14] reported four cases in a series of patients that experienced recurrent instability after an initial elbow dislocation. All patients that redislocated had an associated fracture of coronoid that was not repaired at the time of initial treatment. Terada [15] demonstrated that repair of type I fractures could improve stability. Clinical evidence reported by Pugh [16] corroborates that finding, stating that type I injuries usually represent a capsular injury. Although in the acute setting fixation of small coronoid fragments may not be necessary, all these clinical findings stress the importance of addressing all possible stabilizers when dealing with persistent instability.

The coronoid fracture in the setting of elbow dislocations remains a significant cause of persistent instability, and it remains incompletely solved. It is still unknown what percentage of the coronoid is necessary to maintain elbow stability. However, it is rather clear that in type I fractures the issue is not the bone, but the anterior capsule.

In 2004, Schneeberger [17] demonstrated that elbows with a defect of 50 or 70 % of the coronoid, loss of the radial head, and intact ligaments could not be stabilized by radial head replacement alone; however, additional coronoid reconstruction was able to restore stability.

Because of its critical role in rendering stability, we try to fix all acute Type 3 fractures when possible and reconstruct it in those fractures that are not amenable to repair, such as those with extensive comminution. Type II fractures may be treated nonoperatively if the radiocapitellar joint can be reconstructed, the lateral ligament is repaired and the elbow is found to be stable through a full arc of motion. However, if the radial head is not amenable to fixation, a type II coronoid fracture may need to be fixed in addition to radial head replacement.

## Coronoid Fracture Repair

Repair alternatives include suture lasso technique, screw fixation (anterior to posterior or posterior to anterior) and plate fixation. Grant et al. [18] reported that the suture lasso technique was more stable than the other techniques intraoperatively, both before and after LUCL repair, and at final follow-up. Open reduction internal fixation (ORIF) was associated with a higher prevalence of implant failure, and suture anchors were associated with a higher prevalence of malunion and nonunion. Greater stability with fewer complications can be achieved with the use of the suture lasso technique for fixation of small coronoid fractures (Fig. 14.5). If the fracture is big enough, screw or plate fixation is probably the optimal technique (Fig. 14.6)

## Coronoid Fracture Reconstruction

The most common scenario in the subluxed elbow presenting 3–6 weeks after the initial injury involves absence of a competent coronoid. In this situation there are several reconstruction options. Esser [19] in 1997 described reconstruction with radial head autograft. Moritomo [20] in 1998 published reconstruction with olecranon autograft; and Kohls-Gatzoulis [21] in 2004 and Chung [22] in 2007 reported good outcomes with iliac crest bone autograft.

In 2014, Kataoka et al. [23] compared the three types of osteochondral autografts that have been employed for coronoid process reconstruction: olecranon tip, lateral radial head, or proximal radial head. They concluded that an olecranon graft was most suitable for defects of the coronoid process involving the tip, and a proximal radial head graft was most suitable for defects of the coronoid process involving the anteromedial rim. The olecranon graft seems to provide the highest "covering rate" and reconstruction of 50 % of the height of the coronoid process only required harvest of about 14 % of the olecranon tip and does not seem to cause gross elbow instability secondary to the donor site defect.

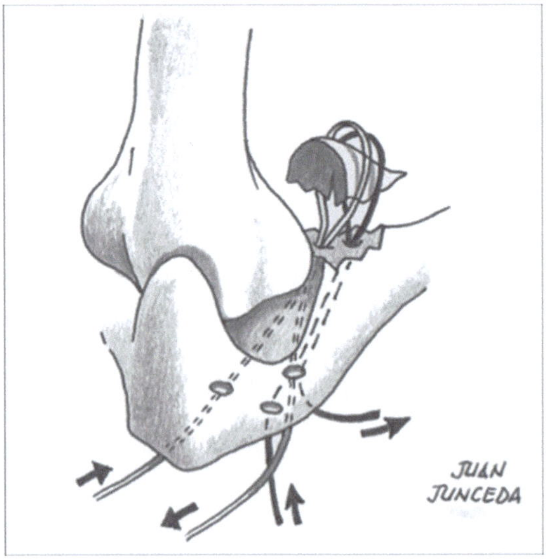


**Fig. 14.5** Suture fixation of small coronoid fractures is seldom required in the acute setting but can be an additional help in subacute cases

Allograft options have also been reported. In 2005, Karlstad [24] published the failure of fresh-frozen radial head allografts in the treatment of Essex-Lopresti injury. This result suggests that allograft reconstruction options may result in less optimal outcomes than autograft. Van Riet et al. reported on six cases of coronoid process reconstruction, three cases using radial head allograft and three cases using radial head autograft [25]. Two of three allograft cases had a poor results based upon the MEPS with mild pain in two cases and severe pain in one. The authors reported that reconstruction of the coronoid process is an option but results are unpredictable.

Time since injury is important in deciding between repair and reconstruction. Ring and others [26] consider repair of the coronoid process 4 weeks after injury as difficult if not impossible in a dislocated or subluxated terrible triad elbow. Papandrea [1] recommends that reconstruction (after a coronoid fracture dislocation) should be done as soon as possible; a delay beyond 7 or 8 weeks is uniformly associated with an unsuccessful outcome (Fig. 14.7).

## Preferred Coronoid Reconstruction Technique

When the coronoid fracture is deemed not reparable, and radial head is available, we prefer to use it for coronoid reconstruction. If radial head

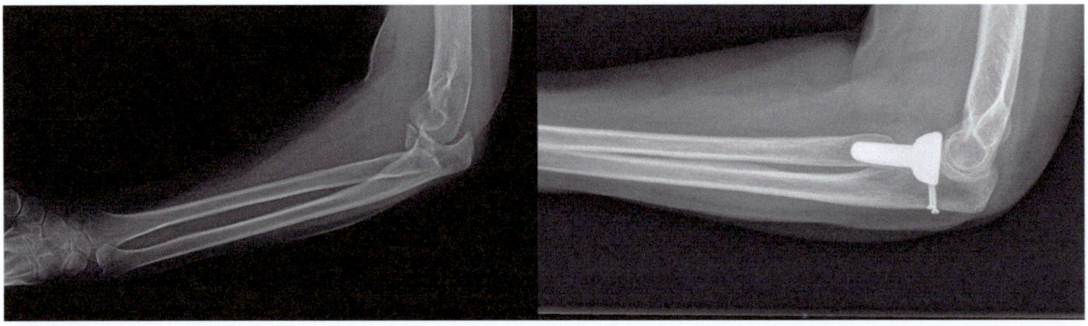

**Fig. 14.6** Radiographs of a 54-year-old patient presenting 10 days after an elbow injury with a subluxed elbow associated with a type II coronoid fracture and a complex radial head fracture. The coronoid was fixed with screws and the radial head was replaced

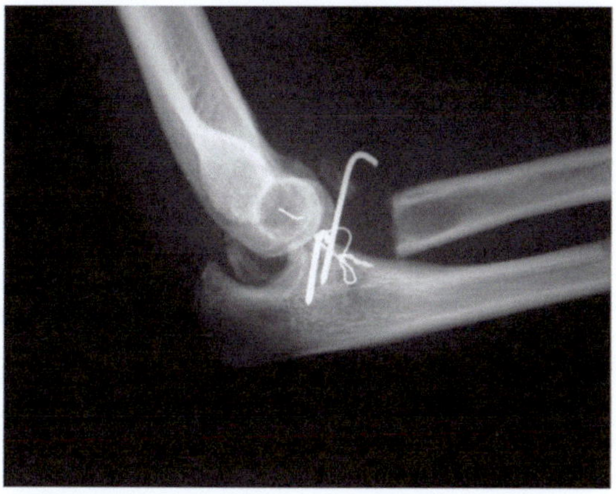

**Fig. 14.7** Persistent elbow instability after an attempt to reconstruct the deficient coronoid with an autograft from the radial head

is not available, as in those patients who may have had radial head replacement in a previous operation or in whom the radial head is severely comminuted, we prefer to use the olecranon tip. We consider allograft to be a reasonable option when neither radial head nor olecranon tip is available, recognizing concerns expressed by Karlstad [24] and van Reit et al. [25].

We generally use a utilitarian posterior incision for skin and lift full thickness flaps. This allows us access to the medial side if it is deemed necessary intraoperatively. It also facilitates posterior-anterior screw placement and/or suture fixation of coronoid fractures and grafting.

## Technique: Radial Head

We enter the radiocapitellar joint laterally through the traumatic rent or through a Kaplan interval, but Kocher is reasonable as well. In cases of delayed presentation and radial head fracture that is in three fragments or more, we resect the radial head with the intention of replacing it "on the way out." This typically gives adequate exposure of the coronoid fracture. Once the decision is made to reconstruct based on the status of the fracture fragment, we assess the radial head fragments. We recognize the findings of Kataoka et al. [23] which suggest using the lateral rim of the radial head to recreate the convexity of the coronoid process and the proximal, concave radial head to reconstruct anteromedial facet fractures; however, we find that in practice we do not have the choice of what part of the radial head we have available to use. Therefore, we seek to recreate the bony buttress and orient articular cartilage toward the trochlea as much as possible.

In a manner similar to Ring et al. [27], we prepare the coronoid fracture bed by creating a flat surface with exposed cancellous bone (callous, hematoma are debrided). We then fashion the radial head graft to have a matching flat surface on which to sit and try to retain at least 50 % of the native radial head width. The proximal radial head (or the lateral radial head) is then oriented toward the trochlea. While holding the graft in place with a dental pick (or large pointed reduction clamp), a k-wire is placed posterior-anterior to hold it provisionally. We then use fluoroscopy and visual inspection to confirm placement. Once it is satisfactory, we place a 2.7 or 3.5 mm screw in a posterior-anterior manner. Suture augmentation through bone tunnels can also be used as needed.

## Technique: Olecranon Tip

If radial head is not available, we prefer to use olecranon tip. An et al. [28] and Bell et al. [29], who found that excision of up to 50 % of the olecranon may not cause gross instability, to determine how much olecranon tip can be harvested. Based on the work of Kataoka et al. [23], only about 14 % is required to replace coronoid fractures of 50 %.

The olecranon tip is approached through a utilitarian posterior approach. The triceps is split from about 2–3 cm proximal to about 1–2 cm distal to the tip. The amount of olecranon harvested depends on the amount require as estimated by visual and radiographic inspection. This is usually about 1.5 cm. A straight osteotome is used to osteotomize the tip, remaining perpendicular to the articular surface. The triceps rent is repaired with a non-absorbable suture.

The bed of the coronoid fracture is prepared as described above. A flat surface is obtained to match the base of the graft. Two holes, approximately 1 cm apart, are made with a 1.0 mm drill in the graft on the back table. Two 1.5 mm holes are drilled approximately 2 cm apart, from the posterior surface of the ulnar through the bed of the coronoid fracture. A heavy, non-absorbable suture is passed through the graft to serve as supplemental fixation and to use as "tow sutures." The graft is oriented such that the articular surface faces the trochlea. The sutures are passed through the holes through the bed of the coronoid fracture to the posterior aspect of the proximal ulna.

While the sutures are pulled tightly, and while holding the graft in place with a dental pick (or large pointed reduction clamp), a provisional K-wire is placed posterior to anterior. Fluoroscopy and gross inspection confirm proper placement, and a 3.5 mm cortical screw is placed in lag fashion. Alternatively, a cannulated screw may be placed over a guide-wire. The suture is then tied over the bony bridge (Fig. 14.8).

After reconstruction of the coronoid with either radial head or olecranon tip, the resected radial head is replaced in a standard manner, the LUCL is repaired and stability is assessed and confirmed with gross inspection and fluoroscopy. If the reduction and fixation are judged to be stable, the patient is placed into a posterior mold splint for 3–5 days to allow for wound healing; the patient is then placed into a hinged elbow brace to begin early, protected ROM. We prefer that exercises be performed while supine to avoid varus and valgus stress on the elbow.

We have a low threshold for placing a hinged external fixator in cases of tenuous fixation or questionable stability. It remains in place for 4–6 weeks, and we encourage early, protected ROM.

## Coronoid Prosthesis

Coronoid prostheses have been described for those injuries in which repair or reconstruction are not achievable. In 2013, Gray [30] demonstrated favorable biomechanics with an anatomic prosthesis compared to the native elbow in a cadaveric model of elbow instability due to coronoid deficiency. More studies are required for in vivo outcomes. Currently there are no coronoid

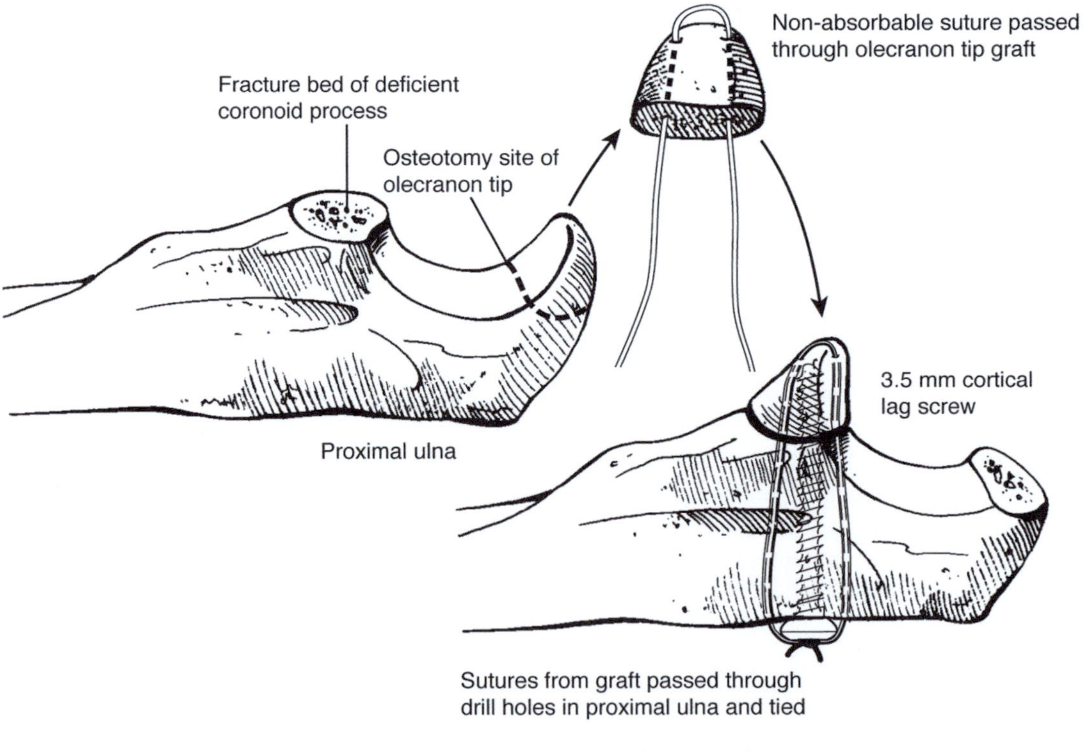


**Fig. 14.8** Coronoid reconstruction utilizing the ipsilateral olecranon tip for a graft source

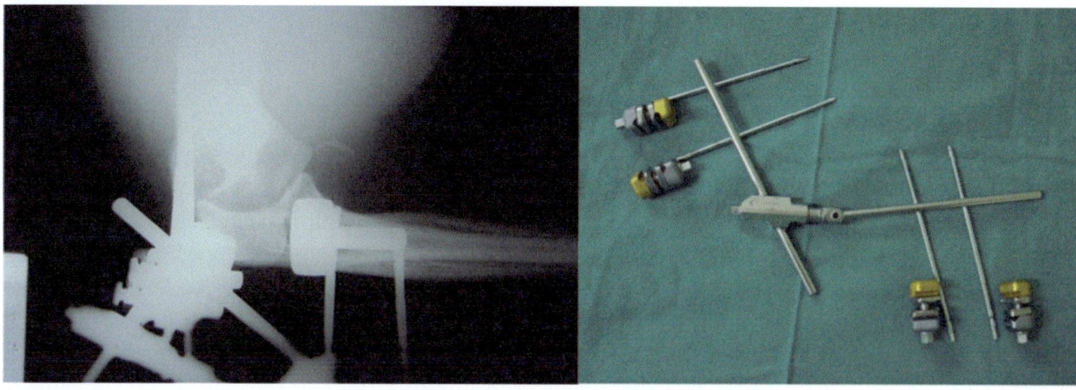

**Fig. 14.9** Patient with persistent elbow instability in Fig. 14.7 treated with radial head replacement, and ligament repair. Intraoperatively the elbow would not be completely stabilized and a static external fixation was placed for 2 weeks. After 2 weeks the external fixator was dynamized to allow motion and kept for 6 weeks

prostheses available for clinical use although reports of custom implants have been made in few case reports.

## External Fixation

Hinged external fixation is useful to maintain a concentric reduction in difficult cases. It allows concentric reduction during active or passive range of movement. It is indicated in cases with poor internal fixation and in cases that may require capsulotomy (Fig. 14.9). The most common complications are pin tract infection and pin failure. We recommend using the hinged external fixation in light distraction and to allow progressive ROM in an effort to balance stiffness and stability with mobility. Static external fixation can also be utilized in cases of tenuous fixation where stability is at risk. Static external fixators allow early healing in a reduced position and are typically removed at 4–6 weeks to then allow therapy to restore range of motion.

## Published Outcomes and Complications

In 1998, McKee et al. [31] reported 16 cases of unstable fracture-dislocations after previous treatment. They performed ligament reconstruction and hinged external fixation with an average 5 weeks elapsed between date of primary injury and reconstruction. The mean Mayo Elbow Performance Score (MEPS) was 84 and average ROM was 105°. They had one patient with residual instability. One patient had and infection, and another had pin failure with infection.

In 2004, Ring et al. [26] reported 13 cases of persistent ulnohumeral instability after a fracture-dislocation of the elbow with adequate articular surfaces and stable alignment of the olecranon. The patients were treated with a hinged external fixator, reconstruction of the coronoid process and radiocapitellar joint and lateral collateral ligament repair. Seven patients had a terrible triad injury pattern and six had a posterior Monteggia injury pattern. The average time to surgery after index injury was 11 weeks. They performed radial head arthroplasty in 11 patients, reconstruction of the coronoid with radial head autograft in six patients and lateral soft tissue repair in 11 patients. All required hinged external fixation. The mean MEPS was 89 and flexion-extension ROM was 99°. Complications included four pin tract infections and three contractures that needed release. Two elbows remained unstable.

Papandrea et al. in 2007 [1] reported 21 cases of coronoid fracture-dislocations that remained unstable after prior treatment. The mean time since previous injury was 11 weeks. They performed nine coronoid reconstructions, ten LUCL repairs and external fixation in 16 cases. The mean MEPS was 71, and the flexion-extension ROM was 96°. Five elbows remained dislocated and three subluxated. The complication rate was 71 %: eight cases of instability, two infections and five contractures.

## Authors' Preferred Treatment

Persistent elbow instability is a challenging problem. Achieving congruence and stability during the index procedure could prevent it. Surgery for persistent elbow instability is a complex procedure requiring wide surgical exposure, comprehensive understanding of elbow pathology and restoration of congruency and stability (Fig. 14.10).

If treatment is unsuccessful, we approach persistent instability as outlined in Fig. 14.11. If the duration of time from the injury to treatment is less than 4 weeks, repair of all bony and ligamentous injuries should be attempted. The coronoid process is repaired using a suture lasso technique, plate or screw fixation. The radial head is either repaired or replaced based upon fracture severity and ability to achieve stable fixation. Finally, the lateral collateral ligament complex is repaired with suture anchors or bone tunnels. If the time from injury is greater than 4 weeks, typically a lateral collateral ligament reconstruction is performed. The coronoid process fracture repair should be attempted but if irreparable then reconstruction with autograft or allograft is performed. The radial head fracture typically needs an arthroplasty at this point in time to maintain

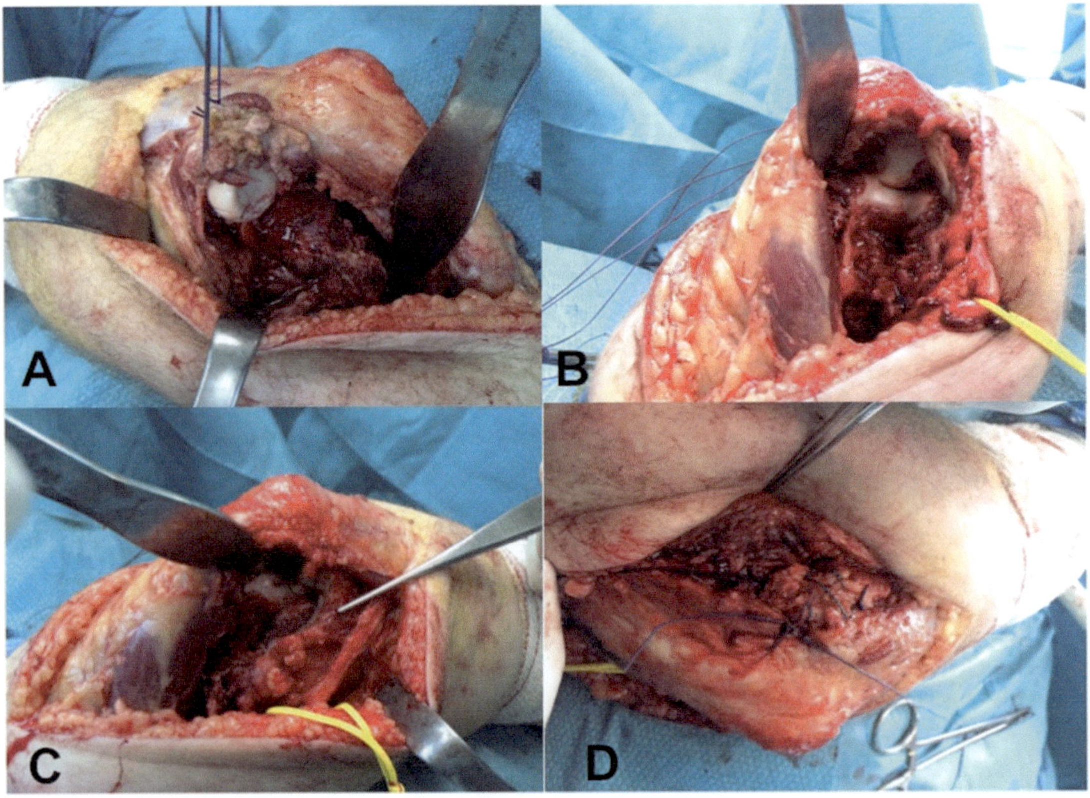


**Fig. 14.10** Intraoperative pictures of a patient with a dislocated elbow treated 8 weeks after the initial injury. (**a**) The lateral compartment is seen dislocated after the lateral collateral ligament is released form the humerus and tagged for further repair. (**b**) Dislocation of the ulnohumeral joint is obvious after triceps reflection. (**c**) The medial collateral ligament is ossified and needs to be released in other to allow reduction. (**d**) After the elbow was reduced and both ligaments repaired, the joint could be stable and no further surgical treatments were necessary

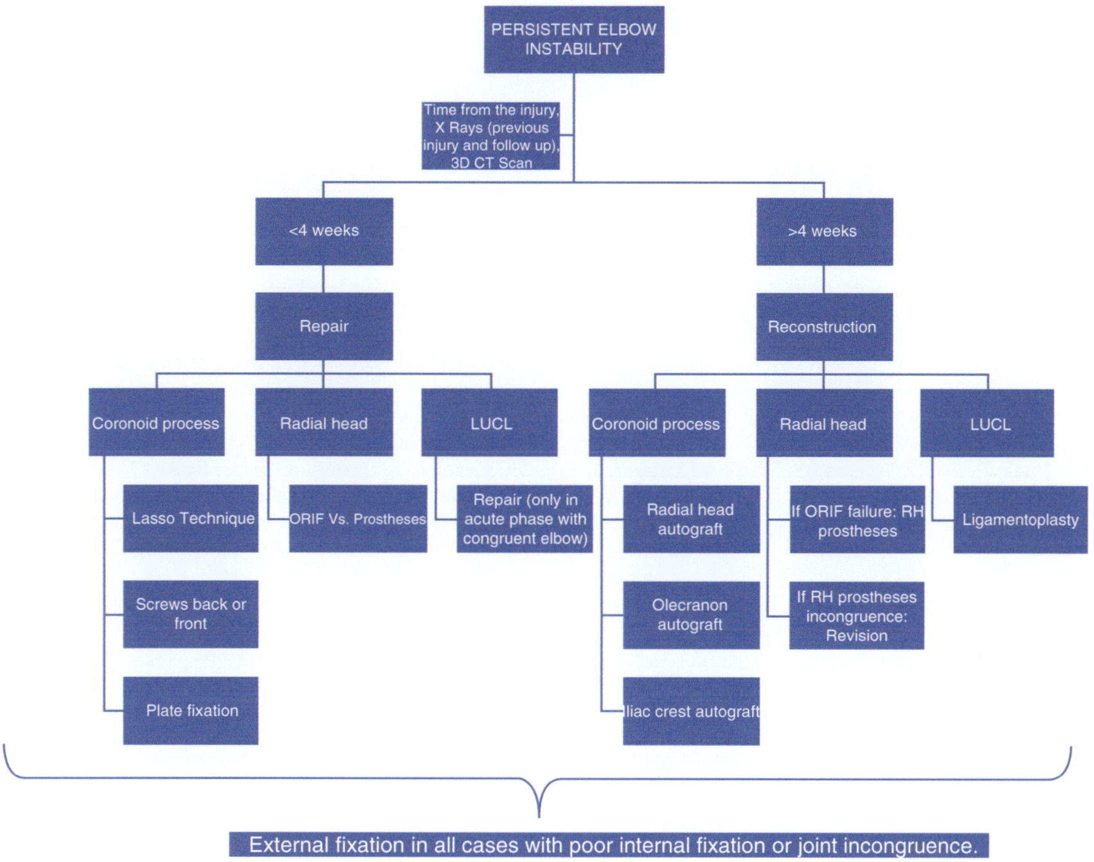


**Fig. 14.11** Treatment algorithm for persistent instability

radiocapitellar joint stability. If a prior ORIF of the radial head has been performed or there is incongruence of a prior radial head arthroplasty, revision radial head arthroplasty achieving a congruent radiocapitellar joint is recommended. Finally, lateral collateral ligament reconstruction is typically required in the setting of a ligament injury older than 4–6 weeks. In both early (<4 weeks) and delayed (>4 weeks) treatment if internal fixation is tenuous or there is persistent subluxation, an external fixator should be placed to restore stability.

## Conclusions

The management of the persistent elbow instability is challenging. The best treatment is an index procedure that addresses the instability and ensures a congruent joint. In cases of persistent instability, a systematic approach is critical. Workup always begins with a detailed history and physical exam, appropriate diagnostic imaging, including X-rays and CT. Finally, treatment should address both bony and ligamentous anatomy to restore stability and a congruent joint to prevent advancement to posttraumatic arthritis.

## References

1. Papandrea RF, Morrey BF, O'Driscoll SW. Reconstruction for persistent instability of the Elbow after coronoid fracture dislocation. J Shoulder Elbow Surg. 2007;16(1):68–77.
2. Morrey, BF; Tanaka, S, and An, KN. Valgus stability of the elbow: a definitions of primary and secondary constrains. Clin Orthop Relat Res. 1991; (265): 187–95.

3. An, KN; Morrey, BF, and Chao, EY. The effect of parcial removal of proximal ulna on elbow constraint. Clin Orthop Relat Res. 1986; (209): 270–9.
4. O'Driscoll SW, Cheng S, Morrey BF, An KN. Biomechanics of coronoid in complex elbow fracture dislocation. J Shoulder Elbow Surg. 1999;8:186.
5. Morrey BF, Askew LJ, An KN, Chao EY. A biomechamical study of normal function elbow motion. J Bone Joint Surg. 1981;63A:872–7.
6. Duckworth AD, Kulijdan A, McKee MD, Ring D. Residual subluxation of the elbow after dislocation or fracture-dislocation: treatment with active exercises and avoidance of varus stress. J Shoulder Elbow Surg. 2008;17:276–80.
7. Mason ML. Some observations on fractures of the head of the radius with a review of one hundred cases. Br J Surg. 1954;5:21–8.
8. Duckworth AD, Watson BS, Will EM, Petrisor BA, Walmsley PJ, Court-Brown CM, McQueen MM. Radial head and neck fractures: functional results and predictors of outcome. J Trauma. 2011;71: 643–8.
9. King GJ, Evans DC, Kellam JF. Open reduction and internal fixation of radial head fractures. J Orthop Trauma. 1991;5:21–8.
10. Morrey BF. Radial head fractures. In: Morrey BF, Sanchez-Sotelo J, editors. The elbow and its disorders. 4th ed. Philadelphia, PA: Saunders; 2010.
11. Regan W, Morrey B. Fractures of the coronoid process of the ulna. J Bone Joint Surg Am. 1989;71: 1348–54.
12. Ablove RH, Moy OJ, Howard C, Peimer CA, S'Doia S. Ulnar coronoid process anatomy: possible implications for elbow instability. Clin Orthop Relat Res 2006;(449):259–61.
13. Cage DJ, Abrams RA, Callahan JJ, Botte MJ. Soft tissue attachments of the ulnar coronoid process. An anatomic study with radiographic correlation. Clin Orthop Relat Res 1995; (320):154–8.
14. Josefsson PO, Gentz CF, Johnell O, Wendeberg B. Dislocations of the elbow and intraarticular fractures. Clin Orthop Relat Res 1989;(246):126–30.
15. Terada N, Yamada H, Seki T, Urabe T, Takayama S. The importance of reducing small fractures of the coronoid process in the treatment of unstable elbow dislocation. J Shoulder Elbow Surg. 2000;9:344–6.
16. Pugh DM, Wild LM, Schemitsch EH, King GJ, McKee MD. Standard surgical protocol to treat elbow dislocations with radial head and coronoid fractures. J Bone Joint Surg Am. 2004;86-A:1122–30.
17. Schneeberger AG. Coronoid process and radial head as posterolateral rotatory stabilizars of the elbow. J Bone Joint Surg Am. 2004;86A:975.
18. Garrigues GE, Wray 3rd WH, Lindenhovius AL, Ring DC, Ruch DS. Fixation of the coronoid process in elbow fracture-dislocations. J Bone Joint Surg Am. 2011;93:1873–81.
19. Esser RD. Reconstruction of the coronoid process with a radial head fragment. Orthopedics. 1997;20:169–71.
20. Moritomo H, Tada K, Yoshida T, Kawatsu N. Reconstruction of the coronoid for chronic dislocation of the elbow. Use of a graft for the olecranon in two cases. J Bone Joint Surg Br. 1998;80:490–2.
21. Kohls-Gatzoulis J, Tsiridis E, Schizas C. Reconstruction of the coronoid process with iliac crest bone graft. J Shoulder Elbow Surg. 2004;13:217–20.
22. Chung CH, Wang SJ, Chang YC, Wu SS. Reconstruction of the coronoid process with iliac crest bone graft in complex fracture-dislocation of elbow. Arch Orthop Trauma Surg. 2007;127(1):33–7.
23. Kataoka T, Moritomo H, Miyake J, Murase T, Sugamoto K. Three-dimensional suitability assessment of three types of osteochondral autograft for ulnar coronoid process reconstruction. J Shoulder Elbow Surg. 2014;23:143–50.
24. Karlstad R, Morrey BF, Cooney WP. Failure of fresh-frozen radial head allografts in the treatment of Essex-Lopresti injury. A report of four cases. J Bone Joint Surg Am. 2005;87(8):1828–33.
25. Van Riet RP, Morrey BF, O'Driscoll SW. Use of osteochondral bone graft in coronoid fractures. J Shoulder Elbow Surg. 2005;14:519–23.
26. Ring D, Hannouche D, Jupiter JB. Surgical treatment of persistent dislocation or subluxation of the ulnohumeral joint after fracture-dislocation of the elbow. J Hand Surg. 2004;29A:470–80.
27. Ring D, Guss D, Jupiter JB. Reconstruction of the coronoid process using a fragment of discarded radial head. J Hand Surg Am. 2012;37(3):570–4.
28. An KN, Morrey BF, Chao EY. The effect of partial removal of proximal ulna on elbow constraint. Clin Orthop Relat Res 1986;(209):270–9.
29. Bell TH, Ferreira LM, McDonald CP, Johnson JA, King GJ. Contribution of the olecranon to elbow stability: an in vitro biomechanical study. J Bone Joint Surg Am. 2010;92(4):949–57.
30. Gray AB, Alolabi B, Ferreira LM, Athwal GS, King GJ, Johnson J. The effect of a coronoid prosthesis on restoring stability to the coronoid-deficient elbow: a biomechanical study. J Hand Surg. 2013;38A: 1753–61.
31. McKee MD, Bowden SH, King GJ, Patterson SD, Jupiter JB, Bamberger HB, Paksima N. Management of recurrent, complex instability of the elbow with a hinged external Fixator. J Bone Joint Surg Br. 1998;80B:1031–6.

# Part IV

# Additional Treatment Strategies for the Unstable Elbow

# External Fixation in the Setting of Elbow Instability

15

Alexander W. Aleem, Matthew L. Ramsey, and Joseph A. Abboud

## Background

The concept of external fixation has been discussed in the medical community for more than 2000 years with Hippocrates using an external "shackle" device for tibia fractures [1]. Today, external fixation devices and techniques have evolved and continue to be an essential part of orthopedic surgeons' armamentarium. External fixation in the setting of elbow instability plays an important role in the management of acute, complex, and chronic instability [2–6].

Hinged external fixation is of specific interest in the elbow, as surgeons have attempted to maintain motion in the joint, which is an obvious limitation of static external fixation [3, 6, 7]. Static fixators are more readily available and significantly easier to apply, but have a limited life span due to pin loosening [4]. An articulating fixator about the elbow is based on normal ulnohumeral kinematics in order to approximate a simple hinged joint. Original descriptions of hinged external devices about the elbow date back to the 1970s, and several improvements have been made to better recreate normal elbow kinematics [8–11]. There are a variety of commercially available hinged external fixators all with the principle of recreating normal elbow kinematics (Fig. 15.1).

The basis of a hinged external fixator about the elbow is to take advantage of the natural kinematics of the elbow joint to convert the joint to a simple hinge joint in a similar manner as total elbow arthroplasty [8, 9]. The elbow does have some rotatory and varus/valgus motion about its center of rotation therefore creating a simple hinge does not completely replicate normal anatomy. Deland et al. performed a cadaveric investigation of five elbows to determine average axis of rotation that served as a best fit for single axis rotation across a full range of elbow motion [9]. They found that this axis is in general centered on the capitellum and trochlea, and the elbow was able to go through a full range of motion in a single plane without disturbing the kinematics of the elbow. This information was used as basis for development of several hinged external fixators.

Stavlas et al. investigated the affects of a hinged external fixator in the ligamentously unstable elbow using a cadaver model [12]. They utilized the Orthofix elbow external fixator (Orthofix, Verona, Italy) on eight human cadaveric elbows. Range of motion and stability of the elbow was tested in three settings: (1) intact

A.W. Aleem, MD
Department of Orthopedic Surgery, The Rothman Institute, Thomas Jefferson University, 1500 Locust St, Apt 2903, Philadelphia, PA 19102, USA
e-mail: alexanderaleem@gmail.com

M.L. Ramsey, MD • J.A. Abboud, MD (✉)
Department of Orthopedic Surgery, The Rothman Institute, Thomas Jefferson University, 925 Chestnut St, 5th Floor, Philadelphia, PA 19107, USA
e-mail: mlramsey2@verizon.net; abboudj@gmail.com

© Springer International Publishing Switzerland 2017
R.Z. Tashjian (ed.), *The Unstable Elbow*, DOI 10.1007/978-3-319-46019-2_15

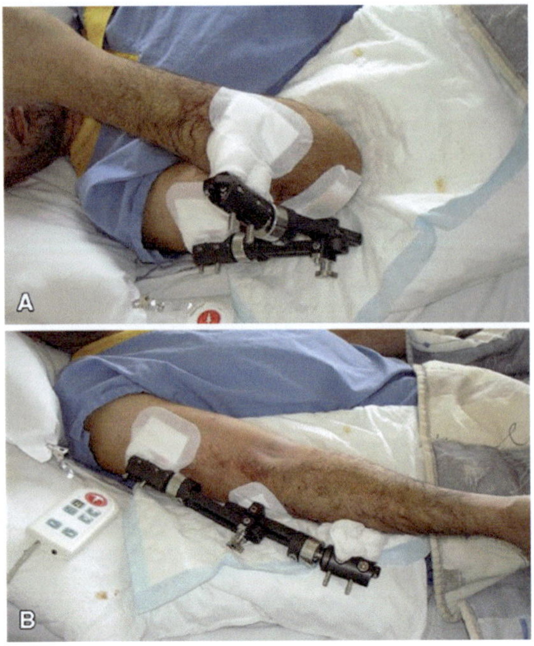


**Fig. 15.1** Clinical picture of commonly used hinged elbow external fixator. (**a**) Flexion, (**b**) Extension (Reprinted with permission from Iordens GI, et al. Clin Orthop Relat Res. 2015;473(4):1451–61)

elbow without the fixator, (2) application of the fixator on the lateral side of the elbow with the lateral collateral ligament (LCL) released, and (3) application of the fixator with the LCL and medial collateral ligament (MCL) released. They found that extension in the ligamentously unstable (LCL and MCL released) elbow was significantly lower at 19.1° compared to 10.5° in the intact elbow. Flexion was not found to be significantly different. They also noted that ligamentously unstable elbows with external fixators were placed in a more varus position through their range of motion and had significant decreases in rotatory and valgus displacement compared to intact joints. The authors concluded that placement of the hinged fixator altered normal elbow kinematics to mimic a hinged joint and decreased motion, notably extension. However, since the extension was still considered at a functional range with fixator placement, they felt that hinged external fixation was still a viable option in unstable elbows to help preserve motion.

With the biomechanics defined that a hinged fixator is a reasonable option to maintain approximate elbow kinematics, numerous authors have reported on the application of hinged fixators in the setting of the unstable elbow. Overall, most studies report good outcomes in the setting of elbow instability using hinged external fixation in cases of acute and chronic elbow instability. Despite limited clinical data on the outcomes of static fixators, static external fixation is also a very reasonable, safe, and in many cases preferred, option in cases of persistent elbow instability. However, complications, including pin loosening and infection, injury to neurovascular structures, and loss of reduction are common. Nevertheless, the use of external fixation is a useful adjunct in patients with complex elbow instability.

## Evaluation

### Acute Injuries

In the acute setting, a thorough history and physical examination must be done. Mechanism of injury information should be obtained, as it can help predict the spectrum of injuries that may have occurred. The neurovascular structures need to be completely and thoroughly evaluated. Additionally, the shoulder and distal forearm should be examined as these structures may be injured concomitantly.

AP and lateral radiographs should be obtained to evaluate the spectrum of injury. Gentle closed reduction of the fracture-dislocation should be attempted, and use of sedation with muscle relaxation can minimize patient discomfort. Generally, in-line traction followed by elbow flexion will reduce the elbow. A post-reduction neurovascular exam should be performed. Post-reduction radiographs should also be scrutinized for widening or nonconcentric reduction, which may represent an entrapped osteochondral fragment. CT scans are extremely valuable for both injury evaluation and surgical planning.

### Chronic Instability

Patients with a history of chronic elbow instability should have a similar initial evaluation of patients with acute instability. A thorough history should be performed focusing on possible missed or unrecognized injury. Additionally, any history of prior procedures attempted at stabilizing the elbow joint should be sought. Physical exam should focus on range of motion of the elbow joint and provocative maneuvers to elucidate any instability. A thorough neurovascular exam should also be performed. AP and lateral radiographs should also be obtained to evaluate if the elbow has a concentric reduction and to evaluate the presence of any arthritis. CT scans are routinely obtained as there are often chronic bony injuries resulting in persistent instability. MRI may also be useful if there is concern for an associated tendon injury or there is a question regarding the status of the ligamentous stabilizers. More information is better in the management of these difficult injuries since the chance for a successful result is completely dependent on the full understanding of the injury spectrum prior to treatment.

## Treatment Algorithm

### Acute Instability

In general, the use of an external fixator, either static or hinged, remains a rare, but useful option for the treatment of acute elbow instability. Surgeons should first determine if they could achieve stability through nonoperative care. If surgical intervention is warranted, surgeons should make all attempts to address all components of bony and soft tissue instability. This includes fixation or replacement of the radial head, fixation of the coronoid, and repair of the lateral and, if needed, medial ligaments. If the elbow remains unstable following surgical fixation, techniques of which are addressed in other chapters, then the surgeon should proceed with placement of an external fixator [2–4]. Persistent instability is most commonly encountered in the acute setting when fracture fixation of the coronoid or proximal ulna is tenuous or coronoid process fragments are irreparable. External fixation may be utilized to stabilize the elbow in the setting where the coronoid is not repaired due to severe comminution or to protect the elbow in cases where the coronoid process is grafted.

For patients with acute gross elbow instability who have sustained poly-trauma or are in a medical condition that prohibits them from undergoing an extensive elbow repair, it is reasonable to proceed with using an external fixator for temporary or definitive stabilization of the elbow [3, 4].

### Chronic Instability

Similarly, for patients with chronic instability, surgeons must first determine if the elbow is salvageable for reconstruction or if they should proceed with arthroplasty. If reconstruction is chosen, surgeons should again attempt to reconstruct all bony and ligamentous components that are responsible for instability. Similarly, if the elbow is not stable through full range of motion after surgical reconstruction, then an external fixator should be placed for added stability. In the chronic setting, fixators are typically adjuncts to when bony stabilizers are compromised, as in the acute setting, and/or the ligamentous stabilizers are compromised and require reconstruction. External fixators can also be used for added stability following total elbow arthroplasty in the setting of chronic instability [3].

## Surgical Management

### Static External Fixator

Placement of a uniplanar static external fixator in the setting of surgical management for either acute or chronic instability is relatively straightforward, but certain pitfalls may still occur. In general, most surgeons recommend placement of two humeral and two ulnar pins.

Lateral humeral pins are most commonly used as they are easier to place based on patient positioning, and are generally placed first. Half pins should be placed without impaling any major muscle-tendon units or jeopardizing neurovascular structures, and should have bicortical purchase. The proximal lateral pin should be placed very carefully, as it will usually be in the vicinity of the radial nerve. Some surgeons recommend making a small incision laterally to ensure that the radial nerve is not injured for humeral pins [13]. In terms of radial nerve location, Kamineni et al. have evaluated the location of the radial nerve in reference to the lateral epicondyle as it exits the posterior compartment of the arm in relation to the transepicondylar axis distance [14]. The average transepicondylar axis distance was 62 mm and the average distance from the lateral epicondyle to the radial nerve was 102 mm. The transepicondylar distance was highly correlated to the distance from the lateral epicondyle to the radial nerve (Pearson correlation coefficient, $r=0.95$). The authors recommended that the absolute safe zone for pin entry into the lateral distal humerus is the area lying within the caudad 70% of a line, equivalent in length to the patients own transepicondylar axis distance, when projected proximally from the lateral epicondyle. If medial pins are placed, an open incision should be made to protect the ulnar nerve [3]. The safest location for pins is likely directly posterior through the triceps muscle (Figure of the static fixator with posterior pins). Carlan et al. evaluated the location of the radial nerve as it crosses the posterior humeral shaft and determined that the nerve as it crosses is within 0.1 mm of the most distal aspect of the deltoid tuberosity [15]. Consequently, the distal aspect of the deltoid tuberosity can be used as a landmark for the location of the radial nerve as it crosses the posterior aspect of the humeral shaft and direct posterior pins should be placed distal to this landmark.

Ulnar pins can be placed in either a dorsal-to-volar or lateral-to-medial direction based on surgeon preference, and should be placed with the elbow concentrically reduced. Again, care should be made to not violate any important neurovascular structures. Half-pins should be bicortical. In general, 4 mm pins are placed in the ulna with the goal of 4–5 cm of spread between the pins. On the humeral side, care must be taken to avoid the radial nerve, and 5 mm pins are generally placed above the radial nerve in the anterolateral aspect of the humerus with the goal of attaining 4–5 cm of spread. Pins can also be placed posteriorly on the humerus (Fig. 15.2). The frame should be applied to the half-pins with the elbow concentrically reduced in its most stable position (generally 90° of flexion and pronation). With a highly unstable reduction, the joint may be temporarily pinned with a stout Kirschner wire [2, 3, 16]. Ring et al. demonstrated equivalent outcomes following cross pinning of a joint compared to external fixation with less device related complications [16]. Caution still needs to be exercised with cross pinning of the joint as the articular cartilage can be injured, the cross pins can break and make removal very difficult and infection can be devastating therefore static external fixation is preferred over cross pinning.

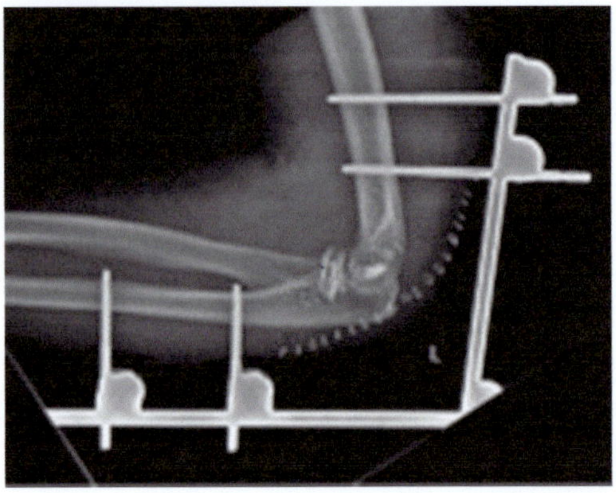

**Fig. 15.2** Static elbow external fixator with posterior humeral pins (courtesy of George Athwal, MD)

## Hinged External Fixator

Placement of a hinged external fixator may depend on the company specifications of fixator used, but certain general principles still apply. All hinged external fixators utilize a central axis pin to center the hinge. This pin must be collinear with the center of rotation of the elbow joint in order to minimize excess forces about the fixator and prevent pin loosening. The center of rotation of the elbow lies in the center of the capitellar circumference on the lateral condyle and just distal and anterior to the medial epicondyle [3, 4, 8, 9]. This should be verified under direct fluoroscopic visualization on the lateral view. On the AP view, the pin should be traversing parallel to the elbow joint line [3, 8, 9]. Perfect placement of the axis pin is very technically challenging, and improper placement can cause more instability. Madey et al. reported misalignment of 5° caused a 3.7-fold increase in motion energy, and a 10° mismatch yielded a 7.1-fold increase in energy [10]. Based on the system used, the axis pin may require unicortical or bicortical fixation.

Once the axis pin has been placed and perfect placement confirmed, placement of humeral and ulnar half-pins follow similar fashion as static fixators. Lateral humeral pins are most common type with each system, and ulnar pins depend on the type of fixator used. Again, it is important to have the elbow concentrically reduced once the frame is applied, and range of motion should be checked under fluoroscopic guidance to ensure that the elbow remains stable throughout [3, 6, 9].

The authors' prefer to address all bony and ligamentous repairs/reconstructions prior to placing any pins needed for the external fixator. Patients are usually supine with the arm on a hand table. Placing the axis pin remains the most technically challenging step in placement of a hinged external fixator. Intra-operative fluoroscopy is needed to ensure proper placement of the pin. In general, we aim to place pins lateral to medial, with the pin centered on the axis of rotation on the lateral epicondyle. Fluoroscopy is then used to confirm placement and ensure that the pin is parallel to the articular surface. We currently have no specific preference on commercial manufacturer of the frame.

## Published Outcomes/Complications

Most studies reporting outcomes of external fixator placement in the setting of elbow instability represent small, retrospective case series for a variety of injuries that discuss both acute and chronic elbow instability. For acute injuries, the focus is generally on complex elbow instability as this spectrum of injuries is likely to have a higher incidence of recurrent instability. Although static external fixators are discussed in several treatment algorithms for elbow instability, there is no published study that investigates outcomes in this setting. Volkov's original report of a hinged external fixator about the elbow described its use in the setting of mobilizing joint contractures and stabilization of complex periarticular fractures [11]. Since then, small case series have expanded these applications to include management of acute and chronic instability. Additionally, several of the studies published utilize devices not available in the USA.

### Simple Acute Instability

Acute simple elbow dislocations are generally treated with closed means and early return to motion [17]. There is however a small subset of patients that have significantly persistent instability, especially posterolateral rotatory instability [18, 19]. Hopf et al. investigated the outcomes of using a hinged external fixator to help stabilize acute simple dislocations. In this series, a specific subset of 26 patients with simple dislocations, who were felt to be at high risk for recurrent instability due to subluxation seen on fluoroscopic exam or provocative physical exam maneuvers following initial closed reduction were included for evaluation. At a mean of 2.5 days from injury, a hinged external fixator was placed without any ligament repair for a total of 6 weeks. The authors found excellent outcomes with an average Mayo Elbow Performance Score (MEPS) of 93.5. They found minimal loss of range of motion compared to the patients' normal contralateral elbow. Overall, 18 joints were found to be clinically stable, and eight had mild evidence of clinical instability. Radiographically, patients were found to have significantly increased varus and valgus instability on dynamic ultrasound examination. Pin site infection occurred in four patients (15.4%), and one patient required surgical debridement of a pin site infection. One patient did sustain an ulnar fracture through a pin site that did not require surgical intervention. Overall, the authors concluded that external fixator placement in unstable simple elbow dislocations provides patients with excellent results. This study is limited, in that they did not have a control group of patients treated by closed means, and not all of these patients were simple dislocations as they found evidence of 3 type I coronoid fractures in their cohort.

## Complex Elbow Instability

The majority of case series investigating the use of hinged external fixators about the elbow focuses on their use in the setting of elbow fracture-dislocations, most commonly terrible triad injuries. The results are all generally good to excellent in regard to clinical outcomes and stability of the joint. Common complications reported include pin site infection and loosening, fracture through pin sites, recurrent instability, and neurovascular injury. Due to the low number of patients, the studies present a fairly mixed cohort of patients in terms of the spectrum of injuries treated.

Early reports of the use of hinged external fixators focused on fixators in the setting of recurrent complex instability following prior surgical management. McKee et al. investigated 16 patients who had all failed prior open repair of their complex instability injuries [20]. Patients averaged 2.1 unsuccessful surgeries before placement of a fixator occurred at an average of 4.8 weeks after injury. Initial surgeries attempted to repair or reconstruct all bony and ligamentous injuries. Fourteen patients had fixators as a subsequent procedure following initial surgical fixation. Two patients had frames placed at the time of their initial surgical repair. They found mixed results with an average flexion–extension range of 105° (65–140). At average 23-month follow-up, MEPS scores ranged from 49 to 96, with 12 patients obtaining good or excellent results. This small cohort had six complications, but only one episode of recurrent instability.

Ring et al. performed a similar analysis in patients with persistent subluxation or dislocation with elbow fracture-dislocations [21]. In their series, 13 patients (seven terrible triad, six posterior Monteggia fracture-dislocations) were treated after 1 month or longer for persistent subluxation or dislocation following initial management. All the posterior Monteggia fracture-dislocation patients had initial surgical management, but only two of the patients with a terrible triad injury were treated with surgical repair initially. Patients were carefully selected to ensure that they did not have radiographic signs of articular wear prior to undergoing surgical management for persistent instability. Fixator placement occurred in the setting of open reconstruction of the elbow with concomitant fixation or reconstruction of the coronoid, radial head, and lateral collateral ligament complex at an average of 2 months post-injury. The results from Ring's series are similar to McKee's with an average arc of motion of 99°, with three patients requiring subsequent elbow contracture release. The majority of MEPS scores were good to excellent, averaging 84, and no patients had recurrent instability. Radiographic posttraumatic arthrosis was present in six patients at final follow-up, with all five of the patients who sustained a prior posterior Monteggia fracture dislocation showing signs of arthrosis. Complications were similar to McKee's report with four patients sustaining pin site infections.

Overall, based on Ring and McKee's studies, surgeons can expect good results with placement of a hinged fixator for failed initial surgical treatment of acute complex instability. The limitations of both these studies include small numbers of patients, and a wide range of injuries treated. The diversity of injuries included in these studies leads to a lack of uniform management making it hard to generalize the results. Complications are common, and are mostly related to pin site infection or breakage. Serious complications including fracture and neurovascular injury are rare, but still occur in ~10 % of patients in these reports.

In an attempt to make a standardized treatment protocol on a more homogenous group of patients, Sorensen et al. published their series of patients treated with a hinged elbow fixator for persistent elbow dislocation [22]. In this series, patients presented both in an acute and delayed manner (>6 weeks after injury) following fracture-dislocation of the elbow including radial head and coronoid fractures. They excluded patients with Monteggia or Essex-Lopresti injuries, leaving a total of 17 elbows available for review. All patients underwent a standardized surgical treatment protocol that consisted of utilizing a posterior approach. Coronoid fractures were addressed first, and able to be repaired in 13 elbows. The coronoid was reconstructed with part of the radial head in one elbow and left untreated in two. The radial head was treated next with repair, retention, or excision. Overall, eight radial heads were resected, three underwent internal fixation, and six were left in the elbow without any fixation. No radial head replacements were performed. The LCL complex was then repaired back to its humeral origin or reconstructed, and placement of hinged external fixator was the final step. Patient results were analyzed based on if treatment occurred within 6 weeks of injury or after 6 weeks of injury. The authors found significant improvements in MEPS scores at final follow-up, with the early intervention group averaging a score of 80.9 and the delayed intervention group averaging a score of 61.6. Nine of 11 patients in the early treatment group had good or excellent results, compared to only 1 of 6 in the delayed group. Range of motion was improved in the early group with an average arc of 100° compared to 84° in the delayed group, but this difference was not statistically significant. They reported no recurrent instability in either group. Overall, 7 of 17 elbows had complications, with four pin site infections, two nerve injuries, one fracture through a pin site, and one report of postoperative complex regional pain syndrome. The authors of this study concluded that early management of persistent instability following fracture-dislocation of the elbow would lead to good or excellent results with the use of a hinged external fixator. The findings from this study may potentially be biased by the fact that very few terrible triad injuries need a fixator after fixation of the bony and ligamentous injuries, and the acute group could have achieved similar results without a fixator. Additionally, the treatment protocols in the study did not adequately address the radial head, as the majority were either excised or left untreated, which may have lead to the delayed group having such poor outcomes.

Building on the theory that patients will obtain good results more reliably if instability is treated in the acute setting, Iordens et al. published a multicenter study evaluating outcomes in acute elbow instability [13]. Patients were initially treated by either open or closed means. Simple dislocations were initially treated with closed reduction, and complex dislocations were treated with open reduction of the bony injuries. External fixators were placed on patients with persistent instability following initial treatment. Persistent instability was defined as recurrent dislocation following closed reduction for simple dislocations. For complex dislocations, if the joint remained unstable during intra-operative examination following repair of the bony injuries, a fixator was then placed in lieu of repairing the ligaments. Overall, they reported 1-year results on 27 patients treated at 11 centers. Fixators were placed at a median of 6 days following injury. The authors reported significant improvements at 1 year follow-up with median MEPS of 100 (range 85–100). The median flexion–extension arc was also excellent at 118° (105°–138°). They did report that patients had a median flexion–extension deficit of 30° compared to their normal contralateral side. Ten patients (37 %) had complications, including pin site infections, fracture through a pin site, and fixator misalignment that required another surgery. Only 1 patient had recurrent elbow instability. It is difficult to draw conclusions from this study, as there was no repair of the ligamentous structures prior to applying the external fixator, which is not the preferred algorithm of treatment.

Overall, the published literature for hinged external fixators in the setting of complex instability shows favorable results. Patient reported outcomes are, for the most part, good to excellent. Patients show a functional range of motion, but all studies consistently report a deficit of motion compared to the normal, contralateral side. The evidence shows that early stabilization will portend more favorable outcomes. Complications related to the fixator are common occurring in 10–40 % of patients.

## Chronic Instability

In general, the published literature on chronic instability and external fixators focuses on the chronically unreduced elbow [3]. These injuries are usually the result of a neglected or irreducible elbow dislocation [3, 23, 24]. Patients typically present with significant clinical deformity, associated fractures, heterotopic ossification, neurologic deficits and severe soft tissue contracture. Surgical management is extremely challenging in these cases.

A variety of small case series have been published describing different treatment methods to treat the chronically dislocated elbow. All described techniques include both lateral and medial ligament reconstruction. Some authors described temporary transfixion of the ulnohumeral joint for added stability, with use of a large caliber Kirschner wires or Steinman pins placed retrograde through the joint [24, 25]. A hinged external fixator device is an attractive option because it can maintain concentric ulnohumeral reduction while simultaneously allowing for immediate motion following surgical reduction [3]. Similarly, a temporary static external fixator for a short period of time can provide enough initial stabilization to allow the joint to remain concentrically reduced after removal.

Jupiter and Ring published their results with utilizing a hinged elbow fixator for a chronically dislocated elbow without associated fractures [26]. In this series of five patients treated at an average of 11 weeks following dislocation, patients were treated with an open medial and lateral release. The joint was then reduced and a hinged fixator was applied. At average 38-month follow-up, all patients maintained a stable, concentric reduction. MEPS scores averaged 89, and the average arc of motion was 123° with full supination and pronation. Three of five patients had complications with two wound complications and one temporary nerve injury.

## New Directions

As discussed previously, two major concerns with using a hinged external fixator about the elbow are the technical challenges to center the fixator directly on the axis of rotation and the high rate of fixator associated complications. The rate of complications is quite concerning. Ring et al. found that intra-articular cross pinning of the elbow joint had less total complications compared to hinged external fixator with equivalent clinical outcomes [16]. Investigators are currently trying to address both of these issues.

Given that most of the complications with external fixators are a direct result of the external pins, Orbay et al. described a new technique using a bent Steinmann pin (Fig. 15.3) as an internal fixator to help stabilize the elbow [27]. In their article, the authors describe placing a bent, stout Steinman pin directly through the axis of rotation of the humerus and then attaching it with screws to the proximal ulna. Patients were allowed unrestricted elbow motion after their surgical wound healed. The first ten patients who underwent this procedure had great results with mean arc of motion of 115°. No patients had recurrent instability. Complications did occur in 4 of 10 patients that required additional procedures including drainage of a hematoma, postoperative infection, removal of the implant, and heterotopic ossification removal. Removal of the implant is not required. Although this technique seems challenging and further investigation is warranted, it can be another useful tool for treating difficult cases of elbow instability.

Placement of the axis pin in most hinged external fixators is the most time consuming and technically challenging part of the procedure. It can also interfere with surgical repair of ligamentous structures, as it needs to be placed in the exact center of rotation of the ulnohumeral joint. Bigazzi et al. recently pioneered a new fixator that uses a specially designed free hinge that auto-centers (Fig. 15.4) on the axis of rotation [28]. In their report of seven patients treated with hinged external fixation for a variety of indications, they found that all patients had correct alignment with no evidence of instability, loss of

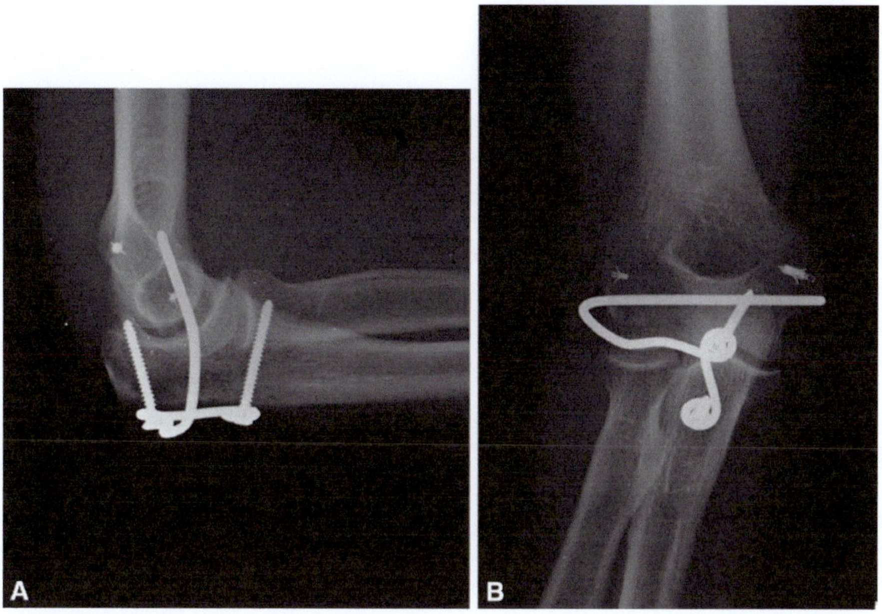


**Fig. 15.3** (**a**, **b**) Bent Steinmann pin for stabilization of elbow joint (reprinted with permission from Orbay JL, Mijares MR. Clin Orthop Relat Res. 2014;472(7):2049–60)

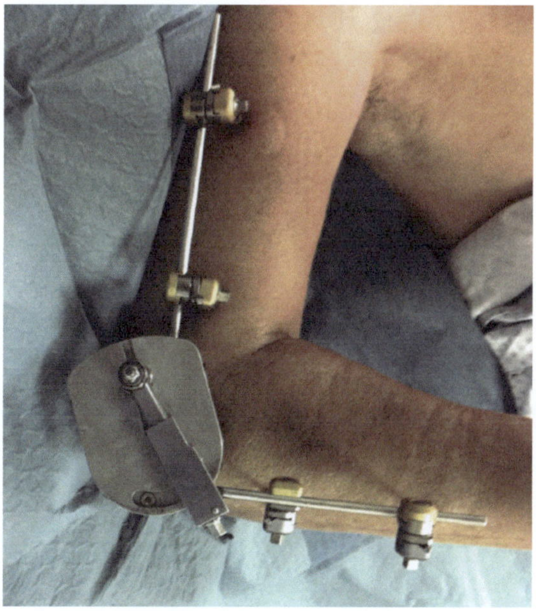

**Fig. 15.4** Autocentering hinged external fixator (From Journal of Shoulder and Elbow Surgery, Vol. 24, Bigazzi P, et al., A new autocentering hinged external fixator of the elbow: a device that stabilizes the elbow axis without use of the articular pin, pp. 1197–205, Copyright 2015, with permission from Elsevier)

fixation, or pin loosening. Further investigation is warranted in this specific technology, but it may allow much more facile application of a hinged external fixator.

## Therapy Protocols

Postoperatively following application of a hinged external fixator in the setting of elbow instability, most authors recommend a brief period of immobilization at 90° for 1 day to 2 weeks [3, 4, 6, 13, 21, 26, 28–31]. After this, most allow for unrestricted active elbow motion in the fixator. Average length of time in the fixator varied between studies, but most averaged between 4 and 6 weeks before removal [3, 4, 6, 13, 21, 26, 28–31]. Additionally, almost all authors recommend the use of indomethacin for 2–6 weeks for heterotopic ossification prophylaxis [6, 7, 13, 21, 22, 26, 30]. After external fixator removal, patients should continue with active and passive range of motion protocols as well as strengthening of the dynamic stabilizers about the elbow.

In our group, the external fixator is also typically removed at approximately 4 weeks and we begin patients in physical therapy to begin active assisted and passive range of motion. Regaining pronation and supination is the main priority, as there is no good surgical option for persistent rotatory stiffness. We generally do not perform any joint manipulation to try to initiate motion. If stiffness in flexion or extensions is still an issue 1 year following initial surgical repair, open surgical release is offered.

## Preferred Treatments/Cases

### Acute Fracture-Dislocation

The authors' of this chapter preferred technique for management of fracture-dislocations of the elbow is to attempt early repair and fixation of all bony and ligamentous injuries. For terrible triads, we agree with previously published protocols to treat the injuries "inside-out" by first addressing the coronoid, then the radial head with fixation or replacement, and finally repair ligamentous structures. External fixators are becoming less frequently used in the setting of acute fracture-dislocation as orthopedic surgeons' understanding of anatomic stability continues to improve [32].

Once all bony and ligamentous stabilizers of the elbow are repaired, the elbow should be taken through a range of motion in supination. Joint stability can be assessed based on clinical findings of gross instability, but fluoroscopy should be used to evaluate for persistent subluxation. If the joint is still not stable in a functional arc of motion, then an external fixator should be placed. It is surgeon preference whether a static or hinged external fixator should be used. Static fixators are more readily available in most hospital settings, and are technically less demanding to place. Unfortunately, due to worries with stiffness, static fixators will likely need to be removed after only 2–3 weeks or possibly require a follow-up lysis of adhesions in the future. Static fixators are somewhat more prone to pin loosening and breakage due to the dynamic forces about the elbow. Hinged fixators may provide patients with quicker motion, but are technically more difficult to place and improper placement can lead to recurrent instability and joint arthrosis. Surgeons should weigh all risks and benefits before deciding which fixator is appropriate. The technical difficulty in placing the axis pin of a dynamic fixator perfectly in line with the center of rotation of the elbow presents a large challenge. Dynamic fixators can act to distract the elbow joint and thus be counterproductive to treatment if the pin is not placed properly. Due to these concerns, the authors of this chapter prefer to use static external fixators in these cases.

### Chronic Unreduced Elbow Dislocation

The external fixator still plays an important role in the setting of a chronically dislocated elbow. Surgical management of these injuries is incredibly difficult, as it requires reconstruction of the deficient elbow stabilizers, while concurrently needing large capsular releases to prevent postoperative stiffness. In these cases, we also recommend the use of an external fixator if the elbow continues to be unstable following all planned surgical fixation and releases. Again, it is up to the surgeon to weigh the risks and benefits of static versus hinged fixation. Similar to the acute setting, given the concerns and technical difficulties of placing a hinged fixator, the authors' prefer to place a static external fixator.

## Case Example

A 52-year-old morbidly obese right-hand dominant woman presented for evaluation of a left elbow injury 1 month after a same level fall. She was initially evaluated in an emergency room, where radiographs demonstrated a fracture-dislocation of the elbow. Closed reduction was attempted and she was placed in a splint. She presented 1 month following injury with persistent dislocation of the elbow (Fig. 15.5a). She underwent surgery 6 weeks following her injury with a combined medial and lateral approach. The radial

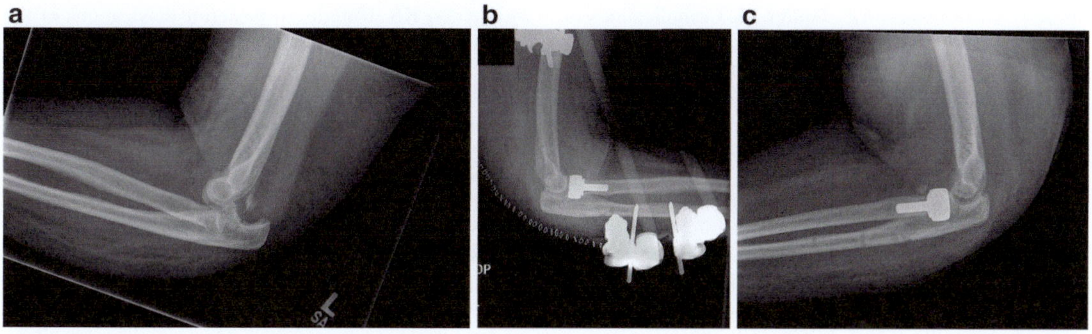

**Fig. 15.5** Case demonstrating use of external fixator. (**a**) Injury film at time of presentation, (**b**) immediate postoperative radiograph demonstrating use of static external fixator, (**c**) postoperative radiograph after removal of fixator

head was replaced, and both the medial and lateral collateral ligament complexes were reconstructed with allograft. Following this reconstruction, the joint was found to grossly stable, but did show subluxation under fluorosocpic exam. Therefore, a static external fixator was placed and her elbow was locked in 90° of flexion with neutral forearm rotation (Fig. 15.5b).

The fixator was left for a total of 4 weeks post-operative, and removed in the clinic. After removal of the fixator, she was found to have a 40° arc of motion in flexion/extension and a 70° arc of motion in pronation/supination. She began physical therapy directed at regaining range of motion. The patient did develop delayed onset ulnar neuritis, which lead to some limitations in fine motor skills. This was not treated with any surgical interventions. At 6 months following surgery, she was found to have a stable elbow joint, with full pronation and supination, and 105° arc of flexion/extension (Fig. 15.5c). Overall, she reported minimal pain in the elbow and was satisfied with her result.

## References


1. Bible JE, Mir HR. External fixation: principles and applications. J Am Acad Orthop Surg. 2015;23(11):683–90.
2. Chen NC, Ring D. Terrible triad injuries of the elbow. J Hand Surg Am. 2015;40:2297.
3. Tan V, Daluiski A, Capo J, Hotchkiss R. Hinged elbow external fixators: indications and uses. J Am Acad Orthop Surg. 2005;13(8):503–14.
4. Tashjian RZ, Katarincic JA. Complex elbow instability. J Am Acad Orthop Surg. 2006;14(5):278–86.
5. Wyrick JD, Dailey SK, Gunzenhaeuser JM, Casstevens EC. Management of complex elbow dislocations: a mechanistic approach. J Am Acad Orthop Surg. 2015;23(5):297–306.
6. Chen NC, Julka A. Hinged external fixation of the elbow. Hand Clin. 2010;26(3):423–33. vii.
7. Stavlas P, Gliatis J, Polyzois V, Polyzois D. Unilateral hinged external fixator of the elbow in complex elbow injuries. Injury. 2004;35(11):1158–66.
8. London JT. Kinematics of the elbow. J Bone Joint Surg Am. 1981;63(4):529–35.
9. Deland JT, Garg A, Walker PS. Biomechanical basis for elbow hinge-distractor design. Clin Orthop Relat Res. 1987; (215):303-12.
10. Madey SM, Bottlang M, Steyers CM, Marsh JL, Brown TD. Hinged external fixation of the elbow: optimal axis alignment to minimize motion resistance. J Orthop Trauma. 2000;14(1):41–7.
11. Volkov MV, Oganesian OV. Restoration of function in the knee and elbow with a hinge-distractor apparatus. J Bone Joint Surg Am. 1975;57(5):591–600.
12. Stavlas P, Jensen SL, Sojbjerg JO. Kinematics of the ligamentous unstable elbow joint after application of a hinged external fixation device: a cadaveric study. J Shoulder Elbow Surg. 2007;16(4):491–6.
13. Iordens GI, Den Hartog D, Van Lieshout EM, Tuinebreijer WE, De Haan J, Patka P, et al. Good functional recovery of complex elbow dislocations treated with hinged external fixation: a multicenter prospective study. Clin Orthop Relat Res. 2015;473(4):1451–61.
14. Kamineni S, Ankem H, Patten DK. Anatomic relationship of the radial nerve to the elbow joint: clinical implications of safe pin placement. Clin Anat. 2009;22(6):684–8.
15. Carlan D, Pratt J, Patterson JM, Weiland AJ, Boyer MI, Gelberman RH. The radial nerve in the brachium: an anatomic study in human cadavers. J Hand Surg Am. 2007;32(8):1177–82.

16. Ring D, Bruinsma WE, Jupiter JB. Complications of hinged external fixation compared with cross-pinning of the elbow for acute and subacute instability. Clin Orthop Relat Res. 2014;472(7):2044–8.
17. Cohen MS, Hastings 2nd H. Acute elbow dislocation: evaluation and management. J Am Acad Orthop Surg. 1998;6(1):15–23.
18. Charalambous CP, Stanley JK. Posterolateral rotatory instability of the elbow. J Bone Joint Surg Br. 2008;90(3):272–9.
19. O'Driscoll SW, Morrey BF, Korinek S, An KN. Elbow subluxation and dislocation. A spectrum of instability. Clin Orthop Relat Res. 1992; (280):186–97.
20. McKee MD, Bowden SH, King GJ, Patterson SD, Jupiter JB, Bamberger HB, et al. Management of recurrent, complex instability of the elbow with a hinged external fixator. J Bone Joint Surg Br. 1998;80(6):1031–6.
21. Ring D, Hannouche D, Jupiter JB. Surgical treatment of persistent dislocation or subluxation of the ulnohumeral joint after fracture-dislocation of the elbow. J Hand Surg Am. 2004;29(3):470–80.
22. Sorensen AK, Sojbjerg JO. Treatment of persistent instability after posterior fracture-dislocation of the elbow: restoring stability and mobility by internal fixation and hinged external fixation. J Shoulder Elbow Surg. 2011;20(8):1300–9.
23. Arafiles RP. Neglected posterior dislocation of the elbow. A reconstruction operation. J Bone Joint Surg Br. 1987;69(2):199–202.
24. Naidoo KS. Unreduced posterior dislocations of the elbow. J Bone Joint Surg Br. 1982;64(5):603–6.
25. Billett DM. Unreduced posterior dislocation of the elbow. J Trauma. 1979;19(3):186–8.
26. Jupiter JB, Ring D. Treatment of unreduced elbow dislocations with hinged external fixation. J Bone Joint Surg Am. 2002;84-A(9):1630–5.
27. Orbay JL, Mijares MR. The management of elbow instability using an internal joint stabilizer: preliminary results. Clin Orthop Relat Res. 2014;472(7):2049–60.
28. Bigazzi P, Biondi M, Corvi A, Pfanner S, Checcucci G, Ceruso M. A new autocentering hinged external fixator of the elbow: a device that stabilizes the elbow axis without use of the articular pin. J Shoulder Elbow Surg. 2015;24(8):1197–205.
29. Cheung EV, O'Driscoll SW, Morrey BF. Complications of hinged external fixators of the elbow. J Shoulder Elbow Surg. 2008;17(3):447–53.
30. Hopf JC, Berger V, Krieglstein CF, Muller LP, Koslowsky TC. Treatment of unstable elbow dislocations with hinged elbow fixation-subjective and objective results. J Shoulder Elbow Surg. 2015;24(2):250–7.
31. Ruch DS, Triepel CR. Hinged elbow fixation for recurrent instability following fracture dislocation. Injury. 2001;32 Suppl 4:SD70–8.
32. Papandrea RF, Morrey BF, O'Driscoll SW. Reconstruction for persistent instability of the elbow after coronoid fracture-dislocation. J Shoulder Elbow Surg. 2007;16(1):68–77.

# The Role of Total Elbow Arthroplasty in the Setting of Elbow Instability

16

Ana Mata-Fink, David Kovacevic, and Theodore A. Blaine

## Background

Elbow instability is a complex problem that can significantly limit functional use and impact activities of daily living. Elbow dislocations are relatively common with an annual incidence of 6 per 100,000 persons [1] and simple elbow dislocations are often successfully treated nonoperatively with low rates of persistent instability [2–4]. In contrast, complex elbow dislocations have an associated fracture and often require surgical management, typically consisting of ligament repair or reconstruction, fracture stabilization, and possibly radial head arthroplasty [5, 6]. Complex elbow dislocations tend to have a worse prognosis than simple dislocations and may require revision surgery [7–11]. Severe complex dislocations in elderly patients are challenging problems as traditional methods of treatment including fracture fixation are often compromised by osteopenic bone and severe comminution. Alternative treatments including elbow arthroplasty may be considered a primary treatment in these patients.

Chronic or recurrent instability is often due to a missed elbow injury or chronic overuse injury. Chronic valgus instability is a common overuse injury in athletes who participate in overhead sports. Posterolateral rotatory instability is often due to a missed injury or treatment failure after a traumatic elbow dislocation [12]. Both of these injuries can be treated surgically with ligamentous repair or reconstruction. Global elbow instability in the setting of chronic instability can be challenging and is typically a result of bone loss of the coronoid and radial head as well as ligamentous insufficiency. In elderly patients, ligament reconstruction and coronoid process reconstruction, which are typical treatments for younger patients with this complicated problem, are at high risk for failure. Alternative treatments in older patients including elbow arthroplasty should be considered to prevent further instability.

Although a less common etiology, distal humerus nonunions can also cause elbow instability. Instability resulting from nonunited distal

**Electronic supplementary material** The online version of this chapter (doi:10.1007/978-3-319-46019-2_16) contains supplementary material, which is available to authorized users. Videos can also be accessed at http://link.springer.com/chapter/10.1007/978-3-319-46019-2_16.

A. Mata-Fink, MD, MS • D. Kovacevic, MD
Department of Orthopedic Surgery, Yale University School of Medicine, PO Box 208071, New Haven, CT 06520-8071, USA
e-mail: amatafink@gmail.com; david.kovacevic@yale.edu

T.A. Blaine, MD, MBA (✉)
Department of Orthopedics & Rehabilitation, Yale University School of Medicine, Yale Physician's Building, 800 Howard Avenue, New Haven, CT 06519, USA
e-mail: Theodore.blaine@yale.edu

© Springer International Publishing Switzerland 2017

R.Z. Tashjian (ed.), *The Unstable Elbow*, DOI 10.1007/978-3-319-46019-2_16

humeral fractures presents only in severe injuries as a flail elbow or gross instability through the fracture site. Approximately 2 % of adult fractures involve the distal humerus [13] and most are treated surgically. Of those treated with operative fixation, 2–10 % result in nonunion [14]. While many distal humerus nonunions can be successfully treated with revision osteosynthesis, some are not reparable. Revision reconstruction is typically reserved for young patients with adequate bone stock for osteosynthesis. Alternative treatments including arthroplasty should be considered for nonunions in elderly patients.

Total elbow arthroplasty (TEA), which was traditionally used for end-stage rheumatoid arthritis, offers the ability to restore joint stability in persistently unstable elbows due to complex comminuted fractures in osteopenic bone, global chronic instability from bony and ligamentous insufficiency, or distal humerus nonunions. TEA has traditionally had high complication rates and early failure rates, but new implant designs have decreased the overall complication rates [15–17]. Recent studies report good outcomes of TEA for elbow instability [18–23]. There continues to be a lifelong lifting restriction after TEA that makes it less appealing for younger patients [16] and the failure rates remain high for young, active patients [24–26]. For this reason, acute open reduction internal fixation for fracture, ligament reconstruction or repair for ligamentous insufficiency, bony reconstruction for structural bone loss, and revision osteosynthesis of distal humerus nonunion is the preferred management strategy in young patients. In older, low-demand patients with elbow instability, TEA should be considered as it can offer a successful outcome with improved pain, function, and elbow stability.

## Evaluation

### History

A thorough history is important in identifying patients with elbow instability that are candidates for total elbow arthroplasty. Persistent instability can present as pain or difficulty using the arm. Difficulty pushing up from a chair is a common complaint of patients with persistent elbow instability. A history of trauma typically reveals a prior elbow dislocation, elbow fracture, or, more commonly, fracture-dislocation.

Symptom duration and previous treatments are important to elucidate. History of prior surgery for distal humerus fracture or complex instability with a concomitant fracture and ligamentous repair or reconstruction for collateral ligament injury needs to be identified. Information regarding treatment of the ulnar nerve during prior surgical procedures and events during the postoperative course, including any history of infection, trauma, or requirement for reoperations, is essential if further surgery is being planned.

Patient age, lifestyle, and expectations are important factors when considering arthroplasty. Despite satisfactory implant survival with modern designs, TEA in young and active patients may result in early failure [24–26]. Precautions after total elbow arthroplasty include significant weight lifting limit with the involved arm [16]. Active patients may have difficulty complying with this restriction. For this reason, TEA is offered primarily to older, low-demand patients.

### Physical Exam

The physical exam should start with inspection of the upper extremity. Previous incisions or scars should be noted and the use of prior incisions should be considered in surgical planning. If a patient has had multiple prior surgical procedures, assistance from a plastic surgeon may be necessary for soft tissue coverage as TEA has a high wound complication rate [27]. Erythema or swelling over the elbow may be worrisome for infection and require further work-up, including inflammatory markers (i.e., peripheral CBC with differential, erythrocyte sedimentation rate, and C-reactive protein) and advanced imaging. Active infection is an absolute contraindication for TEA.

Elbow range of motion and stability should be assessed. Decreased elbow range of motion due to arthritis, heterotopic ossification, or instability is not a contraindication for TEA but lack of elbow flexion due to neurologic dysfunction is a contraindication for surgery [17]. Elbow stability should be tested throughout the flexion-extension arc of motion. Additionally, varus and valgus stress testing should be performed with the elbow flexed 30°. Posterolateral rotatory instability can be assessed with either the chair rise test, posterolateral drawer test or lateral pivot-shift maneuver, which can be performed in the office or with the patient under general anesthesia in the operating room [28]. The clinician should include neurovascular testing to complete the exam as neurologic dysfunction of the upper extremity is a contraindication to TEA [17].

## Imaging

Appropriate imaging is essential and should include orthogonal radiographic evaluation and advanced imaging. Standard radiographs of the elbow typically include AP, lateral, and oblique images. If the elbow is unstable throughout the arc of motion, lateral radiographs in flexion and extension are helpful. Varus and valgus stress radiographs may reveal joint space widening indicative of ligamentous disruption. Elbow radiographs should be inspected for hardware from prior surgery that may need to be removed and fracture healing if there is a history of trauma. Fracture malunions or nonunions of the proximal ulna, radius, and distal humerus should be identified. Overall bone quality should be assessed including fragment size and osteopenia. The ulnohumeral or radiohumeral joints should be evaluated for joint space narrowing consistent with arthritic changes. Finally, bone loss of the coronoid, proximal radius, and distal humerus should be recognized and quantified because deficiency in these locations will commonly result in chronic instability.

Advanced imaging such as MRI and CT should also be considered part of the evaluation. MRI is the best imaging modality for assessing the soft tissues around the elbow. It is useful for identifying ligamentous injury as well as fluid collections or bone edema that may be indicative of infection [29]. CT scan is useful for evaluation of prior fracture healing or nonunion, current bony alignment in the case of malunion, and bone loss. Significant bone loss associated with complex instability is typically seen in the coronoid process, radial head, or articular surface of the distal humerus. CT has also been reported to be useful for preoperative planning or imaged-based navigation in patients with extensive bone loss or atypical anatomy [30].

## Laboratory Studies

Standard preoperative laboratory work-up should include a complete blood count with differential, coagulation markers (INR, PT, aPTT), and a basic metabolic panel. Hemoglobin A1C is typically checked in diabetic patients as those with poor long-term glucose control (i.e., >7.5 %) are at increased risk of wound healing complications and postoperative infection. Type and screen should be obtained on all patients preoperatively in the event an allogeneic blood transfusion is required perioperatively.

In elderly patients in whom there is a concern for malnutrition, pre-albumin, albumin, and transferrin should be obtained. Malnourished patients are at increased risk for wound healing complications and infection [31]. Total elbow arthroplasty has a relatively high rate of wound complication so improving the patient's nutritional status is essential [27, 32], and consideration for referral to and consultation with a nutritionist may be warranted.

Infection should be ruled out in high-risk patients, especially in those patients with elbow instability due to failed osteosynthesis either of the distal humerus, proximal ulna or proximal radius. White blood count, erythrocyte sedimentation rate (ESR), and C-reactive protein (CRP) should be obtained. Aspiration of the ulnohumeral joint, as well as the nonunion site if possible, should be performed prior to consideration of arthroplasty. Cultures should be assessed for cell count, gram stain, and culture held for 2 weeks to rule out P. Acnes. Open biopsy of the surgical site or two-stage surgical reconstruction with initial debridement, biopsy, and hardware removal should be considered in patients with abnormal labs with a dry tap or negative aspiration, or any suspicion of infection.

## Treatment Algorithm

The treatment algorithm for elbow instability is based on age and patient activity. Young patients and high-demand patients should be treated with acute repair of complex dislocations even in the setting of comminution. Repair can often be augmented with external fixation if there is a concern regarding fracture fixation. In the setting of chronic instability with global ligamentous insufficiency or complex dislocations with bony deficits, ligamentous repair or reconstruction and/or bony deficit reconstruction should be performed. Finally, revision osteosynthesis of distal humerus nonunions should be the treatment of choice, even in severe cases, for this patient population. Patients over the age of 65 or low-demand patients with no infection and without significant neurologic compromise to the arm are candidates for TEA for each of these problems. Patients who are not medically fit to tolerate the stress from surgery should be treated conservatively with bracing or splinting.

When considering TEA, infection must be ruled out with laboratory studies and aspiration. An active, chronic infection is a contraindication to TEA and should be surgically treated with hardware removal, irrigation and debridement, placement of a polymethylmethacrylate antibiotic cement spacer, at least 6 weeks of intravenous antibiotics, and consultation with an infectious disease specialist. After clearance of infection, elbow arthroplasty may be considered a second stage procedure. Patients with a flail arm due to neurologic injury are also not candidates for TEA. Some of these patients may benefit from elbow arthrodesis to better position their arm in space [33].

## Nonoperative Treatment Strategies

Most chronic or recurrent elbow instability that may require arthroplasty for treatment is not typically amendable to nonoperative treatment. Chronic bracing or sling wear may be considered in cases of patients that are medically unfit or those not wishing to pursue surgery, although function is typically limited.

Nonoperative management can also be attempted for elbow instability due to distal humerus delayed union or nonunion. Bone stimulators may be used in cases of delayed union and nonunions with limited deformity although with unreliable effectivness [34]. Nounions resulting in instability will typically be severe enough that a stimulator will have a limited effect. Most nonunions of distal humerus fractures are caused by inadequate fixation and require revision osteosynthesis to unite, making bone stimulators unlikely to be beneficial in this group [13, 14].

## Surgical Management/Technique Based/Surgical Pearls

In older, low-demand patients with elbow instability, TEA is an excellent salvage option to alleviate pain, restore stability, and improve range of motion. Surgical considerations when performing TEA are described below (Video 16.1).

### Approach

The skin incision for a TEA is typically a posterior incision that runs along the ulnar border and skirts the tip of the olecranon. Many patients with chronic or recurrent elbow instability have had prior surgical procedures. In those cases, a prior incision may be used. Patients with multiple prior incisions may require plastic surgery consultation to help with soft tissue coverage postoperatively.

It is important that the collateral ligaments are fully released from the humerus. Even in cases of gross elbow instability, there is often a remaining attachment that must be released to obtain optimal visualization.

### Triceps Management

Many approaches have been used with the triceps for TEA including paratricepital (triceps sparing), triceps splitting, and triceps reflection [35]. The two most commonly reported triceps management options in TEA for elbow instability are triceps sparing or triceps reflecting (i.e., subperiosteal elevation) [18, 19, 23]. There does not appear to be a significant difference in functional outcomes between the two approaches [36]. The triceps reflecting approach offers the most extensive visualization of the ulnohumeral joint and is often considered less challenging when there is no bone loss. Patients with distal humerus nonunions may have significant distal humerus bone loss, making visualization of the elbow through a triceps sparing approach less difficult. In a triceps sparing approach, the triceps must be elevated off the humerus. This can be challenging in patients with prior surgeries, as there may be extensive scarring and adhesion formation. Decision for triceps management should ultimately be based on surgeon preference and experience [35].

## Ulnar Nerve and Soft Tissue Management

The rate of ulnar neuropathy after TEA is around 2–5 % [36, 37]. The ulnar nerve should be identified early in the case and mobilized along its length. Once the ulnar nerve has been mobilized, it can be marked with a vessel loop and translated anteriorly away from the elbow. Because of the degree of mobilization, the ulnar nerve is often subcutaneously transposed at the end of the case.

In cases of prior surgery associated with a nonunion, deep cultures and pathology should be sent for gram stain, cultures, and frozen sections. Any significant acute inflammation on frozen sections should alert the surgeon to possible infection. There is no consensus regarding cutoff levels of acute inflammation although any acute inflammation on any frozen sections should be concerning, especially in the setting of a TEA, and strong consideration of placement of a spacer should be made. Cultures should be held for 2 weeks to rule out P. Acnes.

## Implant Choice

TEA implants are either linked or unlinked and have different amounts of constraint (Fig. 16.1). In a linked implant, the ulnar and humeral components are attached. Unlinked components rely on soft tissues for elbow stability. Constraint is the amount of varus-valgus and rotational motion in the ulnohumeral joint. Unlinked implants have less constraint than linked implants. Linked implants are either fully constrained (rigid hinge) or semi constrained (sloppy hinge).

While there appears to be no difference in functional outcome between linked and unlinked TEA for rheumatoid arthritis [38], TEA for elbow instability requires a linked implant as the collateral ligaments are deficient. Fully constrained TEA implants have shown an above average loosening rate and have fallen out of favor [15]. All series of TEA for instability reported on the use of semi-constrained implants with good results [18–20, 22, 23].

Both the humeral and ulnar implants should be stemmed in TEA for instability to improve implant fixation. Cement fixation for the components is recommended. Cement restrictors should

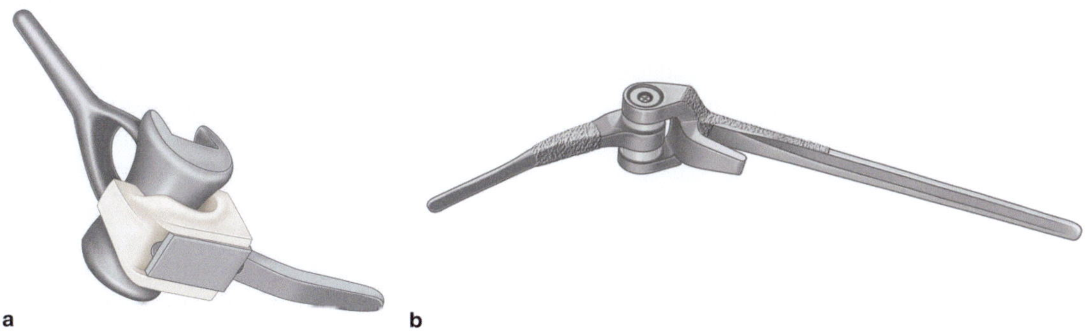

a b

**Fig. 16.1** Unlinked total elbow prosthesis (**a**); linked, semi-constrained elbow prosthesis (**b**) be utilized in both the humerus and ulna to improve cement mantles. In cases of significant bone loss, a TEA prosthesis with an extended flange may not be adequate for reconstruction. In those cases, a tumor prosthesis or an allograft prosthesis composite may be required. The allograft host union rate with these composites is similar to that for allograft prosthesis composites in the hip or knee [39].

## Component Positioning and Humeral/Ulna Preparation

In patients with significant distal humerus bone loss, positioning of the humeral implant can be challenging, as there are few intraoperative anatomic landmarks from which to reference. In such cases, preoperative planning should include full-length radiographs of both the involved humerus and contralateral humerus. The contralateral humerus could be used to measure the total humeral length and a comparison is made to determine the amount of humeral bone of the affected humerus. Intraoperatively, humeral implant length should be based on soft tissue tension. This can be difficult in a flail elbow as soft tissue contractures are common. The "shuck test" can be used to determine humeral stem position when there is distal humerus bone loss. The humeral and ulnar components are placed and linked together. With the arm flexed to 90°, the forearm is distracted distally. This will result in optimal positioning of the humeral component [40]. If needed, the humerus can be shortened by up to 2 cm without causing triceps weakness [23].

Rotational alignment is also challenging with distal humerus bone loss. Inaccurate positioning can affect functional outcomes and lead to accelerated wear [41]. The proximal ulna can be used to assess for rotation alignment of the ulnar component by aligning the posterior aspect of the ulnar component with the flat dorsal aspect of the proximal ulna [42]. The humeral component should be internally rotated approximately 15° in relation to the posterior humeral shaft and, even in cases of severe bone loss of the distal humerus, the shaft can still be referenced [43]. Research has shown that image-based navigation leads to improved alignment compared to nonnavigated implantation although no currently available TEA system has the capability of image-based navigation [30].

Perforation of the canals is at high risk in cases of TEA after failed osteosynthesis. Cannulated flexible reamers can help avoid perforation. Placement of guidewires for reamers under fluoroscopy intraoperative can be used to confirm intramedullary placement and avoid perforation.

## Closure

Wound closure for TEA should be meticulous as there is a relatively high rate of wound complications [27, 37]. If the triceps is reflected, it should be reattached through cruciate drill holes in the ulna [35]. The rate of triceps insufficiency after TEA is 2–3 % [36, 37]. The triceps should be completely repaired to the flexor and extensors isolating the joint from the subcutaneous region. This will help prevent hematoma or seroma development and limit the possibility for wound compromise. The subcutaneous tissue should be closed in layers and the skin should be reapproximated with interrupted nonabsorbable suture. A drain should be placed to prevent seroma or hematoma development in the subcutaneous tissue.

## Postoperative Care

There is no consensus in the literature on postoperative management. Postoperative splinting in extension ranges from none to almost 2 weeks. Longer splinting time appears to be associated with decreased wound problems [37] but decreases postoperative range of motion. In the literature on TEA for elbow instability, splinting ranged from none to 2 days postoperatively with all splinting done in extension [19, 22, 23]. In general, anterior extension splinting should be performed to reduce tension and pressure on the posterior wound to prevent wound complications. For a triceps-on approach, immediate active and passive range of motion exercises are allowed, typically with nighttime anterior splinting to maintain extension. Patients are allowed immediate use of the limb for everyday activities of daily care after the initial splint is removed and then moved to the 5 lb lifting restriction at 6 weeks. If a triceps-off approach is utilized, active extension needs to be protected during the first 6 weeks after TEA to prevent triceps failure. Failure of the triceps to heal is a major complication associated with TEA. In cases of bone loss, exposure is not often a problem; therefore, a triceps-on approach is recommended if possible to prevent triceps failure.

## Published Outcomes/Complications

Elbow instability is an indication for TEA for the carefully selected patient. Most reports of TEA for instability are for distal humerus nonunions in older patients. Early reports did not show favorable results with TEA [44, 45]. More recent studies using modern implants in older patients (over 60 years of age) demonstrate better outcomes (Table 16.1). The largest reported series is from the Mayo Clinic, which updated a previous series to include 91 consecutive patients with 92 elbows treated with TEA for distal humerus nonunion followed for an average of 6.5 years [18, 20]. The authors showed improvement in range of motion, elbow stability, and Mayo Elbow Performance Score (MEPS) in the majority of their patients. Based on the MEPS score, 78 % had a satisfactory (good or excellent) outcome postoperatively. They reported 44 complications, including infection, aseptic loosening, component fracture, periprosthetic fracture, and wound complications. Implant survival without removal or revision was 96 % at 2 years, 82 % at 5 years, and 65 % at 10 and 15 years [18].

Two smaller series out of Europe showed similar results to the Mayo Clinic series. Pogliacomi et al. followed 20 patients treated with TEA for distal humerus nonunion for an average of 65 months [22]. They reported improved MEPS score postoperatively with 90 % of patients having good or excellent outcomes despite a 30 % complication rate. Espiga et al. reported on six patients treated with linked TEA for symptomatic distal humerus nonunion followed for an average of 40 months [19]. They reported acceptable range of motion and improved pain postoperatively. Based on postoperative MEPS score, 67 % of the patients had a satisfactory outcome. There was one complication in their series, difficulty with wound healing that required fasciocutaneous flap coverage 2 months after surgery.

**Table 16.1** Clinical studies on TEA for elbow instability and distal humerus nonunion

| Study (Year) | Number | Avg age, years | Avg follow-up, months | Pre-op ROM, degrees | Post-op ROM, degrees | Pre-op MEPS | Post-op MEPS | Complication rate, % (number) | Reoperation rate, % (number) |
|---|---|---|---|---|---|---|---|---|---|
| Case series | | | | | | | | | |
| Cil et al. (2008) [18] | 92 | 65 | 78 | 37–106 | 22–135 | 29 | 81 | 43 (44) | 35 (32) |
| Espiga et al. (2011) [19] | 6 | 80 | 40 | 43–104 | 15–125 | – | 82 | 17 (1) | 17 (1) |
| Pogliacomi et al. (2015) [22] | 20 | 71.9 | 65 | – | – | 51.3 | 86 | 30 (6) | 15 (3) |
| Ramsey et al. (1999) [23] | 19 | 66 | 72 | – | 25-128 | 44 | 86 | 21 (4) | 16 (3) |
| Case report | | | | | | | | | |
| Murthu et al. (2013) [21] | 1 | 40 | 24 | – | – | 30 | 100 | – | – |

*ROM* range of motion, *MEPS* Mayo elbow performance score, – not reported
Results of Morrey et al. (1995) were not included in this table as the results were included and updated in Cil et al. (2008) [18]

There is one series reported in the literature examining patients treated with TEA for distal humerus nonunion with a primary complaint of elbow instability [23]. Ramsey et al. reported on 19 elbows and showed improvement in MEPS score and range of motion postoperatively. There was no residual elbow instability postoperatively and 16 of the 19 elbows had satisfactory outcomes.

Complications from total elbow arthroplasty were summarized in two systematic review of primary TEA for all indications [36, 37]. The overall reported complication rate varied between 20 and 40 %. The rate of wound complications was 9 %, infection 4 %, and ulnar neuropathy 2–5 %. There was a 5–9 % loosening rate and 4 % rate of implant failure. Given the relatively high complication rate, TEA for instability should be reserved for older, functionally low-demand patients who have failed other treatment options.

## Preferred Treatment/Cases

### Case Presentation

An 83-year-old right hand dominant female presented to the office with a chief complaint of an unstable left elbow. She initially sustained a left closed, simple elbow dislocation after a fall down stairs. The elbow was reduced in the emergency department and she was treated conservatively. She did well for 4 months until she had a recurrent dislocation while carrying a laundry basket. The elbow was again formally reduced. She had persistent pain and instability of the left elbow since the second dislocation, which made it difficult for her to complete her activities of daily living. At this time, she presented to the office with recurrent elbow instability.

On physical examination, she had a grossly unstable elbow that was reduced in flexion and dislocated in extension. Her range of motion in the flexion-extension arc was 0–120° and painful. The elbow was also unstable to varus and valgus stress testing. The arm was neurovascularly intact with normal motor function and sensation of the hand and a palpable radial pulse.

Plain radiographs demonstrated no fracture. Flexion and extension lateral radiographs demonstrated the ulnohumeral joint reduced in flexion and dislocated in extension with posterior heterotopic ossification (Fig. 16.2). She was unable to obtain an MRI, but a CT scan was obtained which revealed recurrent dislocation with periarticular calcification and subcortical capitellar lucency with no significant bone loss.

Treatment options were reviewed with the patient. Given her age and comorbidities, it was unlikely that a medial and lateral ulnar collateral ligament reconstruction would heal and provide her with a stable elbow. She elected to proceed with a TEA. The decision was made to use a

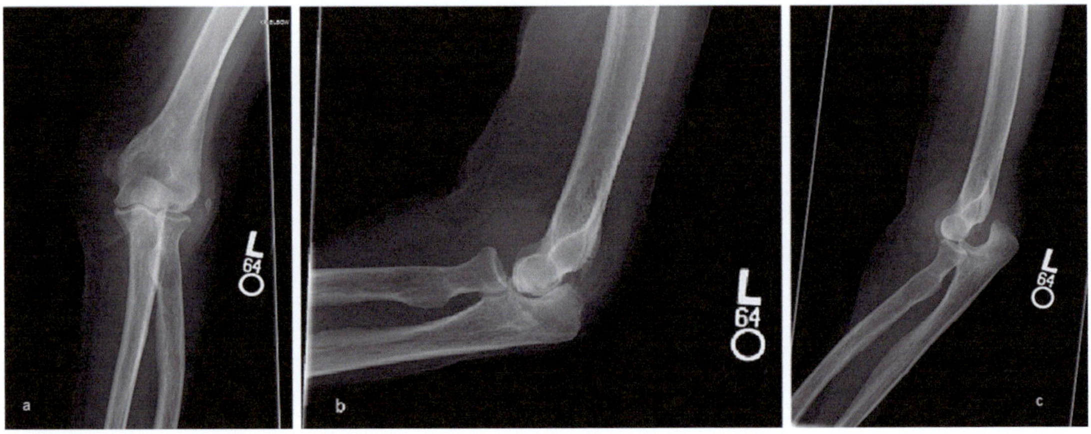


**Fig. 16.2** Preoperative X-rays: AP (**a**), lateral in flexion (**b**), and lateral in extension (**c**)

linked, semi-constrained implant with cement fixation of both the humeral and ulnar components utilizing a triceps sparing approach.

## Surgical Procedure

Tourniquet was used to minimize blood loss. A posterior midline incision was made just medial to the tip of the olecranon. The ulnar nerve was identified and decompressed. The decision was made to proceed with a triceps sparing approach. The triceps was elevated off of the humerus and the remaining collateral ligaments were released.

The humerus was exposed first and prepared for the humeral implant. The proximal ulna was exposed next and prepared for the ulnar implant. The humeral and ulnar components were trialed and anterior capsule was released to improve elbow extension. After trialing the humeral and ulnar components, the implants were cemented into the humerus and ulna. The elbow was reduced and the implants were linked. Elbow range of motion was assessed and found to be 0–135°.

The ulnar nerve was transposed subcutaneously and the incision was closed in layers with a nonabsorbable layer for the skin. The dressing was placed and the arm was splinted in extension with an anteriorly molded splint. The splint was removed approximately 24 h postoperatively. The patient was instructed to minimize elbow range of motion to allow for soft tissue healing. The patient remained in the hospital for one night postoperatively for pain control.

## Postoperative Results

The patient was seen in follow-up 1 week postoperatively for a wound check. Plain radiographs at that time showed appropriate position of the implant with no hardware complications (Fig. 16.3). At that visit, superficial epidermolysis was noted medial to the incision. Antibiotics were given in combination with daily silvadene application to the affected area. This was followed weekly for 3 weeks at which point the wound had healed with no further complications. Sutures were removed 3 weeks postoperatively and she was allowed to start ranging her elbow with no formal physical therapy (Fig. 16.4).

## Conclusion

TEA for elbow instability due to ligamentous insufficiency or distal humerus nonunion should be reserved for older, sedentary, low-demand patients because of the high complication rates, patient satisfaction rates less than 80 %, and a prosthesis failure rate up to 35 % at 10-years after surgery. TEA is a technically demanding surgical

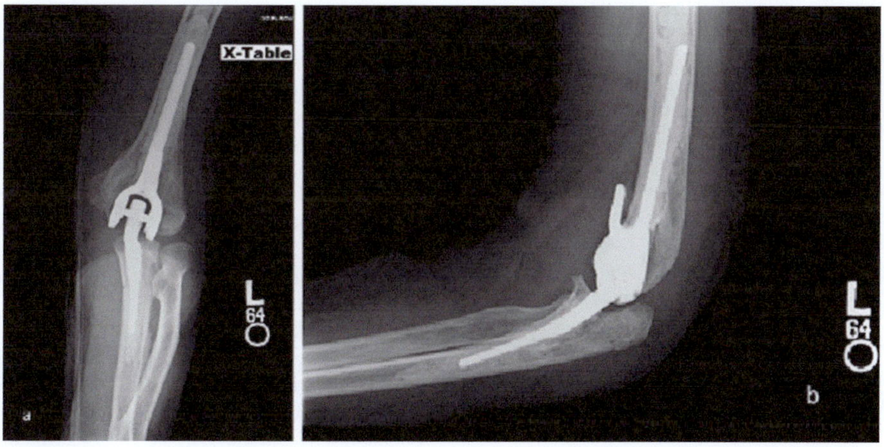


**Fig. 16.3** Postoperative X-rays: AP (**a**) and lateral (**b**)

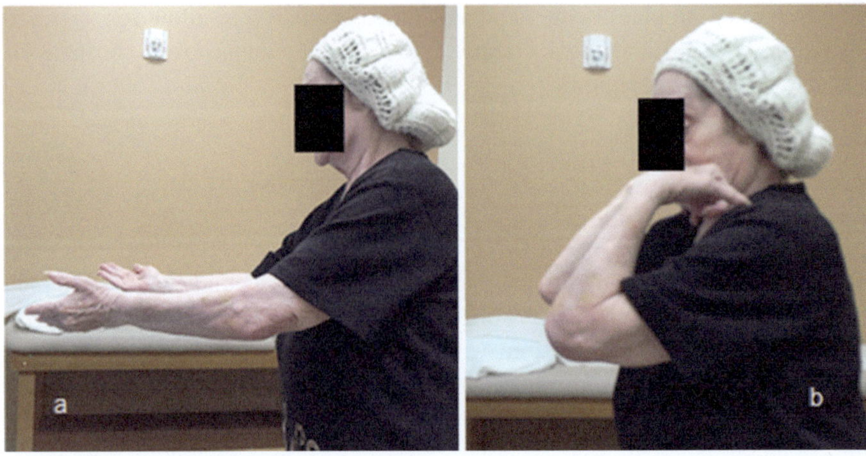


**Fig. 16.4** Postoperative range of motion: extension (**a**) and flexion (**b**)

procedure for even the most experienced orthopedic surgeon; therefore, several principles should be followed to optimize successful patient outcomes and minimize complications. These principles include patient selection, adequate surgical exposure and triceps management, appropriate implant selection and positioning (i.e., linked, semi-constrained cemented prosthesis), careful ulnar nerve decompression with transposition, meticulous wound closure, and appropriate postoperative care.

## References


1. Linscheid RL, Wheeler DK. Elbow dislocations. JAMA. 1965;194(11):1171–6.
2. Josefsson PO, Gentz CF, Johnell O, Wendeberg B. Surgical versus non-surgical treatment of ligamentous injuries following dislocation of the elbow joint. A prospective randomized study. J Bone Joint Surg Am. 1987;69(4):605–8.
3. Josefsson PO, Johnell O, Gentz CF. Long-term sequelae of simple dislocation of the elbow. J Bone Joint Surg Am. 1984;66(6):927–30.
4. Mehlhoff TL, Noble PC, Bennett JB, Tullos HS. Simple dislocation of the elbow in the adult. Results after closed treatment. J Bone Joint Surg Am. 1988;70(2):244–9.
5. Morrey BF. Acute and chronic instability of the elbow. J Am Acad Orthop Surg. 1996;4(3):117–28.
6. Tashjian RZ, Katarincic JA. Complex elbow instability. J Am Acad Orthop Surg. 2006;14(5):278–86.
7. Broberg MA, Morrey BF. Results of treatment of fracture-dislocations of the elbow. Clin Orthop Relat Res. 1987; (216):109–19.
8. Regan W, Morrey B. Fractures of the coronoid process of the ulna. J Bone Joint Surg Am. 1989;71(9):1348–54.
9. Scharplatz D, Allgower M. Fracture-dislocations of the elbow. Injury. 1975;7(2):143–59.
10. Vichard P, Tropet Y, Dreyfus-Schmidt G, Besancenot J, Menez D, Pem R. Fractures of the proximal end of the radius associated with other traumatic lesions of the upper limb. A report of seventy-three cases. Ann Chir Main. 1988;7(1):45–53.
11. Josefsson PO, Gentz CF, Johnell O, Wendeberg B. Dislocations of the elbow and intraarticular fractures. Clin Orthop Relat Res. 1989; (246):126–30.
12. Lee ML, Rosenwasser MP. Chronic elbow instability. Orthop Clin North Am. 1999;30(1):81–9.
13. Pollock JW, Faber KJ, Athwal GS. Distal humerus fractures. Orthop Clin North Am. 2008;39(2):187–200. vi.
14. Helfet DL, Kloen P, Anand N, Rosen HS. Open reduction and internal fixation of delayed unions and nonunions of fractures of the distal part of the humerus. J Bone Joint Surg Am. 2003;85-A(1):33–40.
15. Choo A, Ramsey ML. Total elbow arthroplasty: current options. J Am Acad Orthop Surg. 2013;21(7):427–37.
16. Sanchez-Sotelo J. Total elbow arthroplasty. Open Orthop J. 2011;5:115–23.
17. Sanchez-Sotelo J, Morrey BF. Total elbow arthroplasty. J Am Acad Orthop Surg. 2011;19(2):121–5.
18. Cil A, Veillette CJ, Sanchez-Sotelo J, Morrey BF. Linked elbow replacement: a salvage procedure for distal humeral nonunion. J Bone Joint Surg Am. 2008;90(9):1939–50.
19. Espiga X, Antuna SA, Ferreres A. Linked total elbow arthroplasty as treatment of distal humerus nonunions

in patients older than 70 years. Acta Orthop Belg. 2011;77(3):304–10.
20. Morrey BF, Adams RA. Semiconstrained elbow replacement for distal humeral nonunion. J Bone Joint Surg. 1995;77(1):67–72.
21. Muthu R, Foead AI, Bin Ali A, Devadasan B. Salvage of elbow function in chronic complex elbow fracture dislocation with total elbow arthroplasty: a case report. Med J Malaysia. 2013;68(4):353–5.
22. Pogliacomi F, Aliani D, Cavaciocchi M, Corradi M, Ceccarelli F, Rotini R. Total elbow arthroplasty in distal humeral nonunion: clinical and radiographic evaluation after a minimum follow-up of three years. J Shoulder Elbow Surg. 2015;24(12):1998–2007.
23. Ramsey ML, Adams RA, Morrey BF. Instability of the elbow treated with semiconstrained total elbow arthroplasty. J Bone Joint Surg Am. 1999;81(1):38–47.
24. Fevang BT, Lie SA, Havelin LI, Skredderstuen A, Furnes O. Results after 562 total elbow replacements: a report from the Norwegian Arthroplasty Register. J Shoulder Elbow Surg. 2009;18(3):449–56.
25. Seitz Jr WH, Bismar H, Evans PJ. Failure of the hinge mechanism in total elbow arthroplasty. J Shoulder Elbow Surg. 2010;19(3):368–75.
26. Celli A, Morrey BF. Total elbow arthroplasty in patients forty years of age or less. J Bone Joint Surg Am. 2009;91(6):1414–8.
27. Jeon IH, Morrey BF, Anakwenze OA, Tran NV. Incidence and implications of early postoperative wound complications after total elbow arthroplasty. J Shoulder Elbow Surg. 2011;20(6):857–65.
28. O'Driscoll SW, Bell DF, Morrey BF. Posterolateral rotatory instability of the elbow. J Bone Joint Surg Am. 1991;73(3):440–6.
29. Frick MA. Imaging of the elbow: a review of imaging findings in acute and chronic traumatic disorders of the elbow. J Hand Ther. 2006;19(2):98–112.
30. McDonald CP, Johnson JA, Peters TM, King GJ. Image-based navigation improves the positioning of the humeral component in total elbow arthroplasty. J Shoulder Elbow Surg. 2010;19(4):533–43.
31. Cross MB, Yi PH, Thomas CF, Garcia J, Della Valle CJ. Evaluation of malnutrition in orthopedic surgery. J Am Acad Orthop Surg. 2014;22(3):193–9.
32. Gay DM, Lyman S, Do H, Hotchkiss RN, Marx RG, Daluiski A. Indications and reoperation rates for total elbow arthroplasty: an analysis of trends in New York State. J Bone Joint Surg Am. 2012;94(2):110–7.
33. Koller H, Kolb K, Assuncao A, Kolb W, Holz U. The fate of elbow arthrodesis: indications, techniques, and outcome in fourteen patients. J Shoulder Elbow Surg. 2008;17(2):293–306.
34. Aaron RK, Ciombor DM, Simon BJ. Treatment of nonunions with electric and electromagnetic fields. Clin Orthop Relat Res. 2004; (419):21–9.
35. Morrey BF, Sanchez-Sotelo J. Approaches for elbow arthroplasty: how to handle the triceps. J Shoulder Elbow Surg. 2011;20(2 Suppl):S90–6.
36. Voloshin I, Schippert DW, Kakar S, Kaye EK, Morrey BF. Complications of total elbow replacement: a systematic review. J Shoulder Elbow Surg. 2011;20(1):158–68.
37. Little CP, Graham AJ, Carr AJ. Total elbow arthroplasty: a systematic review of the literature in the English language until the end of 2003. J Bone Joint Surg. 2005;87(4):437–44.
38. Wright TW, Wong AM, Jaffe R. Functional outcome comparison of semiconstrained and unconstrained total elbow arthroplasties. J Shoulder Elbow Surg. 2000;9(6):524–31.
39. Renfree KJ, Dell PC, Kozin SH, Wright TW. Total elbow arthroplasty with massive composite allografts. J Shoulder Elbow Surg. 2004;13(3):313–21.
40. Morrey B, Sanchez-Sotelo J. Revision of failed total elbow arthroplasty with osseous deficiency. In: Morrey B, Sanchez-Sotelo J, editors. The elbow and its disorders. Philadelphia, PA: Saunders Elsevier; 2009. p. 899–910.
41. Lenoir H, Micallef JP, Djerbi I, Waitzenegger T, Lazerges C, Chammas M, et al. Total elbow arthroplasty: influence of implant positioning on functional outcomes. Orthop Traumatol Surg Res. 2015;101(6):721–7.
42. Duggal N, Dunning CE, Johnson JA, King GJ. The flat spot of the proximal ulna: a useful anatomic landmark in total elbow arthroplasty. J Shoulder Elbow Surg. 2004;13(2):206–7.
43. Sabo MT, Athwal GS, King GJ. Landmarks for rotational alignment of the humeral component during elbow arthroplasty. J Bone Joint Surg Am. 2012;94(19):1794–800.
44. Figgie MP, Inglis AE, Mow CS, Figgie 3rd HE. Salvage of non-union of supracondylar fracture of the humerus by total elbow arthroplasty. J Bone Joint Surg Am. 1989;71(7):1058–65.
45. Mitsunaga MM, Bryan RS, Linscheid RL. Condylar nonunions of the elbow. J Trauma. 1982;22(9):787–91.

# Elbow Fusion for The Unstable Elbow

# 17

April D. Armstrong

## Background

Elbow fusion is an operation that is, for the most part, limited to young active individuals that really have no other reconstructive options for the elbow. The patients' have either sustained severe trauma to the elbow or they have failed multiple previous surgical interventions to the elbow, which has resulted in severe bone loss and instability of the elbow. These individuals are not typically good candidates for total elbow arthroplasty. Limitations after total elbow arthroplasty include a five-pound lifetime lifting restriction and the younger patient can have a difficult time abiding by these rules often resulting in multiple revision surgeries. A resection arthroplasty is not always a great functional solution as well since it often leaves the elbow very unstable and the patients describe difficulty with positioning the hand in space and using the arm with any type of resistance. The advantage of an elbow fusion is that it provides permanent stability to the elbow, which better positions the hand in space for functional resistance but it comes with a great cost in that the patient no longer has full capability of the elbow. The decision to fuse the elbow in a more flexed or extended position is made jointly by the surgeon and the patient, but obviously will compromise activity in one of the planes of functional activity depending on the position chosen.

A.D. Armstrong, BSc(PT), MD, MSC, FRCSC (✉)
Penn State Milton S. Hershey Medical Center, Bone and Joint Institute, Mail Code EC 089, 30 Hope Drive, Building A, Hershey, PA 17033, USA
e-mail: aarmstrong@hmc.psu.edu

## Evaluation

The key to evaluation for these patients is to be certain that the patient has realistic expectations and that they are properly educated about what it means to have a fused elbow. You must also understand their motivation for an elbow fusion and what they are expecting to achieve. This procedure has a drastic end result from a functional standpoint but it also has great advantage. They will stop the endless surgical interventions and have the potential to obtain good pain control and stability of the elbow but it comes at the cost of losing some elbow function and the ability to do selected activities. You must look at the entire patient; look at their hand dominance, job requirements, and their hobbies and understand why they would not be a candidate for a total elbow arthroplasty or a resection arthroplasty or other reconstructive options. Often times these patients have had multiple previous surgical interventions and therefore it is important to obtain all previous operative notes, clinic notes, laboratory studies, EMG studies, or advanced imaging such as MRIs or CT scans. You also need to have a good understanding of the associated comorbidities

© Springer International Publishing Switzerland 2017

R.Z. Tashjian (ed.), *The Unstable Elbow*, DOI 10.1007/978-3-319-46019-2_17

that will weigh in on your decision to fuse and their risk for surgery.

On physical examination you want to be sure that there is no ongoing concern for infection since this will compromise your ability to achieve union. You want to assess the soft tissue and bone quality. Many times these patients have had multiple procedures and so you want to be sure that you will have enough soft tissue coverage to allow for healing. The bone can be shortened in order to facilitate soft tissue coverage. If the patient has had a previous soft tissue procedures such as a free flap, then you will want to consult with your plastic surgery colleagues to be sure you are clear on the development of the soft tissue planes for the procedure and in most cases it would be wise to have them involved at the time of the surgical procedure. Bone loss is very common and you will need to determine the viability of the bone and the ability to approximate the bone to allow for solid healing. If you have removed previous hardware, then the fusion plate should extend two cortical widths past the last screw hole to prevent later fracture. Neurovascular status should be assessed. The hand should ideally be functional; however, an argument can be made that even just having a stable forearm and nonfunctional hand to act as an opposing pain free limb can also increase overall function. In these situations it can be helpful to discuss prosthetic options with a physical medicine and rehabilitation specialist who can advise the patients' on the risks and benefits of amputation and potential for future prosthetic options.

## Treatment Algorithm

### Nonoperative Strategy/Therapy Protocols

Usually patients have attempted to wear removable orthoses to help provide some external stability to the elbow but unfortunately these are not really well tolerated. They tend to create pressure sores around the elbow and can be bulky and uncomfortable. Resection arthroplasty does not relieve pain entirely and patients describe achiness or even more severe pain because of the lack of ligamentous and bony support. The resection arthroplasty can be very dysfunctional as it does not allow them to work with their arm over their head due to triceps insufficiency and it does not provide stability to allow for activity against resistance. Younger patients find it difficult to function with a resection whereas older individuals who are more sedentary may have an easier time coping.

When deciding to electively fuse an elbow, it is critical to allow the patient to experience in real time what it would be like to live with a permanently stiff elbow. Some authors talk about using an orthosis; however, this can still be misleading to a patient if they, even occasionally, remove the splint to perform an activity. Preferably, the patient should be rigidly casted for 1 week ideally. If they are casted in a rigid position, then this will truly give them the sense of what it would be like to live with their elbow permanently fused and what it would be like to perform activities of daily living with no "opt out." This can be very helpful for the patient to decide if this is a feasible option for them and to decide on the actual position. The optimal fusion position has been discussed before in previous articles [1–4]. With the original description of elbow fusion, patients were typically fused at 90° [5]. It has been concluded that there is no single optimal elbow fusion position to cover all activities of daily living [1, 4]. O'Neill et al. found that 90° allowed most individuals to take care of personal hygiene needs and that a 70° angle made reaching for objects easier [1]. Tang et al. reported functional activity scores for healthy individuals who were locked in elbow braces at increments of 20° [2]. They reported that functional scores for personal hygiene and activities of daily living were more optimal at 110° compared to 90°; however, they agreed that their functional tasks measured had a bias towards activities that require more elbow flexion. Groot et al. concluded that the optimal elbow arthrodesis position should bias toward either the flexion domain or the extension domain depending on the patient's preference [3]. The patient should try different fusion angle options to see what works best for them. With the rise of technology and computer use, often times an elbow fused around 70° is optimal and it tends to be less obvious clinically when the patient is ambulating since their arm can still rest down by their side whereas with a fusion at 90° it is more obvious that the elbow is contracted.

## Surgical Management/Technique/ Surgical Pearls

It is important to plan preoperatively for these cases to firstly decide on the optimal fusion angle, which is individual to the patient, and also to plan the actual fusion technique. The author has had success using a large 4.5 LCD plate, which is pre-bent to the optimal angle of fusion position determined preoperatively by the patient. The plate is given to one of our machinists who pre-bend the plate in a controlled fashion to the specified angle; this can also be done in the operating room but the 4.5 plate is a very stout plate and can be difficult to bend with the intraoperative plate bender. Depending on the bony deformity, it is best to think how the bones will align with one another with the most surface area for healing, i.e., a chevron, oblique, or a step cut for example.

## Surgical Technique

The patient is in a supine position. The author prefers this position as it allows one to visualize the elbow in a normal anatomic position. An argument could be made to place the patient in a lateral position, which would allow easier access for application of the plate. A midline posterior incision is preferable provided that there are no special soft tissue considerations. Thick fasciocutaneous flaps are elevated medially and laterally. The ulnar nerve is formally transposed or decompressed in situ. The author prefers formal subcutaneous transposition. The triceps is mobilized using a splitting approach. The radial nerve is identified and protected proximally between the long and lateral heads of the triceps muscle. The split is carried through deeper medial head of the triceps through its midline being careful to protect the ulnar nerve medially and then carried down to the joint and down to the crest of the ulna. The bones ends are cut to expose bleeding bone to maximize surface are for healing and the intramedullary canals are cleared of any debris or sclerotic bone to maximize healing potential. The plate can be used as a template to help shape the cut of the two bone ends. Once the bones have been shaped to optimize contact at the correct angle, a large interfragmentary compression screw is used perpendicular to the cut angle to allow compression at the fusion site. Large fragment clamps can also be placed perpendicular to the cut surface to compress the site before the screw is tightened. The 4.5 plate is then placed along the posterior cortex of the humerus and the ulna to complete the fusion with eight cortices above and below the fusion site. The area is then packed with autogenous bone graft. The bone graft is classically harvested from the iliac crest but the author has also harvested from the ipsilateral proximal tibia. The triceps split and the soft tissues across the olecranon crest are then closed over the plate to optimize blood supply to the area. The subcutaneous tissue and skin are closed in standard fashion. The patient is provided with a simple sling but is not allowed any weight bearing or resisted activity until there is bony fusion. At 4–6 months post op the patient undergoes a CT scan looking for evidence of bony bridging across the fusion site based on evidence of more solid healing on the plain film images. Once bony healing across the osteotomy site is confirmed, the patient can start a gentle strengthening program. The patient is instructed to maintain full shoulder wrist and hand range of motion.

## Published Outcomes/Complications

The outcome literature for elbow arthrodesis is limited to small series and case reports [6–16]. The first reported cases were in 1926 where they describe an elbow arthrodesis in a 28-year-old female who has developed tuberculosis of the elbow and after subsequent irrigation and debridement procedures developed a dysfunctional flail elbow. The patient improved their function after an elbow fusion. The second case reported in this paper was for a 17-year-old male who had a flail elbow due to poliomyelitis [5]. In 1967, Koch et al. reported on 17 cases of elbow arthrodesis performed at the Mayo Clinic [17]. They attempted various techniques and reported successful fusion in 8 out of 17 cases. They reported that the most successful technique utilized tibial graft in the humeral canal with additional autogenous bone and temporary fixation with a Steinmann pin that was later removed. McAuliffe et al. in 1992 reviewed retrospectively 15 patients who had an elbow arthrodesis utilizing an AO compression plate technique [18]. Arthrodesis was successful in 14 out of 15 patients. They described eight patients having exposed plates due to severe soft tissue loss. These plates were later removed after healing and then allowed for soft tissue closure. The authors reported two forearm fractures that were thought to be related to ghost screw holes below the fusion plate and they recommended extending the fusion plate beyond previous screw fixation. Koller et al. in 2008 reported outcomes for 14 patients; 11 patients had a compression plate technique and the remaining three had an external fixation technique [19]. Successful union was reported in 11/14 patients. Complication rate was 43 % (6/14) resulting in revision surgery for skin breakdown, deep infection, implant failure, and delayed union. Sala et al. report an Ilizarov technique for elbow fusion in four patients with success of fusion in 3/4 patients [20].

## Cases

### Case #1: Severe Trauma

This is a 32-year-old male who was involved in a motor vehicle collision and he has sustained severe trauma to his elbow with a near amputation. He had significant loss of bone and also soft tissue loss requiring soft tissue reconstruction by the plastic surgery service. The patient had also lacerated his radial nerve and required tendon transfers later in his recovery for loss of function. He elected to undergo an elbow fusion since he was a manual laborer and would not be able to function with a five-pound lifetime lifting restriction that would be required for an elbow replacement. He presented, at the time of the trauma, with deficient distal humeral and proximal ulnar bone. The bone was lost at the scene of the initial accident (Fig. 17.1). He was initially placed in an

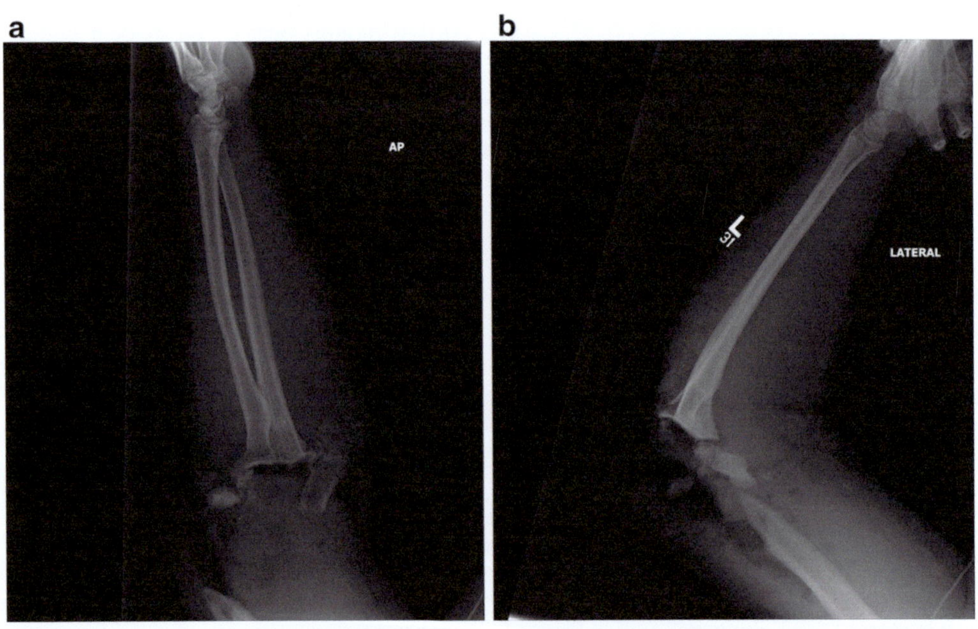


**Fig. 17.1** AP (**a**) and lateral (**b**) image showing severe acute loss of distal humeral and proximal ulnar bone

external fixator and antibiotic beads were placed for infection prevention (Fig. 17.2). After multiple washout procedures he was ready for his bony reconstruction. His bones approximated best with an oblique cut of the distal humerus to match the deficient proximal ulna. The area was compressed with a large interfragment screw and then further stabilized posteriorly with a large 4.5 plate (Fig. 17.3). The patient felt that a fusion closer to 90° would be better for him since he was a laborer and needed to carry heavy objects. CT scan at 4 months shows bony union of the fusion site (Fig. 17.4). He continues to function in a manual labor occupation.

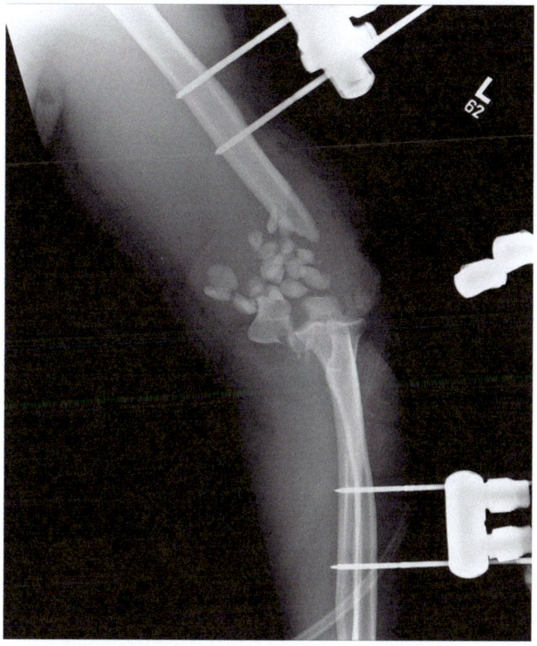


**Fig. 17.2** AP image showing external fixation and antibiotic beads

## Case #2: Chronic Elbow Pain

This patient, at the age of 23, was diagnosed with a giant cell tumor of the distal humerus and underwent a total elbow arthroplasty with a tumor prosthesis and allograft reconstruction. Unfortunately, she then required multiple total elbow revision procedures and then developed an infected total elbow replacement and presented at the age of 38 years with a long stem total elbow replacement, that was infected with cement extending to the humeral head, and severe humeral bone loss (Fig. 17.5). She then underwent an explanation of the implant with removal of all infected cement and placement of antibiotic spacers (Fig. 17.6). She had the usual IV antibiotic treatment and was cleared of her infection but could not live with pain and instability created by the resection. After a series of cast treatments she decided that she was more functional with her elbow in a more extended position, likely

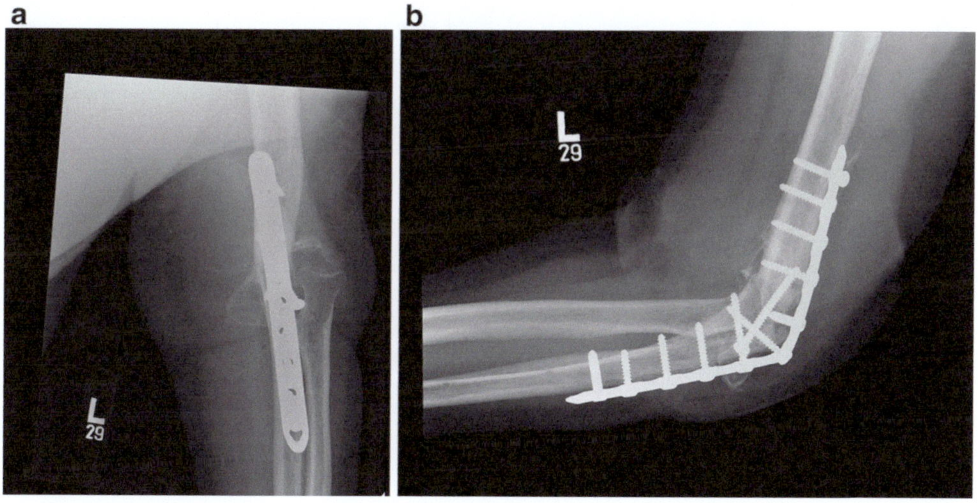


**Fig. 17.3** AP (**a**) and lateral (**b**) plain image of healed elbow fusion

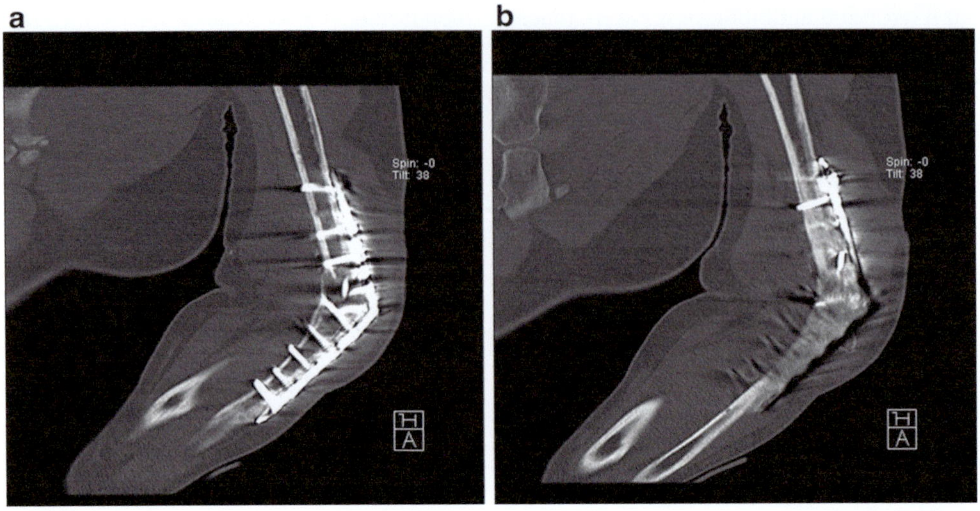


**Fig. 17.4** Two representative lateral CT scan images (**a**, **b**) showing healed fusion

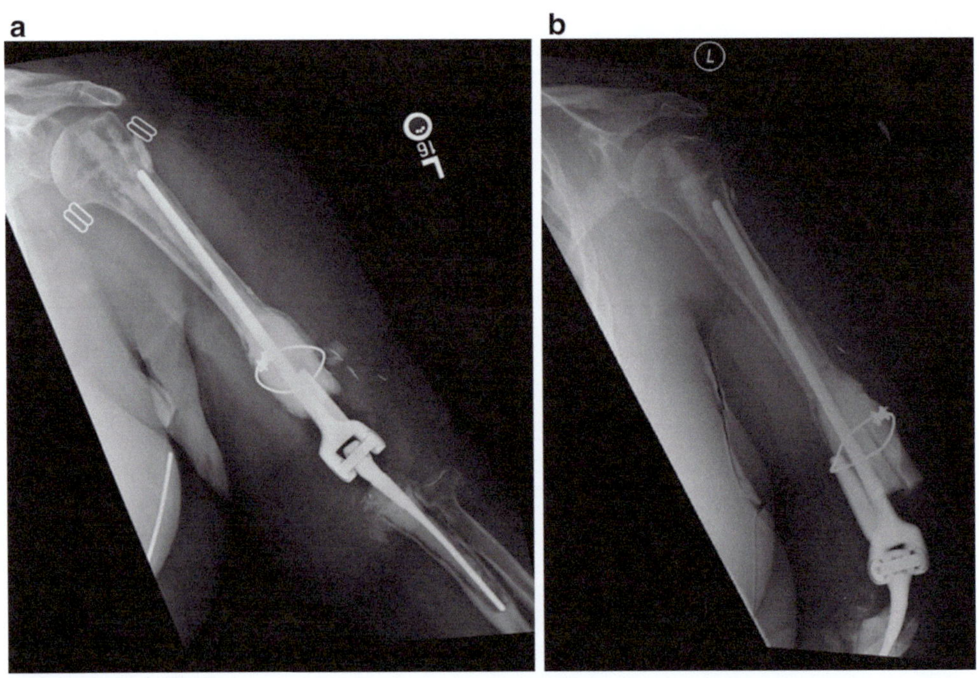


**Fig. 17.5** Presentation plain film images (**a**, **b**) showing long stem cement total elbow arthroplasty

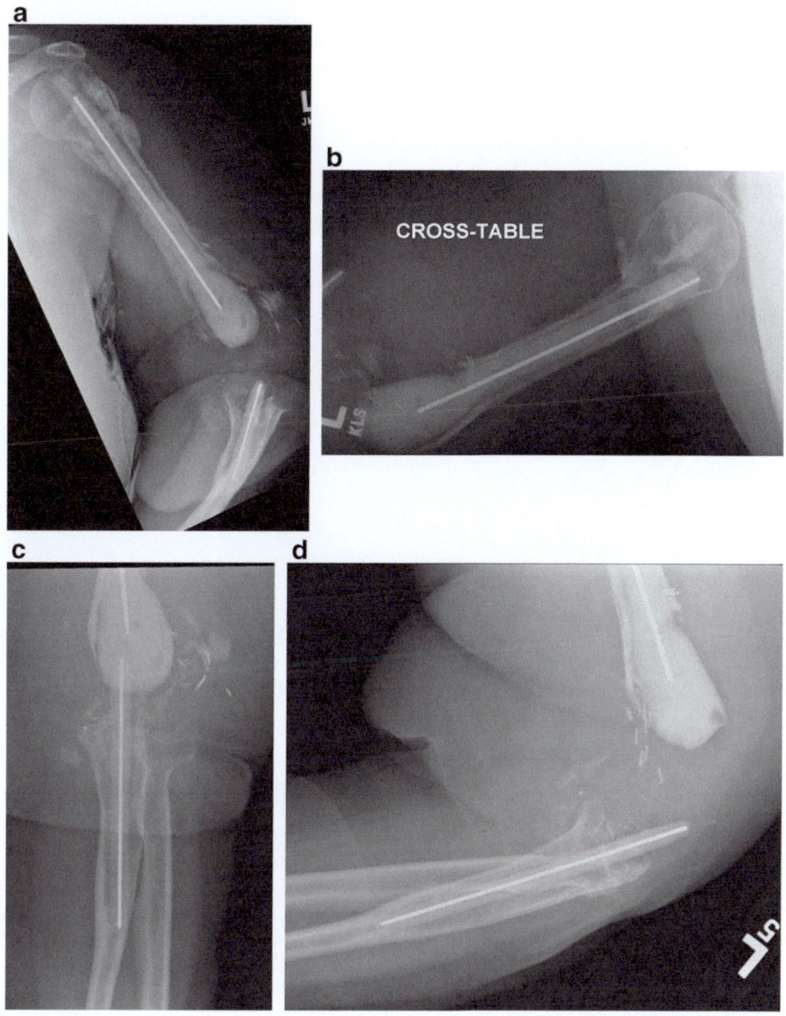


**Fig. 17.6** Plain film images (**a**–**d**) showing resection of total elbow arthroplasty and antibiotic spacers

due to the fact that she had severe shortening of her humerus. At age 40 she underwent a fusion of the elbow at 40° (Fig. 17.7). An oblique cut of the bone allowed for an appropriate fusion surface that was initially compressed with a large interfragment screw (Fig. 17.8). You will note that the antibiotic cement spacer for the humerus was kept in situ thinking that it was providing support to the bone since it was already osteopenic. Her pain control improved and her ability to touch her head with good control and use her arm overhead improved due to the stability of the elbow.

## Conclusions

In conclusion, an elbow fusion is a reasonable consideration in the young patient when all other reconstructive options for a severely damaged elbow have failed. It has the advantages of providing stability to the elbow and improving pain; however, it comes at a considerable loss of selected function of the extremity depending on the angle of fusion. The patients must be carefully chosen and must also be fully informed

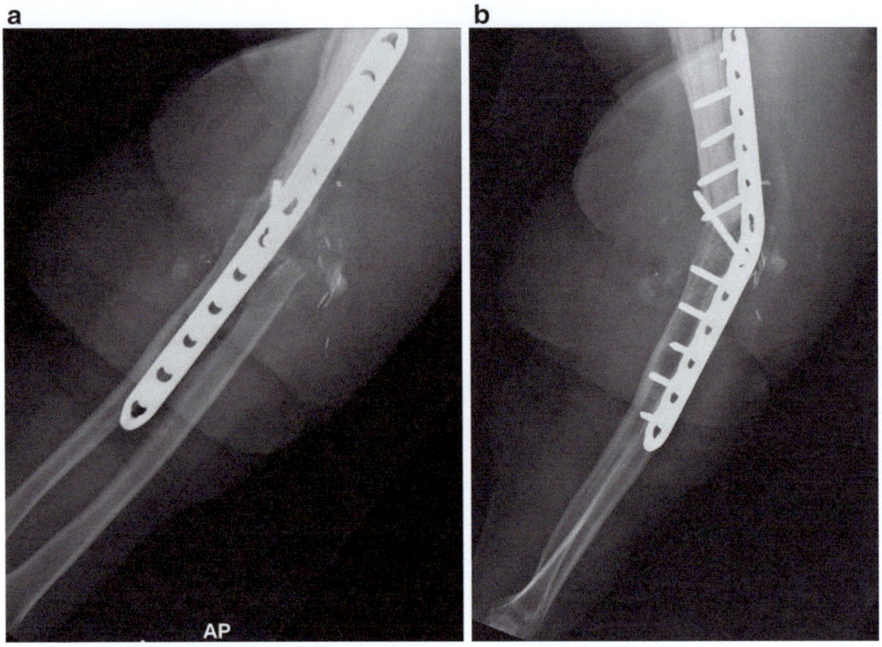


**Fig. 17.7** AP (**a**) and lateral (**b**) showing healed fusion of elbow joint

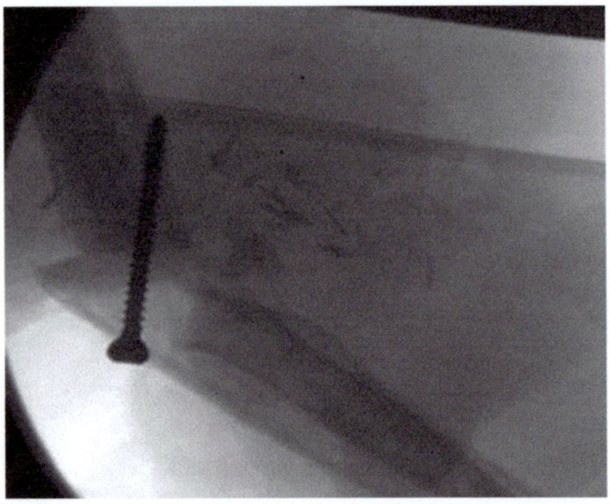

**Fig. 17.8** Intraoperative image showing interfragment screw placement across fusion site to allow for compression

about the potential risks and benefits of this procedure. Preoperative planning with the use of casting to determine optimal fusion angle can be very helpful for elective cases. Stable plate fixation with compression at the fusion site is the authors' preferred surgical technique.

## References


1. O'Neill OR, Morrey BF, Tanaka S, An KN. Compensatory motion in the upper extremity after elbow arthrodesis. Clin Orthop Relat Res. 1992;(281):89–96.
2. Tang C, Roidis N, Itamura J, Vaishnau S, Shean C, Stevanovic M. The effect of simulated elbow arthrodesis on the ability to perform activities of daily living. J Hand Surg Am. 2001;26(6):1146–50.
3. de Groot JH, Angulo SM, Meskers CG, van der Heijden-Maessen HC, Arendzen JH. Reduced elbow mobility affects the flexion or extension domain in activities of daily living. Clin Biomech. 2011;26(7):713–7.
4. Nagy 3rd SM, Szabo RM, Sharkey NA. Unilateral elbow arthrodesis: the preferred position. J South Orthop Assoc. 1999;8(2):80–5.
5. Ashhurst AP. Arthrodesis of the elbow. Ann Surg. 1926;83(1):104–10.
6. Kovack TJ, Jacob PB, Mighell MA. Elbow arthrodesis: a novel technique and review of the literature. Orthopedics. 2014;37(5):313–9.
7. Lerner A, Stein H, Calif E. Unilateral hinged external fixation frame for elbow compression arthrodesis: the stepwise attainment of a stable 90-degree flexion position: a case report. J Orthop Trauma. 2005;19(1):52–5.

8. Orozco R, Giros J, Sales JM, Videla M. A new technique of elbow arthrodesis. A case report. Int Orthop. 1996;20(2):92–9.
9. Otto RJ, Mulieri PJ, Cottrell BJ, Mighell MA. Arthrodesis for failed total elbow arthroplasty with deep infection. J Shoulder Elbow Surg. 2014;23(3):302–7.
10. Staples OS. Arthrodesis of the elbow joint. J Bone Joint Surg Am. 1952;34-A(1):207–10.
11. Gellman M. Arthrodesis of the elbow a preliminary report of a new operation. J Bone Joint Surg Am. 1947;29(4):850–2.
12. Rashkoff E, Burkhalter WE. Arthrodesis of the salvage elbow. Orthopedics. 1986;9(5):733–8.
13. Bilic R, Kolundzic R, Bicanic G, Korzinek K. Elbow arthrodesis after war injuries. Mil Med. 2005; 170(2):164–6.
14. Ozer K, Toker S, Morgan S. The use of a combined rib-latissimus dorsi flap for elbow arthrodesis and soft-tissue coverage. J Shoulder Elbow Surg. 2011; 20(1):e9–13.
15. Vaishya R, Singh AP, Singh AP. Arthrodesis in a neuropathic elbow after posttubercular spine syrinx. J Shoulder Elbow Surg. 2009;18(4):e13–6.
16. Song DJ, Wohlrab KP, Ingari JV. Anterior ulnohumeral compression plate arthrodesis for revision complex elbow injury: a case report. J Hand Surg Am. 2007;32(10):1583–6.
17. Koch M, Lipscomb PR. Arthrodesis of the elbow. Clin Orthop Relat Res. 1967;50:151–7.
18. McAuliffe JA, Burkhalter WE, Ouellette EA, Carneiro RS. Compression plate arthrodesis of the elbow. J Bone Joint Surg Br. 1992;74(2):300–4.
19. Koller H, Kolb K, Assuncao A, Kolb W, Holz U. The fate of elbow arthrodesis: indications, techniques, and outcome in fourteen patients. J Shoulder Elbow Surg. 2008;17(2):293–306.
20. Sala F, Catagni M, Pili D, Capitani P. Elbow arthrodesis for post-traumatic sequelae: surgical tactics using the Ilizarov frame. J Shoulder Elbow Surg. 2015; 24(11):1757–63.

# Index



© Springer International Publishing Switzerland 2017
R.Z. Tashjian (ed.), *The Unstable Elbow*, DOI 10.1007/978-3-319-46019-2

MIX
Papier aus verantwortungsvollen Quellen
Paper from responsible sources
FSC® C105338

If you have any concerns about our products,
you can contact us on
**ProductSafety@springernature.com**

In case Publisher is established outside the EU,
the EU authorized representative is:
**Springer Nature Customer Service Center GmbH**
**Europaplatz 3, 69115 Heidelberg, Germany**

Printed by Libri Plureos GmbH
in Hamburg, Germany